Improving Anesthesia Technical Staff's Skills

Nabil A. Shallik
Ahmed Ismail • Othman Al Hariri
Editors

Improving Anesthesia Technical Staff's Skills

Springer

Editors
Nabil A. Shallik
Department of Clinical Anesthesiology
Weill Cornell Medical College
Doha, Qatar

Ahmed Ismail
Department of Anesthesia, ICU
Perioperative Medicine HMC
Hazm Mebareek General Hospital
Doha, Qatar

Othman Al Hariri
Department of Anesthesia, ICU
Perioperative Medicine HMC
Hamad Medical Corporation
Doha, Qatar

ISBN 978-3-030-88848-0 ISBN 978-3-030-88849-7 (eBook)
https://doi.org/10.1007/978-3-030-88849-7

This Springer imprint is published by the registered company Springer Nature Switzerland AG
The registered company address is: Gewerbestrasse 11, 6330 Cham, Switzerland

Preface

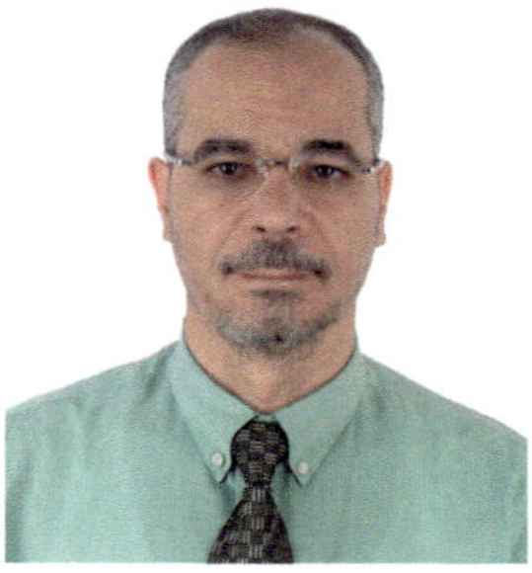

Knowledge sharing is one of the best things a man can do for humanity. So, we are excited to introduce our new book entitled *Improving Anesthesia Technical Staff's Skills*.

In combination, knowledge and technology have the immense power to improve healthcare services. This is achieved by excellent use of the best technology for the management of medical diseases and treatment of patients.

It is not uncommon to find anesthesia technicians, anesthesia technologists, or anesthesia nurses working solo in several countries across the globe due to lack of specialist anesthesiologists; therefore, this book will be of value, and it will give them a piece of fast and concise information to act properly and safely.

Enhancing the knowledge and skills of anesthesia technicians, technologists, and anesthesia nurses will improve the preparedness for surgical cases of any kind of clinical condition. This in turn will help to learn how to manage and avoid surgical and anesthetic complications.

This book covers both basic and advanced topics and includes an evidence-based scientific background that is designed to help to apply theoretical knowledge to real patient situations.

Our goal is to provide concise, easy-to-use, and up-to-date introduction to the practice of anesthesiology.

Producing an educational resource of this size and complexity would not be possible without the tireless effort of our authors and a broad array of experts.

We would like to express our gratitude to the staff at Springer Nature who works tirelessly to produce this handbook.

We would like to express our sincere gratitude to Mr. **Abil Luez**, who assisted in the capture of most of the book's images. A special thanks to the

Department of Anaesthesia, ICU and Perioperative Medicine, Hamad Medical Corporation, and Departmental leaders, (Drs. **Mohamed Hilani, Yasser Hammad**, and **Mashael Al-Khelaifi**) for their tireless support, encouragement, and guidance.

Finally, a special thanks to my family (Dr. Hanan, Mohamed, Nada, and Anas).

Doha, Qatar Nabil A. Shallik

Preface

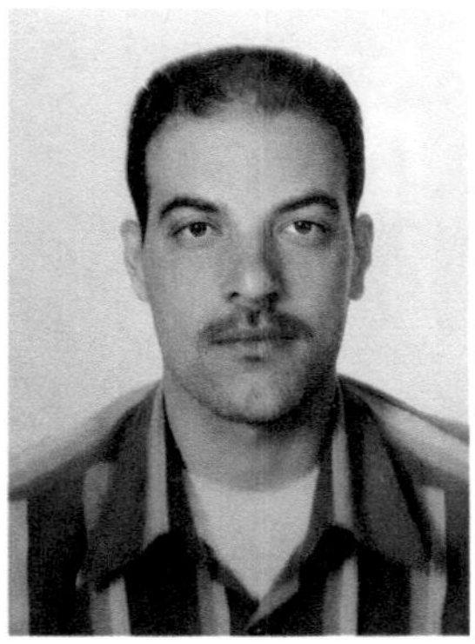

Currently, there is a strong demand for healthcare professionals. One of the most exciting works in the medical field is that of an anesthesia technician.

The anesthesia technician and technologist are responsible for ensuring that everything is in order and that the whole team is prepared for the operation.

While the anesthesiologist's work is finished until the procedure is performed, as an anesthesia technician, it is your obligation to keep track of all anesthesia supplies and equipment, refilling medications, cleaning, sterilizing instruments, and preparing the operating room for the next procedure.

In our experience, we have gathered a lot of knowledge and wisdom on the topic, and I am excited to present the first edition of our book *Improving Anesthesia Technical Staff's Skills*.

Although this book is specifically targeted at anesthesia technicians and technologists, anesthesia residents, anesthesia nurses, researchers, fellows, and anesthesiologists can be other target readers. Also, our book ends with suggestions and predictions for the future.

The book is a joint project by top anesthesiologists, anesthesia technicians, and technologists. The book focuses on cutting-edge techniques as well as clinical, technological, and non-technical skills.

It emphasizes the dependability of modern techniques against traditional clinical methods for predicting problems peri-operatively within the operating room. Anesthesia technical personnel receives one-of-a-kind instruction in technical and non-technical skills and improved management of operating room and OR utilization.

We also will scratch the quality initiatives that anesthesia technical staff will lead, and also the major roles of anesthesia technical staff during accreditation processes such as ACGME-I and Joint Commission International (JCI) accreditation and re-accreditation. In this way, our book is exclusive.

Despite our best efforts to prevent any kind of misinformation, we encourage our readers to contact us if they find any, such as spelling or grammar errors.

My wife and sons deserve special thanks for their unwavering support in the writing process, for their contributions to this one-of-a-kind book, and to all the contributing authors and chief editor Dr. Nabil Shallik for their contributions.

Doha, Qatar Othman Al Hariri

Preface

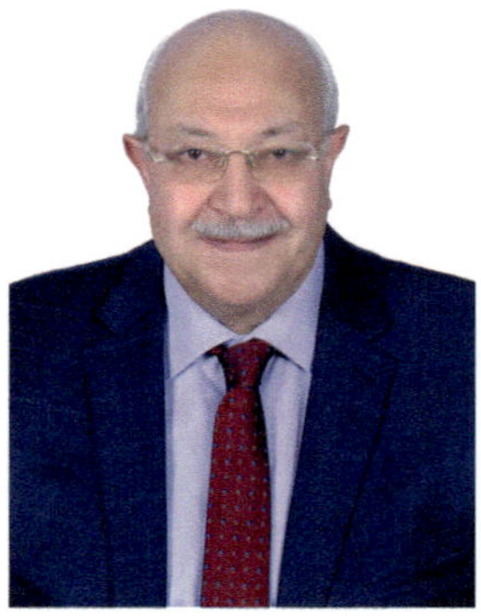

Sharing knowledge is beneficial for humanity. We strongly believe in that, so we are thrilled to introduce our new book titled *Improving Anesthesia Technical Staff's Skills*.

As you discover the exciting world of anesthesiology, we hope that you find our new book.

This book will serve as a ready reference for those embarking on anesthesia technical job. Its intent is not to be a heavy book that can only be stored on a bookshelf, but a pocket-sized reference that can be carried, be easily navigated, and be available whenever a conceptual gap compromises the anesthesia technical staff's knowledge. This book is intended for new trainees in the field of anesthesia technical job as well as senior technical staff.

While we did our best to prevent any misinformation of any form, we would urge our readers to inform us of any such error, including spelling or contextual errors. We also would advise that this book certainly does not replace professional or expert guidance and consultation.

We would like to express our sincere gratitude to Smitha and Springer team, who assisted in the production and editing of this handbook.

Finally, a special thanks to our families.

Doha, Qatar — Ahmed Ismail

Contents

Abbreviations

AAGBI	Association of Anaesthetists of Great Britain and Ireland
ABHR	Alcohol-based hand rub
ACLS	Advanced cardiac life support
ACRM	Anesthetists Crisis Resource Management Courses
ADE	Adverse drug event
AE	Adverse events
AF	Atrial fibrillation
AGSS	Active Anesthesia Gas Scavenging Systems
AHRQ	Agency of Healthcare Research and Quality
AIMS	Anesthetic Incident Monitoring Study
ALS	Advanced life support
ANTs	Anesthesia technical staff
APL	Adjustable pressure-limiting
APRV	Airway pressure release ventilation
APSF	Patient Safety Foundation
ASA	American Society of Anesthesiologist
ASATT	American Society of Anesthesia Technologists and Technicians
AT	Anesthesia technician
BBB	Blood brain barrier
BIPAP	Biphasic positive airway pressure
BIS	Bispectral Index
BLS	Basic life support
CDC	Centres for Disease Control
CFT	Clot formation time
CHGIS	Chlorhexidine gluconate-impregnated sponge
CI-CO	Cannot intubate/cannot oxygenate
CMV	Continuous mandatory ventilation
COPD	Chronic obstructive pulmonary disease
COVID-19	Corona virus disease of 2019
CPD	Citrate phosphate dextrose
CPR	Cardiopulmonary resuscitation
CRM	Crew resource management
CRRT	Continuous renal replacement therapy
CT	Clotting time
CVC	Central venous catheter
DAS	Difficult Airway Society
DIC	Disseminated intravascular coagulation

DISS	Diameter index safety system
DLT	Double lumen tube
DO_2	Oxygen delivery
DVT	Deep vein thrombosis
EAC	Epsilon aminocaproic acid
ECG	Electrocardiography
ECMO	Extra-corporeal membrane oxygenation
ECT	Electroconvulsive therapy
EMS	Emergency medical service
$EtCO_2$	End tidal carbon dioxide
ETT	Endotracheal tube
FDA	Federation of Drug Administration
FFP	Fresh frozen plasma
FiO_2	Fraction of inspired oxygen
FIVE	Flexible intubation video endoscope
FONA	Front of neck airway
GA	General anesthesia
GVHD	Graft-vs-host disease
HAI	Hospital-acquired infection
HCW	Healthcare workers
HEPA	High-efficiency particulate air
HFNO	High flow nasal oxygen
HH	Hand hygiene
HICS	Hospital incident command system
HME	Heat moisture exchange
HMEF	Heat moisture exchanger filter
ICS	Intensive Care Society
ICU	Intensive care unit
IHI	Healthcare improvement
IJV	Internal jugular veins
IM	Intramuscular
IN	Intranasally
IO	Intraosseous
IPA	Isopropyl alcohol
IPSGs	International Patient Safety Goals
IV	Intravenous
JCI	Joint Commission International
LA	Local anesthesia
LASA	Look alike-sound alike
LAST	Local anesthesia systemic toxicity
LET	Liposomal encapsulated cream
LMA	Laryngeal mask airway
LT	Laryngeal tube
MAC	Minimal alveolar concentrate
MH	Malignant hyperthermia
MOI	Management of information
MRC	Minimum required concentration
MRI	Magnetic resonance imaging

N_2O	Nitrous oxide
NAP4	National Audit Project 4
NIOSH	Occupational Safety and Health
NIR	Near-infrared
NIST	Non-interchangeable screw thread
NMBA	Neuromuscular blocking agent
NMDA	*N*-methyl-D-aspartate
NORA	Non-operating room anesthesia
NSAID	Nonsteroidal anti-inflammatory drugs
NTS	Non-technical skill
OFPD	Oxygen failure protection device
OR	Operating room
OSA	Obstructive sleep apnea
PACU	Post-anesthesia care unit
$PaTCO_2$	Partial pressure of carbon dioxide
PCA	Patient-controlled anesthesia
PCEA	Patient-controlled epidural analgesia
PD	Pharmacodynamics
PEA	Pulseless electrical activity
PEEP	Positive end expiratory pressure
PFS	Prefilled syringe
PICC	Peripherally inserted central catheters
PK	Pharmacokinetics
POC	Point of care
POCT	Point of care test
POCUS	Point of care ultrasound
PPE	Personal protective equipment
PPM	Part per million
PPV	Positive pressure ventilation
PRBC	Packed red blood cells
Psig	Pound-force per square inch gage
PSV	Pressure support ventilation
QI	Quality improvement
RBC	Red blood cell
RES	Reticuloendothelial system
ROTEM	Rotational thromboelastometry
RSI	Rapid sequence induction
SADs	Supraglottic airway devices
SALAD	Suction-assisted laryngoscopy airway decontamination
SaO_2	Oxygen saturation
SC	Subcutaneous
SIMV	Synchronized intermittent mandatory ventilation
SLA	Service level agreement
SUDs	Single-use devices
SVR	Systemic vascular resistance
SVT	Supraventricular tachycardia
TB	Mycobacterium tuberculosis
TCI	Target-controlled infusion

TD	Transdermal
TEE	Transesophageal echocardiogram
TEG	Thromboelastogram
TF	Tissue factor
THRIVE	Trans-nasal humidified rapid insufflation ventilatory exchange
TIVA	Total intravenous anesthesia
TOF	Train of four
TPA	Tissue plasminogen activator
TRALI	Transfusion-related acute lung injury
TSI	Technical sensitive indicators
URTI	Upper respiratory tract infection
US	Ultrasound
UVGI	Ultraviolet germicidal irradiation
VA	Veno-arterial
VF	Ventricular fibrillation
VFE	Viral filtration efficiency
VT	Ventricular tachycardia
VV	Veno-venous
vWF	von Willebrand factor
WAG	Waste anesthetic gas
WHO	World Health Organization

Introduction

The field of anesthesia continues to expand, and anesthesia providers keep themselves updated on the latest medical knowledge and skills. In addition to these, technology has come to play an important role in modern anesthetic practice. In most countries, anesthesia technicians or technologists (ATs) occupy an important role in safe anesthesia practice. While it is important to have quality medical technology, a trained person is also important in order to safely use this technology. ATs provide important support to physicians for adequate and safe delivery of anesthesia. Their role includes not only the technical aspects of anesthesia machines and delivery but also various non-technical skills such as communication, cognition, and social and personal skills.

Our goal is to create a book which will discuss in a simple yet complete manner the various roles and responsibilities of an AT and to highlight key lessons. We believe that this book will also be useful to anesthesia nurses, medical students, anesthesia physicians, and anesthesia residents.

Book Overview

This book contains a concise, practical, and simple approach to all relevant topics for ATs to safely deliver a good anesthetic care. Care has been taken to confirm the accuracy of the information presented and to describe generally accepted practices.

Nevertheless, the authors, editors, and publishers can make no warranties that the information contained herein is totally free from error, not least because clinical standards are constantly changing through research and regulation.

Each chapter provides a list of additional complementary topics that are available on a given topic to give the reader the opportunity to supplement their knowledge. We believe that this will appeal to all ATs, and we sincerely hope that the practical nature and quality of this text will contribute to the reader's learning and benefit patients in the ever-growing field of anesthesia.

How to Navigate Inside the Book?

It may be useful to read each chapter as an independent topic with the goal of eventually linking pieces of information together as one progresses through the book. A topic discussed briefly by one author is often explored in more detail by another. As you will see, the experts take you by the hand and tell you not only what to do but also why.

Overview of Chapters

- **Introduction:** After the introduction, we have included below the key points covered in each chapter.
- **Chapter 1:** Non-technical Skills for Anesthesia Technician
  The first chapter discussed non-technical skills for ATs which includes cognitive, social, and personal resource skills that complement technical skills and hence contribute to safe and efficient performance of tasks. The importance of this lies in the fact that a systematic study of medical errors has shown that a considerable percentage of these errors are caused by factors related to non-technical skills. Being able to communicate effectively as part of a team is essential for good ATs, and standard communication practices keep every team member in a shared mental model.
- **Chapter 2:** Role of Anesthesia Technician in Operating Theatre Including Quality Projects and JCI Accreditation
  This chapter explains the roles and responsibilities of ATs. This is usually a very extensive list and includes but is not limited to acquiring, preparing, and use of supplies; preparing medications; assisting the licensed anesthesia care provider with different types of anesthesia; vascular access; airway management including difficult airways; resuscitation; troubleshooting of anesthesia equipment; and performing point-of-care laboratory tests. Additionally, the AT should be comfortable using sophisticated blood collection equipment or even intra-aortic balloon pumps to support patients with severe congestive heart failure depending on the country of practice. Additionally, the importance of performing quality improvement projects and maintenance of Joint Committee International (JCI) standards are discussed.
- **Chapter 3:** Pharmacology of the Most Common Anesthesia Drugs
  This chapter discusses the most common drugs used for induction, maintenance, and emergence from anesthesia. Dosage, side effects, and special features of various drugs have also been discussed.
- **Chapter 4:** Pharmacy, Drugs Labeling, and Storage
  This chapter deals with important pharmacy practices to ensure safe use of medication.
- **Chapter 5:** Checklists: To Get Things Done Right—All the Time
  The development of a variety of checklists is needed to enable the ever-increasing need to improve patient safety and reduce morbidity and mor-

tality as well as improve workflow, teamwork, and communication within the operating room. Such anesthesia machine, medication, and crisis checklists have developed over decades of development of anesthesia practice and the experience of unfortunate lapses, errors, and patient harm.

- **Chapter 6:** Essential Anesthesia Monitors and Equipment in the Operating Theatre
  One of the responsibilities of the AT is to assist in preparation of the anesthesia or induction room. This includes making sure of the availability of, preparing and maintaining functioning equipment including patient monitoring devices. The AT also assists with acquiring, preparing, and maintaining anesthesia delivery systems before, during, and after anesthesia. This chapter highlights the various relevant types of monitoring equipment as well as other commonly used equipment in anesthesia practice.
- **Chapter 7:** Infection Control and Prevention in Operation Theatre
  It is of utmost importance to create a safe and clean environment to treat each surgical patient and a safe working environment for the staff. While not exclusively a role for the AT, this chapter is included as it also comprises essential knowledge and standards for practicing anesthesia. With patient safety in mind, in this chapter we discuss means of cleaning, disinfection, sterilization of the theater, and other parts of the mechanisms of development of infection and the mechanism of action of commonly used disinfecting and sterilizing agents. We discuss standards of cleanliness present in operating theaters. Additionally, we cover the management of new emerging infectious threats such as COVID-19 and rare diseases such as prions.
- **Chapter 8:** Anesthesia Machines and Anesthetic Breathing System
  This chapter explains in detail the various commonly used anesthesia machines and Anesthetic Breathing Delivery Systems including the Mapleson systems, modifications of the Mapleson system, and the modern circle system. Our focus will be on essential features required to differentiate each system as well as ways to check for appropriate function and ways to check for problems and fixing them. We will also discuss the components, features, working mechanism, standards, and checklists of the modern anesthesia machine. As always manufacturer recommendations are important.
- **Chapter 9:** Airway Management and Equipment
  Airway management is a key competence and core skill in Anesthesia, Intensive Care, Resuscitation, and Emergency Medicine practice. Many critical incidents in relation to patient care still occur because of challenges in securing the patient's airway in a safe manner. Also, recent evidence suggests that while equipment availability and its preferred, efficient and timely use is important to prevent such incidents, most critical incidents actually come from non-technical issues that include problems in communication, lack of training, less than adequate adoption of a pre-procedural strategy, handover, and team work. This chapter highlights the importance of non-technical skills. This chapter also provides an overview

of available airway management equipment, underlining the position of each device or class of devices in a decisional tree and in the context of a human-based planning and procedural process.

- **Chapter 10:** Scavenging, Medical Gas Pipelines, and Vacuum Systems
While anesthetic and medical gases are an essential part of daily anesthetic practice, these tend to accumulate in the theater environment with each patient expiration. Unless safely removed, these cause pollution and can be hazardous and detrimental to the patient and staff working in the operating theater. For this reason, a sophisticated scavenging system has been developed. In this chapter we discuss the important types of scavenging systems and try to simplify it by discussing its major components, types, safety precautions, and ways to diagnose and troubleshoot if there are issues in its safety and features.
- **Chapter 11:** Operating Room; Complications, and Emergencies
An AT is an immediate source of skilled assistance to the anesthesia physician in case of any intraoperative patient complication. The role by the AT during any emergency condition has to be immediate, effective, and efficient with appropriate knowledge and skills. In this chapter various emergency conditions have been discussed, e.g., difficult intubation and airway spasm and its management following the Difficult Airway Society (DAS) Guidelines; pulmonary aspiration; total spinal anesthesia; allergic reactions; acute medical conditions such as bronchospasm, pneumothorax, and malignant hyperthermia; and local anesthetic systemic toxicity and others. Further clinical scenarios such as hemorrhage control with transfusion complications, cardiac arrhythmias, and cardiac arrest management following the Resuscitation Council of United Kingdom guidelines, will be discussed with more details in this book. Malignant hyperthermia is a rare clinical condition, because of its serious effect on patient's health. It has been discussed in this chapter.
  The operating theater is also a place with multiple electrical equipment and combustible materials including liquids, and thus fire safety and safety in use of LASER devices have been discussed so that the AT can manage properly in case of such a scenario.
- **Chapter 12:** Vascular Access: From Cannulation to Decannulation
Peripheral vascular access is commonly performed in the anesthesia room, and various sizes and models of peripheral venous cannula have been discussed in this chapter. Additionally, safe fixation of the cannula, safe precautions, and other standards have also been discussed. Specialized vascular access such as arterial line, central venous cannula, dialysis catheter, and peripherally inserted central line have also been discussed. A good performance of these techniques requires good knowledge of basic vascular anatomy, location of the vein or artery with landmark, palpation and ultrasound guidance, and good technique. There is also a discussion of safety care bundles.
- **Chapter 13:** Hypothermia and Its Management
One of the important physiological parameters for human beings to remain in good health is a constant core body temperature of around 37 °C (36.3–37.3 °C). Patients under general anesthesia may lose heat due to inhibition

of thermoregulatory mechanisms and exposure to a cool theater environment or may also gain heat if the environment is hot. Changes in core body temperature increase the risk of infection, bleeding as well as arrhythmias. This chapter discusses temperature control in the operating room, means of active and passive warming of patients, and temperature monitoring techniques.

- **Chapter 14:** Transfusion of Blood and Other Products
Many patients may require transfusion of blood and other products during anesthesia and surgery. ATs have to be familiar with the different types of blood products, their transfusion practices, other safety practices such as verification of patient and blood products, blood transfusion reactions, and also use of filter infusion sets and blood warmers and other equipment. The Anesthesia and Surgical team including the nurses should be trained in the management of massive bleeding. Each institution should have their own massive transfusion protocol including the essentials of clinical monitoring and safety and treatment thresholds.
- **Chapter 15:** Regional Anesthesia for Anesthesia Technologists
Regional anesthesia is a specialized field and is gradually gaining prominence. Many institutions have dedicated regional nerve block rooms in the preoperative area. ATs have helped in the effort to expand the range of anesthetic services that can be provided. With regard to regional anesthesia, ATs can help with the setup of equipment, instruments, and monitors. Additionally, they can also help the anesthesia physician with local anesthesia drug prescription, preparing, and injecting and handling as per institution rules.
- **Chapter 16:** Transportation of the Anaesthetized and Critically Ill Patient
Transfer of the anesthetized and/or critically ill patient has seen a surge in number in recent years, and there has been a lot of research into developing suitable transfer guidelines and protocols to reduce adverse events and avoidable mishaps related to transfers. Nowadays, facilities that may be involved in patient transfer must ensure that trained personnel, appropriate equipment, training, and a governance structure are available and set in place. With advanced medical technology, patient monitoring and other equipment are more robust, portable, and intuitive making transfers safer for even very ill patients.

The editors and I are extremely proud to welcome contributions from colleagues around the world who are among the highest-ranked researchers and practitioners in the field of anesthesia, ICU, and pain management.

Please enjoy reading of this high standard book.

1 Non-technical Skills for Anesthesia Technician

Ahmed Elgeziry, Narjis Mumtaz,
Abdul Vahab Thodika, and Khalid Abu Mallal

Contents

1.1 Introduction

The concept of non-technical skill was first adopted by aviation which was the first high-risk industry to recognize that technical competence alone was not enough to guarantee safe performance. It is becoming more widely acknowledged that safe and efficient task performance requires a combination of technical expertise and NTS.

A. Elgeziry (✉) · N. Mumtaz · A. V. Thodika
Department of Anaesthesia, ICU and Perioperative Medicine, Hamad Medical Corporation, Doha, Qatar
e-mail: ageziery@hamad.qa; avahab@hamad.qa

K. A. Mallal
Department of Cardiac Anesthesia, Heart Hospital, Doha, Qatar
e-mail: Kabumallal@hamad.qa

N. A. Shallik et al. (eds.), *Improving Anesthesia Technical Staff's Skills*,
https://doi.org/10.1007/978-3-030-88849-7_1

Between 1959 and 1989, more than 70% of commercial plane crashes were attributed to deficiencies in the flight crew's NTS rather than solely mechanical failures. In 1979 NASA psychologist John Lauber coined the term Crew Resource Management (CRM). This training program was implemented in United Airlines in 1981. In few yew years it became the global gold standard in aviation industry. This made remarkable positive changes in communication and team culture in aviation. Most of the safety measures in healthcare are adopted from aviation.

There is an increasing body of evidence that failings in NTS such as poor communication or lack of teamwork are prominent factor leading to adverse events in the operating room.

Recognizing that the human error is a factor in perioperative anesthetic mortality was evident in the Lancet commission on the relative safety of the use of ether and chloroform in the 1890s, which described the failure of situation awareness, decision-making, and teamwork.

Lunn and Mushin in 1982, also related anesthetic mortality to the lack of skilled anesthetic assistance. Recently, the Fourth National Audit Project (of the Royal College of Anesthetists and the Difficult Airway Society) reported on major complications of airway management in the UK. This report clearly identified contributory NTS factors including failure of communication, decision-making, and social failures which included leadership and support. Failure by staff who are considered lower in hierarchies to speak up has been associated with an increased risk of accidents, both in in health care and in aviation as well.

An Australian database of 5837 reports the Anesthetic Incident Monitoring Study (AIMS), revealed187 incidents caused by insufficient assistance contributed towards an incident, on the other hand, 808 instances where skilled assistance had contributed to minimize the adverse incident. Hence emphasizing the fact that poor NTS of anesthesia technician can be associated with poor outcomes for patients including arrhythmias, iatrogenic coagulopathy, anesthetic awareness, and admission to intensive care.

A good example of proper utilization of NTS by an anesthesia technician "speaking up" and guiding a new trainee anesthetist when he was about to induce anesthesia for a patient violating the fasting guidelines. Under the pressure from the surgeons, the anesthetist was about to proceed with an anesthetic for appendicectomy without the fasting time being completed. His response was to insert a nasogastric tube and proceed. The technician suggested that the trainee must discuss the situation with his consultant before proceeding. Here, he/she showed leadership, teamwork, decision-making, and communication in guiding a doctor to accept her concerns and phone the consultant. She demonstrated situation awareness and proper understanding of the pressure a new trainee might be suffering which would lead him to deviate from the fasting guidelines.

Examples of behaviors that are relevant to anesthesia technician non-technical skills include, but not limited to, collection of information from team to prepare equipment to be ready at the appropriate time, anticipation when colleagues will need assistance/extra equipment, and can help as an extra of eyes to see the relatively hidden problems and communicate them to the anesthetist, and function as a second check on the anesthetist's decision-making when involved in re-evaluations.

It is extremely important to develop a taxonomy of NTS specifically for the anesthesia technician in order to have a common vocabulary aiming to facilitate discussion and also make learning more effective rather than expecting them to passively learn these skills over time with mere exposure to his colleagues in operating room.

Applying proper NTS cannot totally eliminate harm to patients; however, the likelihood of it happening can be significantly minimized by providing staff, who are considered as lower in the theater hierarchy, with the authority and capability to discuss or question the operation room team regardless to their position.

1.1.1 Current Situation

Today, the riskiest industries (such as nuclear, military, and power) have realized that safety depends not only on the academic knowledge and application of practical skills. However, it heavily depends on basic human behavior, common sense, and attitude of the individuals in the team.

Clinicians have been using these non-technical skills informally since ages, however, only recently have they been identified as skills that need to be acquired consciously for safe and effective patient care. With rapid expansion of clinical knowledge and technological advances, clinical teaching and training has also greatly evolved.

Modern day clinical anesthesiologists accept the need for a more formal education and training of these skills. As much as the lack of technical skill can lead to harm in delivery of patient care, absence of non-technical skills, like lack of communication, situational awareness, and ineffective teamwork, can lead to a greater chance of avoidable errors and serious adverse events.

Anesthesia is a safety driven specialty. The aim of emphasizing on incorporation of non-technical skills is to promote excellence in anesthetic management of patients in the operating room. Similar tools are available for surgeons and scrub nurses as well.

1.1.2 Introducing Non-technical Skills to Anesthesia

Many different models of the Crew Resource Management have been adapted from the aviation industry to the health care systems, two most prominent ones being the ACRM: Anesthetists Crisis Resource Management Courses in the US and ANTs: Anesthetists Non-technical skills in the United Kingdom.

Over the years, many anesthesiology residency programs have incorporated the teaching of non-technical skills to not only anesthesia residents, but to anesthesiology technicians and nurse anesthetists. This has led not only to increased awareness about safe delivery of anesthesia care among anesthesiologist but the very vital part of the team, the anesthesiology technicians. Gaba et al. were the first ones to introduce Anesthesia Crisis Resource Management (ACRM) in September 1990 in the USA.

Non-technical skills system is not a new invention to anesthesiology, but a re-discovery and conscious realization of known skills, behaviors, and efforts that need to be brought into our conscious practice. Delivery of safe anesthesia over the years has been ensured by the subconscious use of these skills.

When we think of Anesthesiologists, we think of the sleep guardians, the know-it-all physicians, who work in a seamlessly perfect manner, know the answers to all. They are the first ones to look up to in times of panic and distress. What makes them so efficient and effective? It is in fact the integration of non-technical to the technical skills which makes the delivery of anesthesia a predictably safe job.

Anesthesiology technicians as the "crew" in the Anesthesiology *Crew* Resource Management (ACRM).

When Anesthesiology Crisis Resource Management (ACRM) was adapted from the aviation's Crew Resource Management (CRM) model, the word "crew" was replaced with "crisis" to make it more applicable and familiar with the anesthesiology background. Later, the developers recognized and emphasized the very vital role of the "crew" that function together with the anesthesiologists, in the team in order to help with the smooth and safe delivery of anesthetic care. Hence these "crew," namely, anesthesia technicians, anesthesia technologists, nurse anesthetists, were considered an important part in the training and teaching of these non-technical skills along with their technical skills training curriculum.

1.1.3 The Core Components

For a greater understanding and usefulness of anesthesia non-technical skills, they have been categorized into four main groups and 15 elements defined further (Table 1.1).

As we run through each one of those elements, we will realize that all four main technical skills are very much intercalated and inseparable when it comes to practical clinical scenarios. Efficient communication skill and a clear common lan-

Table 1.1 Categories and elements of anesthesia non-technical skills

Category	Elements
Task management	Planning and preparing
	Prioritizing
	Providing and maintaining standards
	Identifying and utilizing resources
Team working	Coordinating activities with team members
	Exchanging information
	Using authority and assertiveness
	Assessing capabilities
	Supporting others
Situational awareness	Gathering information
	Recognizing and understanding
	Anticipating
Decision-making	Identifying options
	Balancing risks and selecting options
	Re-evaluating

guage are the backbone for all these elements. It must be applied timely.

Let us dive right in!

The following table shows broadly the categories and elements of anesthesia non-technical skills.

1.2 Task Management

Managing resources and organizing tasks to achieve goals, be they individual case plans or longer-term scheduling issues.

It has four skill elements: planning and preparing; prioritizing; providing and maintaining standards; and identifying and utilizing resources. Task Management is a very important part of the routine of the anesthesiologist and the anesthesia technician. From the time of planning before starting a case till the debriefing after the case is over, every team member should be sharing all the information. This is called *Shared mental model.* All team members should be on the same page.

Team briefing sessions to be done before staring a case. Team leader and all the members should attend this. This is the time to know the team members. In big institutions, the members of team keep changing. Patient details are exchanged between team members. In case the anesthetist is not conducting briefing, being a responsible team member, the anesthesia technician should suggest and take the initiation. Adequate planning for the case, preparedness, organization of drugs and other equipment, machine checks, availability of resources (for example: Blood ready at blood bank), notifying the team members of any troubles or issues with the same, having a plan B are all indispensable components of the usual job of the anesthesia team. It is imperative that the anesthesia technician be aware of the patient, discuss the plan with the anesthetist, determine all requirements, any special requirements, have good knowledge base about the possible clinical situations that could arise, and have a backup plan in mind to be able to contribute as an effective team member. Inability to do so may lead to breaks in the smooth provision of patient care and may add to disorganization. For major cases, if multiple members are in the team *assignment of roles and responsibilities* are done during this planning. These roles should be clear to everyone. The assignment is very important for the smooth workflow and to avoid chaos in emergencies. That will make the concerned member accountable for the assigned task. Ideally, the senior anesthetist will assign the roles knowing the capabilities and weakness of team members. But anesthesia technician also can suggest and initiate. For example: *I will give medication, you give cricoid pressure, let him prepare and assist fibro optic scope.*

1.3 Team Working

Working with others in a team context, in any role, to ensure effective joint task completion and team satisfaction; focus is particularly on the team rather than the task. Any task that involves more than one person needs effective and efficient teamwork and coordination of all team members. There needs to be an element of respect, acknowledgement and each individual needs to feel valued and important. An easy exchange of vital information about key events, important observations and their communication in a clear manner helps towards achieving a common goal.

When we speak of a team, we need to acknowledge the presence, role, and place of the team leader and how all input needs to be channeled in a positive way for smooth completion of a task. The team leader needs to possess a certain degree of authority in order to effectively and confidently lead the rest of the members especially in states of panic and emergency when these virtues are most needed. Hierarchy and power struggle often add to the challenge and are an important topic that we will discuss in the chapter later.

Clear communication is most important for the best coordination in teamwork. There are lot of barriers for the communication in teamwork. Difference in language, accent, culture, nonverbal communication style, and hierarchy are few among them. We should make sure the correct information is conveyed. *Checkback* and *closing the loop* strategy is used to ensure this. This is practiced for any type of communication in operation theater.

Example:

Anesthetist: Give injection Paracetamol

Technician: Injection Paracetamol 1 gm IV infusion over 15 mts?

Anesthetist: Yes, that is correct

Now, Because of the checkback, the team knows the information is correctly conveyed. If there was a misunderstanding it is easily correctable at this point.

Technician: Injection Paracetamol given.

Now the loop is closed.

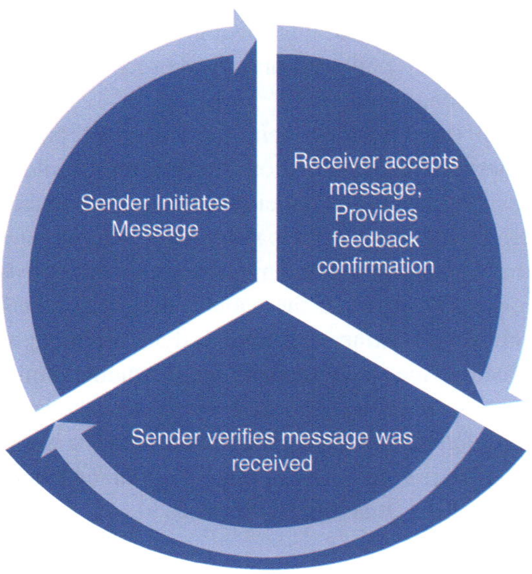

1.4 Closed Loop Communication

In the operating room, the anesthesia technician serves as an important part of the team to deliver quality anesthesia care to the patient. He needs to play an active part in communicating with other team members to relay important information, close loops with all team members and communicate with the anesthesiologist in a clear manner about case plans so he/she can be a strong support for the anesthesiologist in crisis.

1.4.1 Good Practice

We reiterate here a very common scenario where the anesthesia technician serves as a very important team member. Often it happens that good anesthesia technicians can pre-emptive with each step during airway management, what the anesthesiologist might need and would provide equipment in hand before even asking. Part of it is attributed to good knowledge about airway algorithms but it is mainly the conscious exercise of the non-technical skills, namely the quality of supporting team members, acknowledging their needs, anticipating specific requirements, and thus contributing towards efficient and smooth execution of the task at hand.

These virtues are a product of the non-technical skills learnt over years and of experience. It is, however, sometimes intimidating for some to step up as equals in the team and point out errors in the functioning or to provide suggestions to other team members that might be deemed as superiors. However, with the modernization of systems and the flattening of this hierarchy, good systems have now started to acknowledge the importance of each team member as being an important part of the matrix.

1.4.2 Poor Practice

Teamwork requires training, re-realization, and practice. Absence of a sense of responsibility or a conscious effort to own their place in the team may lead to an aura of indifference and thus break the chain of support that may lead of safety concerns.

Often times we witness a display of poor teamwork either by virtue of lack of communication or not closing loops in communication. For example, not giving a proper hand over while going off for a break, assuming they would return just in a while, attaching a new bag of saline and leaving it on, assuming more fluid needed to be given, and not confirming with the anesthetist. This kind of attitude not only conveys indifference and lack of interest but may jeopardize patient safety. That open IV line could result in fluid overload in a patient with kidney failure, had the anesthesia technician not been aware of patient history, and had the anesthesiologist not been aware of the running IV line and replacement of the empty saline bag.

Hence, we learn that it is not only appreciated but also very important to have a sense of belonging in the team and recognize individual importance that contributes to the safety of the patient.

1.5 Situational Awareness

Developing and maintaining an overall dynamic awareness of the situation based on perceiving the elements of the theater environment: patient, team, time, displays, equipment, understanding what they mean and thinking ahead about what could happen soon.

The OR is a constantly changing, dynamic environment and distractions are common and often. Often, beeping of alarms, surgeon's chit-chat, a joke here and there, may prove to be distracting enough to lose that attention to the surrounding and may lead to missed actions, like missed medication timed muscle relaxant dose, low volume ventilator alarm indicating near empty vaporizer.

On part of the anesthesia technician, in addition to the anesthesiologist, it demands a great deal of alertness, vigilance and a constant look out for any abnormal or unwanted change in the OR environment and appropriate actions taken or at times, alerting the anesthesiologist for appropriate action to be taken.

Anticipation is an art, that needs to be learnt, and is the key to that "extrasensory perception" that good anesthesia technicians seem to possess. Struggling with passing the ET tube, the anesthesia trainee lifts his head and witnesses the magical appearance of a hand with a bougie! Voila! What did I do to deserve you? (He thinks in his head!).

Let us look at few examples of good and bad practice demonstrating situational awareness.

1.5.1 Good Practice

Let us take the example of a usual list of laparoscopic appendectomies, one after the other. This is one of the instances where anesthesia seems just too easy. Mundane. Simple. Boring maybe? The same recipe, same drugs, same sequence. Patient is wheeled in, identified, pre-op checks done, monitors attached. As the anesthesiologist handles the airway and begins to pre-oxygenate the patient, the anesthesia technician assists by injecting the drugs. On a usual case, this usually goes by without much of talking in between the anesthetist and the anesthesia technician. Being a vigilant anesthesia technician, she had seen the patient in the pre-op handling area, found the patient to be septic, observed the patient to be tachycardic, and slightly hypotensive on the monitors. Right before injecting the usual full dose of the anesthetic, she had a glance at the anesthetist and closed the loop by reconfirming that the fluid was well and running and that she would give a slow incremental dose of the anesthetic in order to avoid the sudden and precipitous drop in BP following induction. The anesthetist confirmed and they proceeded with induction.

In this scenario, there were a lot of points where a lack of attention, recognition of situation, vigilance, and anticipation could have led to errors and harm to the patient. However, we saw that the anesthesia technician took the proactive approach, observed the patient, dissociated herself from routine, and used a dynamic thought process. She anticipated the hemodynamic implications of giving too much of the anesthetic in *that patient* and then closed loop with the anesthesiologist and hence displayed an excellent example of situational awareness.

Another example was one recalled by an anesthesiologist where the anesthesia technician was relieved by one of his colleagues for a break. On his way to the lounge from the operating room, he heard a call for help from the same room he left, and without second thought rushed back to lend a helping hand. To note and appreciate here is the fact that he realized that the colleague he handed over to for the break might not be as completely aware of the patient, situation, and the equipment placement as he was and it would not hurt to give a helping hand in an emergency situation.

Another problem while performing complicated critical cases is deviation from the actual goal. A patient with ongoing bleeding, the anesthetist tries to put an arterial line to monitor the hypotension efficiently. He attempts to do it multiple times without success and the concentration is deviated to this task for long time. At this time, he forgets about bleeding, fluid resuscitation, blood products, and all. It is the duty of the anesthesia technician as the responsible member of the team to alert the anesthetist and bring his attention back to the goals.

1.5.2 Poor Practice

On the contrary, poor display of situational awareness, of lack thereof can be observed from the example of a anesthesia technician who assists a difficult intubation, and then leaves the intubation trolley as is, does not sort it out or clear and rearrange it. He returns the video scope, does not check for availability of spare similar sized tubes, not anticipating the need for reusing that equipment in case of an accidental extubation upon proning of the patient for a back surgery.

Here, the anesthesia technician did not focus on the fact that proning will be required for back surgery. Proning carries a risk of extubation and hence, timely re-arrangement of the airway trolley post intubation, would indeed help him and the anesthesiologist in case they needed to re-intubate the patient. The availability of a neat, sorted trolley, with possibly an extra ETT of similar size and definitely that video scope he already moved out of the room would be paramount.

Hence, we learn that constant awareness of the environment, preparedness with knowledge of the patient, situation, surrounding, and anticipation of the possible problems that could arise and a pre-emptive plan of its solution are important virtues for any anesthesia care provider.

1.6 Decision-Making

Making decisions to reach a judgment or diagnosis about a situation, or to select a course of action, based on experience or new information under both normal conditions and in time-pressured crisis situations.

When it comes to decision-making anesthesia per se lies in the category of a complex dynamic world where naturalistic decision-making is required.

Currently, hierarchy plays a role in decision-making. If the team leader is not compliant, other team members will hesitate to make suggestions and opinions. Anesthesia technician should actively involve in the discussion. They should act as advocate of the patient, should raise the concern assertively, and *speak up* on behalf of the patient. Whenever you raise a concern, make sure it is conveyed. During emergency and stress situations, many communications are unnoticed and unregistered. Therefore, get the response for your suggestions. There are situations where a senior experienced anesthesia technician is not comfortable about the decision and management. If the response is not satisfactory even after repeated alert, it is his responsibility to stop the line and seek parallel solution like inform a senior anesthetist. Patient safety is the most important goal. In a good team hierarchy should not be a hindrance to raise concern and speak up. To achieve this, everyone in the team including the senior most anesthetist should be aware of the NTS and team strategies.

Decision-making comprises of identifying options available, balancing risks, and benefits of each and then deciding upon suitable options and then re-evaluating those decisions.

1.6.1 Objective Evaluation of ANTs

A four-point scoring system has been developed in order to rate anesthesia non-technical skills in trainees/nurses and to provide effective feedback (Table 1.2).

Therefore, in a given scenario, the non-technical skills can be evaluated according to the quality of performance; 1–4 from the worst to the most perfect, such scoring system can give an objective evaluation and facilitate feedback and reinforce learning.

Table 1.2 Scoring system for anesthesia non-technical skills evaluation (Flin et al. 2003b)

Rating label	Description
4-Good	Performance was of high standard, enhancing patient safety; it could be used as a positive example
3-Acceptable	Performance was satisfactory but could be better
2-Marginal	Performance was inadequate, considerable improvement is required
1-Poor	Performance is compromising patient safety, prompt remediation is required
N-Not observed	Skill was not observed

1.6.2 Teaching ANTs

Gaba et al. were the first one to introduce Anesthesia Crisis Resource Management (ACRM) in September 1990 in the USA.

Even though there is widespread acknowledgment of their importance, medical education yet does not formally teach non-technical skills as a part of their curriculum. Most of these non-technical skills are acquired subconsciously from peers. New or junior anesthesia technicians or trainees learn from their senior peers as role models. However, there is a great deal of influence, positive or negative, from the culture and work ethic of the workplace, its people and the systems in place.

Contrary to classroom and skills lab teaching of medical knowledge and technical skills, respectively, ANTS need to be taught and learnt *in the workplace*. Many models have been set in place across multiple institutes, one of them being the peer-learning model, where anesthesiology residents, fellow anesthesiology technicians teach these non-technical, cognitive and behavioral skills to their junior peers. However, in order to achieve this goal, we need to identify the peer group capable of teaching these skills. Having said that, it is not non-technical skills alone, but their incorporation into technical skills to particular situations for anesthetic excellence.

Simulation can help learners to gain and practice these skills in an artificial, controlled, safe and stress-free environment with proper design, the anesthesia nurse can gain the necessary elements of both technical and non-technical skills and merge them together in harmony and synergism.

1.6.3 Importance of Non-technical Skills

- To promote excellence in anesthesiology practice.
- Important to mitigate the effect of errors in the safe delivery of patient care.
- Accounts for most of the human factor related errors.

National Audit Project 4 (NAP4) was a prospective study of all major airway events. The analysis showed that human factors were a relevant influence in every major airway case. The current Difficult Airway Society (DAS) guidelines have incorporated a section on human factors.

Following the analysis of cases from NAP4. The NAP5 audit reviewed accidental awareness during general anesthesia. The findings were that 73% of the awareness cases were avoidable with miscommunication being the main contributing factor to the incidents.

1.6.4 Challenges

The introduction of ANTS system does have some obstacles.

- Relative lack of clinicians' familiarity with anesthesia non-technical skills and their ability to evaluate it objectively and provide valuable feedback.
- Most senior anesthetists are unfamiliar with a formal approach to the ANTS jargon, even though they realize the importance of those skills, e.g. they were found to be unaware of the term *situational awareness,* however, it would be second nature for them to be continually vigilant.
- Cultural setup. Culture of hierarchy in the OR. Theater hierarchy. Anesthesia technicians are considered lower down in the theater hierarchy.
- Lack of standard duration of training.
- Lack of agreement on what is considered safe anesthesia practice.
- Hiding errors. Need to establish a "reporting culture" and moving away from blame and shame culture.
- Good systems try to flatten the hierarchy to enable effective team work. So that even the most junior team member or the least qualified individual can raise concerns without feeling intimidated.

1.6.5 Room for Improvement

Need to be taught as a part of formal medical education.

Two days training shown to be effective.

Take-Home Message

The systemic study of medical errors has shown that considerable percentage of these errors are caused by factors related to non-technical skills.

Standardized communication practices keep every team member in shared mental model.

Adequate importance needs to be given to these skills in order to provide a safe clinical practice, hand in hand with technical skills.

Anesthesia technician plays a pivotal role in operating room and should have a high level of both technical and non-technical skills.

Suggested Reading

Beaty D. The naked pilot: the human factor in aircraft accidents. Wiltshire: Airlife Publishing Ltd; 1995.

Catchpole KR, Mishra A, Handa A, McCulloch P. Teamwork and error in the operating room: analysis of skills and roles. Ann Surg. 2008;247:699–706.

Commission on Anaesthetics. Report of the Lancet commission appointed to investigate the subject of the administration of chloroform and other anaesthetics from a clinical standpoint. Lancet. 1893a;141:693–708.

Commission on Anaesthetics. Report of the Lancet commission appointed to investigate the subject of administration of chloroform and other anaesthetics from a clinical standpoint. Lancet. 1893b;141:761–76.

Commission on Anaesthetics. Report of the Lancet commission appointed to investigate the subject of the administration of chloroform and other anaesthetics from a clinical standpoint. Lancet. 1893c;141:899–914.

Commission on Anaesthetics. Report of the Lancet commission appointed to investigate the subject of the administration of chloroform and other anaesthetics from a clinical standpoint. Lancet. 1893d;141:971–8.

Commission on Anaesthetics. Report of the Lancet commission appointed to investigate the subject of the administration of chloroform and other anaesthetics from a clinical standpoint. Lancet. 1893e;141:1112–8.

Dyke M. When is it right to say no? Br J Theatre Nurse. 1999;9:584–7.

Fioratou E, Flin R, Glavin R, Patey R. Beyond monitoring; distributed situation awareness in anaesthesia. Br J Anaesth. 2010;105:83–90.

Flin R, Maran N. Basic concepts of crew resource management. Best Pract Res Clin Anaesthesiol. 2015;29(1):27–39.

Flin R, Patey R. Non-technical skills for anesthetists: developing and applying ANTS. Best Pract Res Clin Anaesthesiol. 2011;25(2):215–27.

Flin R, Goeters K, Amalberti R, et al. The development of the NOTECHS system for evaluating pilots' CRM skills. Hum Fact Aerosp Saf. 2003a;3:95–117.

Flin R, Glavin R, Maran N, Patey R. Anaesthetists' non-technical skills (ANTS) system handbook v1. 0. University of Aberdeen; 2003b.

Flin R, O'Connor P, Crichton M. Safety at the sharp end. A guide to non-technical skills. Aldershot: Ashgate; 2008.

Flin R, Patey R, Glavin R, Maran N. Anaesthetists' non-technical skills. Br J Anaesth. 2010;105(1):38–44. https://doi.org/10.1093/bja/aeq134.

Gaba DM. Crisis resource management and teamwork training in anaesthesia. Br J Anaesth. 2010;105(1):3–6.

Gaba DM, Howard SK, Fish KJ, Smith BE, Sowb YA. Simulation-based training in anesthesia crisis resource management (ACRM): a decade of experience. Simul Gaming. 2001;32(2):175–93.

Gawande AA, Zinner MJ, Studdert DM, Brennan TA. Analysis of errors reported by surgeons at three teaching hospitals. Surgery. 2003;133:614–21.

Glavin RJ. Excellence in anesthesiology: the role of non-technical skills. Anesthesiol J Am Soc Anesthesiol. 2009;110(2):201–3.

Harmer M. The case of Elaine Bromiley. 2005 Available from http://www.chfg.org/wp-content/uploads/ElaineBromileyAnonymous.

Helmreich RL, Foushee HC. Why crew resource management? Empirical and theoretical bases of human factors training in aviation. In: Wiener EL, Kanki BG, Helmreich RL, editors. Cockpit resource management. San Diego, CA: Academic Press; 1993. p. 3–45.

Jones C, Fawker-Corbett J, Groom P, Morton B, Lister C, Mercer S. Human factors in preventing complications in anaesthesia: a systematic review. Anaesthesia. 2018;73:12–24.

Kluger MT, Bukofzer M, Bullock M. Anaesthetic assistants: their role in the development and resolution of anaesthetic incidents. Anaesth Intensive Care. 1999;27:269–74.

Lingard L, Espin S, Whyte S, et al. Communication failures in the operating room: an observational classification of recurrent types and effects. Qual Saf Health Care. 2004;13:330–4.

Lunn JN, Mushin WW. Mortality associated with anaesthesia. Oxford: Nuffield Provincial Hospital Trust; 1982.

Maharaj A. Non-technical skills for the anaesthetist making the implicit, explicit. University of KWAZUKU-NATAL, No. 07; 2018.

Runciman WB, Sellen A, Webb RK, et al. The Australian Incident Monitoring Study. Errors, incidents and accidents in anaesthetic practice. Anaesth Intensive Care. 1993;21:506–19.

Rutherford JS, Flin R, Mitchell L. Non-technical skills of anaesthetic assistants in the perioperative period: a literature review. Br J Anaesth. 2012;109(1):27–31. https://doi.org/10.1093/bja/aes125.

Smith AF, Mishra K. Interaction between anaesthetists, their patients and the anaesthetic team. Br J Anaesth. 2010;105:60–8.

The Royal College of Anaesthetists. 4th National Audit Project. Major complications of airway management in the UK. 2011.

2 Role of Anesthesia Technician in Operating Theatre Including Quality Projects and JCI Accreditation

Y. Hammad, S. Bali, and A. Feki

Contents

Y. Hammad (✉)
ICU and Perioperative Medicine, Weill Cornell Medical College in Qatar, Hamad Medical Corporation, Doha, Qatar
e-mail: yhammad@hamad.qa

S. Bali · A. Feki
Department of Anesthesia, ICU and Perioperative Medicine, Hamad Medical Corporation, Doha, Qatar
e-mail: sbali@hamad.qa; afeki@hamad.qa

N. A. Shallik et al. (eds.), *Improving Anesthesia Technical Staff's Skills*,
https://doi.org/10.1007/978-3-030-88849-7_2

2.1 Background

The term of anesthesia tech. is often applied to technicians and technologists, However, the differences in qualifications and application between them are substantial.

The most common level of education for anesthesia technician, and that required for certification, is an associate degree, although certificate programs and bachelor's degrees in anesthesia technology do exist.

Associate degree programs typically take about 2 years to complete, and clinical experiences or internships are likely to take place near the end of that period.

Depending on the requirements, anesthesia tech. require a minimum of 1 year of academic education program after the completion of general high school certificate, from a recognized anesthesia education institute/university and some on-the-job training.

Most of this training practice should be learned in the hospital directly under the supervision of qualified preceptors. Anesthesia technician will have less responsibilities than anesthesia technologist but will still be responsible for keeping the anesthesia equipment clean and operating properly.

For an anesthesia technology program, this will be in addition to the above, other courses such as:

- Introduction to anesthesia technology.
- Anatomy and physiology.
- Medical terminology.
- Pharmacology related to anesthesia technology.

Other programs may also be required outside of the context of the anesthesia technology program such as life support training, infection prevention and control, and environmental safety.

Both anesthesia technician and technologist are assistants to licensed anesthesia providers working in a surgical arena in a hospital, clinic or maternity unit, and any other facility as part of their scope of services. But anesthesia technologist will have more responsibility than a technician although they will do a lot of the same things as a technician. He may be tasked with monitoring a patient's vital signs while they are under anesthesia.

2.2 Scope of Service

Anesthesia Tech. provide their services in all surgical centers, including all hospital services and off-site sites where anesthesia services are provided and works with all types of anesthesia-related care for surgical procedures, diagnostic and therapeutic [1].

The Anesthesia Tech. works in general in the operating theater, nonoperating room anesthetizing areas, and office-based settings, and provide his anesthesia service for all surgical specialties, including, but not limited to general, obstetric, trauma, cardiac, orthopedic, gastrointestinal, dental, and plastic surgery.

Anesthesia Tech. work areas may include:

Operating rooms (OR)	Emergency room (ER)
Obstetrics suites (OB)	Endoscopy areas
Interventional and/or diagnostic radiology	Dental suites
Post anesthesia care unit (PACU)	Ambulatory surgery suites
Intensive care unit (ICU)	Animal and research laboratories
Catheterization laboratory	Magnetic resonance imaging (MRI)

Anesthesia Tech. provide also anesthesia care to patients in urban, suburban, and rural areas, and are sometimes the sole anesthesia professionals delivering care to the military, rural, and medically underserved populations and serve as leaders, educators, mentors, and administrators.

2.3 Scope of Practice

The scope of practice is the legally authorized parameter concerning the clinical evaluation, intervention, and level of care functions that a healthcare practitioner can provide to a patient.

The basic intent of the scope of practice is to ensure that a health care practitioner has the appropriate training, knowledge, and experience to care for a patient. The scope of practice is mainly found or defined in:

- Legislation and government laws
- Accreditation standards
- Job descriptions
- Hospital policies and procedures
- Legal opinions

Job descriptions, legal opinions, and policies and procedures can define the operational duties and responsibilities of a specific position; however, the definition cannot exceed the laws that govern the scope of practice of the certified practitioner.

The following defines the scope of practice for the certified anesthesia tech* in compliance with education and training standards:

- *Airway Management and Ventilation*: Anesthesia Tech. are required to demonstrate knowledge, comprehension, and support the application of anesthetic principles and guidelines in relation to airway management during patient care.
- *Fluids, Whole Blood, and Blood Component Management*: Anesthesia Tech. are required to demonstrate knowledge, comprehension, and practical assistance with relation to fluid, whole blood, salvaged blood, and blood component management during patient care.
- *Pharmacology:* Anesthesia Tech. are required to demonstrate knowledge of pharmaceuticals and their practical use by the anesthesia provider during patient care.
- *Pathophysiology and Anesthesia Management:* Anesthesia Tech. are able to demonstrate knowledge, comprehension, and practically apply the following factors in relation to pathophysiology and anesthesia management during patient care.
- *Utilization of Biotechnology and Monitoring Equipment:* Anesthesia Tech. demonstrate knowledge, understanding, and practically apply anesthesia devices and ancillary equipment in relation to the use of biotechnology

during patient care in collaboration with the anesthesia care provider.

- *Critical Events Management in Anesthesia:* Anesthesia Tech. demonstrate knowledge and participate in the management of critical events during patient care, and support the application of anesthetic principles related to the management of critical events by identifying signs and symptoms and properly assisting in emergency situations with an appropriate treatment plan for a critical event specific to all age groups.
- *Equipment Guidelines:* Anesthesia Tech. are to demonstrate knowledge, understanding, and operational familiarity in relation to critical and non-critical equipment during patient care. In general, anesthesia tech. should demonstrate knowledge and aptitude with multiple devices and equipment. Furthermore, an understanding of maintenance standards and regulations should be demonstrated.
- *Regulatory Compliance:* In carrying out their practice, the Anesthesia Tech. will maintain and organize the environment, equipment, supplies, and anesthesia personnel to facilitate the functions of the department.
- *Management or Supervisory Roles:* In the practice of Anesthesia Tech. it may be necessary to develop a hierarchical position to maintain and organize the staff of anesthesia technology staff. When establishing a leadership role, the selected person must demonstrate an exemplary ability to organize and coordinate the functions of the department. It is recommended that such individuals have many years of experience and/or obtain an appropriate higher university degree [2].

2.4 The Responsibilities

Anesthesia Tech. are a vital part of any medical facility's anesthesia care team. They ensure that the anesthesia equipment is clean and functional and, most importantly, use their technical knowledge to protect the safety of the patient.

Anesthesia Tech. essential role is to assist Anesthesiologists in the acquisition, preparation and application of the equipment and supplies required for the administration of anesthesia. Outlined below are the common duties and responsibilities for each position. However, as stated above, job duties may differ depending upon where the Anesthesia Tech* works.

Generally, Anesthesia Tech. perform the same functions and provide this service by preparing and maintaining patient monitoring devices and anesthesia delivery systems before, during, and after anesthesia.

The common responsibilities of anesthesia tech* may include, but are not limited to, the following services:

2.5 Prior to Anesthesia

Anesthesia Tech. prepare equipment needed for the patient to safely undergo anesthesia. This involves [3]:

- Ordering and stocking routine anesthesia consumables supplies.
- Obtain the necessary equipment that anesthesia provider may need.
- Setting up the anesthesia equipment for which they are responsible.
- Preparing anesthesia drugs under the direction of the anesthesiologist.
- Checking and setting up the anesthetic machine.
- Preparing intravenous drugs.
- Preparing intravenous therapy administration equipment.
- Preparing a range of devices to maintain the patient's airway (e.g. laryngeal masks and endotracheal tube).
- Communicating with the patient when they arrive into the operating theatre.
- Establishing peripheral intravenous access.
- Applying anesthetic monitoring to help assess the patients' condition whilst under anesthesia. This may include electrocardiography (ECG), blood pressure, and oxygen saturation devices. The monitoring of other parameters such as anesthesia depth monitors (EEG, Bispectral index (BIS), etc.) may also be necessary.

2.6 During Anesthesia

The Anesthesia Tech. role includes assisting with:

- Inducing and maintaining adequate anesthesia.
- Assisting with line placements and intubations or spinals and epidurals.
- Assisting with IVs and airway devices.
- Establishing and securing an airway.
- Making sure that patients are positioned in such a way NOT to cause discomfort or injury during their procedure.
- Monitoring and maintaining patients' vital signs and anesthesia depth.
- Connecting and operating equipment that monitors patients' vital signs during surgery.
- Temperature monitoring and regulation.
- Collection and analysis of patient (blood) samples.
- Acquiring and administering transfusion fluids and equipment.

2.7 After Anesthesia

Anesthesia Tech. assist the anesthetist with:

- Waking the patient.
- Removing airway devices.
- Transferring patients to post-operative care units.
- Cleaning, Sterilizing, Disinfecting, anesthesia equipment and medical monitoring devices.
- Maintaining equipment and troubleshooting as necessary.
- Performing first-level maintenance on anesthesia equipment.
- Helping to transfer patients to post-op care units (PACU).
- Testing and maintaining equipment ahead of surgery.
- Managing operating room supply inventory [4].

2.8 The Advanced Roles

There are currently many recognized schools offering anesthesia assistant programs and a graduate degree specializing in anesthesia, where a graduate anesthesia assistant with advanced practical training and a diploma is capable of practicing anesthesia independently in some countries, and under the direct supervision of an anesthesiologist in others.

The institutions will further define the local scope of practice through their boards of directors and accreditation committees, which may include the following.

2.9 Preoperative/Pre-procedure

- Provide patient education and counseling.
- Perform a comprehensive history and physical examination, assessment, and evaluation.
- Conduct a pre-anesthesia assessment and evaluation.
- Develop a comprehensive patient-specific plan for anesthesia, analgesia, multimodal pain management, and recovery.
- Obtain informed consent for anesthesia and pain management.
- Select, order, prescribe, and administer pre-anesthetic medications, including controlled substances.

2.10 Intraoperative/Intra-procedure

- Implement a patient-specific plan of care, which may involve anesthetic techniques, such as general, regional and local anesthesia, sedation, and multimodal pain management.
- Select, order, prescribe, and administer anesthetic medications, including controlled substances, adjuvant drugs, accessory drugs, fluids, and blood products.

- Select and insert invasive and noninvasive monitoring modalities (e.g., central venous access, arterial lines, cerebral oximetry, bispectral index monitor, and transesophageal echocardiogram (TEE)).

2.11 Postoperative/ Post-procedure

- Facilitate emergence and recovery from anesthesia.
- Select, order, prescribe, and administer post-anesthetic medications, including controlled substances.
- Conduct post-anesthesia evaluation.
- Educate the patient related to recovery, regional analgesia, and continued multimodal pain management.
- Discharge from the post-anesthesia care area (PACU) or facility.

2.12 Pain Management

- Provide comprehensive patient-centered pain management to optimize recovery.
- Provide acute pain services, including multimodal pain management and opioid-sparing techniques.
- Provide anesthesia and analgesia using regional techniques for obstetric and other acute pain management.
- Provide advanced pain management, including acute, chronic, and interventional pain management.

2.13 Quality Improvement and Health Management

Quality improvement in the healthcare environment is the continuous review of patient processes and outcomes with the goal of gradually improving patient care and the efficiency of resources used such as time, personnel, equipment, and supplies.

2.14 Quality Improvement in Anesthesia Services

The aims for quality improvement in anesthesia services were outlined and adopted by many organizations, including the Institute for Healthcare Improvement (IHI) [5]. These aims serve as a basis on which quality is evaluated and improved and are described as follows:

- Safety.
- Effectiveness.
- Patient centeredness.
- Timeliness.
- Efficiency.
- Equity.

In other words, the goal of quality improvement is to improve patient outcomes and reduce health care costs. Additionally, risk management attempts to reduce or prevent patient injury or other negative patient experiences and what to do in the event of a negative event. Thus, to reduce future risks, it should introduce the event into a quality improvement process where the root cause of the event can be analyzed and can lead to policy or procedural changes to reduce the likelihood of similar injuries in the future.

The anesthesia Tech. who is an integral part of the perioperative team can also play an important role in quality improvement and risk management by:

- Following quality assurance processes and procedures.
- Helping to provide a safe, clean, and well-functioning anesthetic work environment by awareness of, response to and reporting of perioperative events.
- Identifying improvement opportunities while performing their tasks.
- Reporting unintended events, they have witnessed or been involved in through an organization's incident reporting system.
- Participating in critical event reviews and quality improvement projects.

2.15 Role of Anesthesia Tech. in Quality Improvement and Risk Management

Improving the quality of anesthesia should be an integral part of the system in which the anesthesia service is provided. Improving the quality of anesthesia services often involves reorganizing the way we work. Therefore, the challenge for the Anesthesia Tech. is to combine the effectiveness of perioperative care (especially the operating room) with safety and the best possible quality in preoperative logistics tasks.

Anesthesia Tech. can organize their quality improvement and patient safety efforts around three key areas:

- Translating evidence into practice,
- Identifying and mitigating hazards, and.
- Improving culture and communication.

While each of these areas requires different tools and programs, they help all healthcare organizations to assess progress in patient safety and quality, improve the delivery of anesthesia services, as well as a positive effect on professional satisfaction of practitioners and organizational commitment.

Anesthesia Tech. have always supported the continuous quality improvement of patient care through:

- Identification of complications and serious adverse events.
- Systematic collection of data on daily anesthesia practice, educational products, and efforts to improve the standardization of anesthesia equipment.
- Participation in a system to support and continually improve the quality of anesthesia services provided to patients and their families, fellow employees, physicians, and other customers.
- Participation in quality improvement and risk management activities of the anesthesiology department.
- Assistance in the development of action plans in response to professional staff feedback regarding improvement opportunities.
- Acquiring basic and possibly advanced life support (BLS–ALS) certifications.
- Participation in the development and continuous updating of departmental policies and procedures directly related to Anesthesia Tech. and performance duties.
- Participates in overtime coverage situations as reasonably requested.

The following activities are listed to highlight certain common areas in which Anesthesia Tech. can participate and even lead in terms of quality improvement and risk management.

2.15.1 Infection Prevention

Anesthesia tech. play a key role in reducing the risk that a patient will develop a postoperative infection each time the anesthesia equipment and work area are cleaned and configured for an incoming patient.

The anesthesia tech. must follow a formal protocol when dealing with contaminated items. Cleaning surfaces and equipment and installing a new enclosure reduces the chances of missing a milestone in the process.

An assessment of the room renewal process can identify opportunities for improvement in the cleaning and configuration process.

2.15.2 Anesthesia Equipment Checkup

Often, investigations of equipment-related injuries reveal that staff was poorly trained or not trained at all on the equipment in question. Part of this responsibility lies with management; however, each Anesthesia Tech. should endeavor to be trained on all of the equipment they use and to stay up to date on product information. Therefore, anesthesia equipment is another important area for both quality improvement and risk management.

The Anesthesia Tech. using patient care equipment must be properly trained before using the equipment. Inappropriate or improper use of equipment is a common source of harm to patients. In addition to cleaning and restocking, adhering to a routine configuration and equipment verification protocol to detect signs of leakage, wear, damage, and malfunction before use, can identify problems before they can cause problems, and therefore reduce patient injury.

When defective or malfunctioning equipment is involved in a patient care event or is suspected of causing injury to a patient, the anesthesia tech. should be aware of the associated policies and procedures as follows.

If the equipment is in use:

- Equipment must be immediately removed from service.
- If possible, leave the device "as it is." Without removing anything attached to the device supplies or accessories involved.
- Store the entire configuration in a safe place.
- Avoid changing settings or connections.

Preserving the equipment in this way will allow the medical equipment technician and risk management team to assess the equipment and its potential contribution to any patient injury. In addition, it may be necessary to return properly stored material to the manufacturer or even a regulatory body for further investigation.

If the equipment is defective but was not in use:

Some of the same considerations mentioned above may still apply:

- Identify the equipment as defective and in need of maintenance by clearly labeling the equipment with a label "Equipment Requires Service."
- Inform the manager or the appropriate technician of the defective equipment.
- As before, and even if a patient has not been injured, it may be necessary to:
- Keep the equipment in the state it was in when it was defective in order to facilitate an investigation by internal personnel, the manufacturer or a regulatory body.
- Make sure the equipment is not returned to service before it has been repaired and inspected.
- After repair, each local establishment will have an inspection and certification policy for the equipment before putting it back into service.

2.15.3 Assisting with Medication Administration

Regardless of whether Anesthesia Tech. can administer medication directly to the patient or not, most Anesthesia Tech. will assist in the preparation of medication. Therefore, careful labeling of syringes and infusions and verbal confirmation of the name, dose, and the route of medication with the anesthesia provider before administration may prevent a patient from receiving the wrong drug or the wrong dose.

The Anesthesia Tech. should check and confirm the right patient is receiving the right medication at the right dose in the right way to avoid serious injury that can occur from medication administration errors.

2.15.4 Witnessing or Involvement in an Unexpected Event

During performing their duties, Anesthesia Tech. may be involved in or attend an event that has injured or almost injured a patient or a worker. This event, which can be anything from a "near miss" to an "adverse event," must be reported to allow for early intervention and corrective action before an injury occurs.

Events reporting track the frequency of an event, so the more an event is reported, the more it becomes apparent that there is a system problem that needs to be resolved. Reporting an event with an adverse outcome will also prompt timely intervention and treatment of the patient.

2.15.5 Reporting of Adverse Events

Reporting usually includes filling in an incident or accident report form and notifying a supervisor. And most organizations have a process for reporting injuries or other adverse events and near misses for quality improvement and risk management. Therefore, most health care facilities have laws in place to protect the reporting and investigation of near misses and adverse events from being used in lawsuits as long as it is done for the purpose of quality improvement.

That is why, it is very important that individuals confine their discussion of the event within the approved reporting and review process. Therefore, Anesthesia Tech* should check with their organization's supervisor, quality management or risk management department to find out which method is used to report incidents and whether there is a specific statement or wording that should be included in the documentation, for example: "For quality improvement purposes only."

2.15.6 Critical Event Reviews and Root Cause Analysis

When there are more than two people or more than one team or service involved in the event, it is often unclear why or how an adverse event occurred. When individual accounts of the events are looked at separately, it can be confusing for the reviewer to set clear timelines and be clear about the details.

At this point, the Anesthesia Tech. if involved or a witness, will be called by the reviewer for a meeting called "review of critical events or root cause analysis of participants." This meeting will facilitate the compilation of each person's story by describing or organizing the occurrences that took place before, during, and after the event in order to identify the underlying cause(s) that led to the event, in order for the root cause is understood, a new process is put in place, and may also results in purchasing of new equipment, a better training of staff, or changes in policies, procedures, and communication methods to prevent the event from happening again.

2.16 Quality Improvement Anesthesia Tech. Team

Establishing a quality improvement project with other team members is the best way to improve any project. This is clearer and is especially true when making improvements that involve or intersect more than one work team or department.

The reasons behind using teams for quality improvement projects are two important reasons: first, people support what they are helping to create and second, decisions are best made at the levels where they carried out.

The project team will be responsible for identifying what is causing the problems or preventing the objective from being achieved within the current framework. And based on the results, the team will then describe the steps and compiled them into formal recommendations which will be submitted to the management group which will allow the desired objective to be achieved.

The role of Anesthesia Tech. in quality improvement projects is twofold:

- To carry out interdisciplinary processes to meet organizational Quality Improvement (QI) goals and to
- Measure, improve, and control Technical-sensitive indicators affecting patient outcomes specific to anesthesia practices.

All levels of Anesthesia technical staff from the Anesthesia technician to the chief of technicians play a part in promoting quality improvement within the healthcare provider organization. Here is an explanation of the involvement each level of the Anesthesia Tech* should have in promoting quality improvement:

2.16.1 The Chief of Technicians

The Chief technician should steer the technician participation in quality improvement. As a member of administrative leadership, the Chief of technicians must integrate technical practices into the organizational goals for excellence in patient outcomes through the communication of strategic goals to all levels of technicians' staff.

2.16.2 The Anesthesia Technologist

Is responsible for communicating and processing the organization's Quality Improvement goals and processes to the anesthesia technicians, identifying specific technical sensitive indicators (TSI) that need improvement according to his or her particular anesthesia unit and facility, and coordinating Quality Improvement processes to improve these at the unit level.

2.16.3 The Anesthesia Technician

The Anesthesia Technician may be the key to quality patient outcomes, carrying out the protocols and standards of care shown by evidence to improve patient care.

2.17 Anesthesia Tech. Familiarity with the Improvement Frameworks

The Anesthesia Tech. improvement path can be made more effective and efficient thanks to a structured approach and sufficient knowledge of the following different improvement models:

2.17.1 PDSA Cycle Methodology

The commonly used project methodology is called the PDCA/PDSA cycle, which is the acronym of the four components: Plan, Do, Check or Study, and Act.

- *Plan:* Make a plan for the test of change. Include predictions of results and how data will be collected.
- *Do:* Test change on a small scale. Document data, observations, and problems that occur.
- *Check/Study:* Use data gathered from previous stages to build new knowledge and make predictions.
- *Act:* Adopt the change or use the knowledge gained to plan or modify the next test of action.

2.17.2 Lean Methodology and Six Sigma

The Lean Production and Six Sigma model focuses on creating more value for the patient with fewer resources. Therefore, the ultimate goal is to eliminate all waste so that each step adds value to a process. Other key components of Lean include reducing workflow irregularities and eliminating the overload of people and equipment. Five principles govern Lean improvement:

- Define the value that the customer (Patient) is seeking.
- Identify and map the value stream.
- Smooth the flow between value-added steps.
- Create a pull between steps.
- Pursue perfection by continuing the process until you have achieved ultimate value with no waste.

2.18 Role of Anesthesia Tech. in Joint Commission International Accreditation

2.18.1 Joint Commission International Accreditation

Accreditation is defined as a process by which an organization grants recognition based on a demonstrated ability to meet predetermined criteria or established international standards. Therefore, the majority of healthcare organizations seek accreditation to demonstrate a satisfactory level of quality to government regulatory agencies and healthcare insurers.

In this regard, Joint Commission International (JCI) is one of the world's leading patient safety organizations that seek a world where every patient receives the highest quality of care possible through a set of demanding standards that represent the most current thinking in patient safety and quality improvement.

2.18.2 What Is JCI Accreditation?

The Joint Commission International (JCI) is a non-profit organization based in the USA founded in 1951, to improve patient safety and the quality of health care in the international community by providing education, publications, advisory services, and international accreditations and certifications. JCI works in partnership with hospitals, clinics, and academic medical centers, health systems and agencies, government ministries, universities, and international advocates to promote rigorous standards of care and provide solutions to achieve peak performance.

The Joint Commission is governed by a council made up of doctors, nurses, administrators, employers, health insurers, ethicists, quality experts, and consumer advocates. The board receives input from a national physician and hospital associations as it develops "standards" that will be used in the accreditation process.

The standards cover key functional areas within hospitals, including medication safety, patient treatment, infection control, patient rights, advocacy, etc. Hospitals are required to report on a selection of 57 different quality measures. Later, the Joint Commission began to place more emphasis on performance measures that have the greatest impact on patient outcomes, calling for performance measures to be supported by solid scientific evidence demonstrating an impact on results and that the measure accurately assesses the evidence-based process.

One of the ways the Joint Commission International exercises its influence is by setting standards and goals for organizations seeking accreditation. Recent examples include the Universal Protocol for Preventing Wrong Site, Wrong Procedure, and Wrong Person Surgery and the International Patient Safety Goals.

2.18.3 The International Patient Safety Goals

International Patient Safety Goals (IPSGs) help accredited organizations address specific areas of concern in some of the most problematic areas of patient safety.

Goal One: Identify patients correctly.

Goal Two: Improve effective communication.

Goal Three: Improve the safety of high-alert medications.

Goal Four: Ensure safe surgery.

Goal Five: Reduce the risk of health care-associated infections.

Goal Six: Reduce the risk of patient harm resulting from falls [6].

The process by which the Joint Commission performs a site assessment and review is called a "survey." The survey is an inspection by a team from the Joint Commission to assess the organization's compliance with current standards set forth by the Joint Commission and an assessment of the organization's quality improvement activities.

In addition to that, the Joint Commission will [7]:

- see the survey as an opportunity to provide education and advice on "good practices" to a hospital, which will help improve the quality of the organization,
- examine facilities,
- review performance measurement information generated by the organization,
- interview staff and management,
- examine identifying information,
- examine quality improvement processes,
- perform detailed reviews documentation in medical records, and,
- review the organization's policies and procedures.

Each hospital and healthcare facility that applies for JCI accreditation takes approximately 2 years to prepare. Meanwhile, the entire organization works together to develop and implement the new high quality and patient- safe policies, practices, and procedures that are required to meet JCI standards. These standards evaluation methods are:

- Designed to stimulate and support sustained quality improvement.
- Created to reduce risk.

- Focused on building a culture of patient safety.
- Developed by health care experts from around the world—and tested in every world region.
- Developed by health professionals specifically for the health care sector.
- Applicable to individual health care organizations and national health care systems.

The perioperative arena in which anesthesia tech. work is a key area that comes under scrutiny when hospitals go through the accreditation process. In addition, many anesthesia technicians may wish to participate in a training program that can be accredited [8].

2.19 Planning for a Successful JCI Accreditation Visit

As surveyors trace a patient's experience in a healthcare organization, they observe the doctors, nurses, and anesthesia tech*. Therefore, awareness of expectations and extensive preparation for the visit will facilitate a successful and rewarding visit.

To ensure a successful accreditation visit, careful preparation is essential. Here are some preparation suggestions:

- Establish a plan with a timeline for all preparation activities.
- Demonstrate awareness of the standards.
- Focus on the intent of each standard.
- Identify areas of partial or no compliance with standards.
- Develop a plan to achieve compliance with identified areas.
- Implement and evaluate the plan.
- Incorporate standards into day-to-day work.
- Assist in the education of all staff on the standards and ways the organization meets them.
- Keep at least a year's track record of evidence.
- Read literature relevant to accreditation of setting.
- Network with others who have gone through the accreditation process.

Preparing for accreditation requires the ability to compare and contrast. Compare the standards of the Joint Commission with the performance of the organization. Are they similar or different? If there is a similarity, what evidence of this similarity can be made obvious to the Joint Commission visitors? If different, what can you do to become compliant?

Anesthesia Tech. should be aware that JCI surveys can be carried out unannounced and could be conducted be during the evening, night, and weekend hours at hospitals, and maybe interviewed or observed by a Joint Commission surveyor to check for compliance with Joint Commission standards and the organization's policies and procedures. Hence Anesthesia Tech. must be knowledgeable of Joint Commission International accreditation policies and procedures, sentinel events, national safety goals, the care environment, and other JCI mandates directly related to anesthesia and patient safety, and should identify the anesthesia-related areas in need of improvement and address any issues that have been raised ("requests for improvement") prior to the official survey throughout the year in order to be ready once the actual survey occurs.

It is a common practice for the surveyor to ask for the employee file of anyone he or she speaks with to verify that the education experience and training are suitable for the work being performed. The surveyor will also inspect specific patient care areas in the facility. This may include physical research for outdated products and medications, check if all employees are wearing the appropriate attire (including ID badge) for their workspace, and verify if the workspace is compliant to safety standards.

JCI surveyors may also review specific documentation in areas of patient care, including documentation generated by or involving anesthesia tech*. For example, surveyors can consult the documentation on:

- Quality control results for a point-of-care testing device,
- Maintenance records for anesthesia equipment, or.

• Documentation in an employee's file demonstrating competence and training [9].

2.20 Role of Anesthesia Tech. in JCI Accreditation Survey

During the survey, the Joint Commission team follows a patient tracer through selectins a specific patient and follows that patient's documentation throughout the duration of the hospital stay. With this tracing methodology, team members can talk to those involved in the patient's care and check medical records to ensure all patient documentation is complete. A negative survey by the Joint Commission can be catastrophic for a healthcare facility that could lose funding and/or be closed. Therefore, hospitals take accreditation very seriously, and every department feels under the microscope when a survey is in process, including the anesthesia department.

Hence, anesthesia tech. has an important role and responsibility during a JCI survey, and can either positively or negatively impact a survey, as their workspace, operating room turnover, infection control procedures, equipment storage, equipment quality control logs, training logs, etc., can all come under scrutiny during a survey. Anesthesia Tech. knowledge of standards and the accreditation process will significantly be important to the facility and the organization and will be much crucial during the JCI survey.

During JCI Accreditation Survey, Anesthesia Tech. should be relaxed and confident, and have to understand the surveyor question, seek help when needed, and show evidence If required, and have to:

- Maintain Anesthesia unit clean and tidy, equipment is in proper place, clean with ready to use tag and valid PPM (planed, preventive, maintenance) stickers and exits and fire hose reel are not blocked.
- Demonstrate knowledge about the vision, mission, and values of the organization.
- Demonstrate knowledge about Accreditation Standards and JCI Requirement Categories.
- Be aware of the six International Patient Safety Goals.
- Know the requirements for staff performing the point of care test (POCT).
- Demonstrate knowledge of medication management and use, narcotics administration and registration Medication management and use (MMU).
- Demonstrate awareness of patient and family bill of rights and responsibilities (PFR and PFE).
- Demonstrate knowledge about Hospital Management Standards such as Quality Improvement and Patient Safety (QPS), Prevention and Control of Infections (PCI), and Facility Management and Safety (FMS).
- Demonstrate knowledge about Management of Information (MOI).
- Show understanding to the various responsibilities and authority of individuals in the organization.
- Demonstrate knowledge about their role in quality improvement program and during a major incident.
- Demonstrate awareness of fire and safety and know how to handle hazardous materials and how to dispose infectious wastes.
- Demonstrate knowledge of sentinel events / untoward events/near misses and how to deal with such situations.

Knowledge of the standards and the JCI accreditation process will provide Anesthesia Tech. with the opportunity to develop their skills and knowledge and significantly increase their values for the organization and they will be highly valued by their facility's management team. On the other hand, Joint Commission certification improves the quality of patient care by reducing variations in clinical processes. The focus on clinical practice guidelines helps organizations establish a cohesive approach to care, reducing thus the risk of error. This helps to maintain a consistently high level of quality, using effective data-driven performance improvement.

2.21 Conclusion

The Anesthesia Tech. are an allied health care professional who plays an important role in performing many critical tasks such as diagnosing illnesses, maintaining equipment, and caring for patients. Without Anesthesia Tech., the operating theatre could not function.

The Anesthesia Tech. help anesthesiologists by performing a variety of important tasks. Generally, Anesthesia Tech. assist in the administration of anesthesia and monitoring of patients. Anesthesia Tech. are highly skilled, with a deep understanding of anesthesia techniques, instruments, dosages, and technology.

Anesthesia Tech. work in operating theaters, but he/she also employed in emergency rooms, intensive care units (ICUs) or outpatient surgery clinics. He/She plays a role in all stages of anesthesia (before, during, and after anesthesia).

Before anesthesia is administered, the Anesthesia Tech. might be responsible for cleaning and testing machines, preparing instruments and medications, and applying monitoring equipment.

When the patient is under anesthesia, Anesthesia Tech. can help ensure that dosages are correct, monitor the patient's vital signs, or help establish and secure the airways so the patient can breathe easily.

After the procedure, the Anesthesia Tech. will help wake the patient up and transfer them to the postoperative care units. With all of these responsibilities, Anesthesia Tech. need a lot of training. In addition to an in-depth knowledge of drugs, equipment, dosages, and anesthesia techniques, AT should understand anatomy and physiology and know how to respond in all types of patient situations.

Therefore, if we want to summarize the role of the Anesthesia Tech. in a short sentence: "It's crucial **work in a growing field**" [10].

References

1. AANA. Scope of nurse anesthesia practice. AANA. 2015. https://www.aana.com/docs/default-source/practice-aana-com-web-documents-(all)/scope-of-nurse-anesthesia-practice.pdf?sfvrsn=250049b1_2.
2. ASATT. American Society of Anesthesia Technologists and Technicians scope of practice. 2015. Retrieved from www.asatt.org: https://www.asatt.org/images/pdfs/ASATTScopeofPracticeFinalNov2015.pdf.
3. Team S-B. The role of an anesthesia tech before and after surgery. 2015. Retrieved from Sanford-Brown: https://www.sanfordbrown.edu/Student-Life/blog/May-2015/The-Role-of-an-Anesthesia-Tech.
4. Description UH Anesthesia technician. 2019. Retrieved from whealth.org: https://www.uwhealth.org/files-directory/position-descriptions/technologists-technicians/anesthesia.tech.510034.pdf.
5. Zezo D. Quality improvement in anesthesia practice and patient safety 2020. Retrieved from Anesthesia Key: https://aneskey.com/quality-improvement-in-anesthesia-practice-and-patient-safety/.
6. JCI Team. International patient safety goals. 2021. Retrieved from Joint Commission International: https://www.jointcommissioninternational.org/standards/international-patient-safety-goals/.
7. Solutions L. Preparing for your joint commission visit. 2017. Retrieved from lippincottsolutions: http://lippincottsolutions.lww.com/blog.entry.html/2017/09/26/preparing_for_yourj-61xz.html.
8. Resources J. Joint Commission International for Hospitals. Oak Brook, IL: Joint Commission Resources; 2021.
9. Wolterskluwer. Preparing for your Joint Commission visit. 2017. Retrieved from Wolterskluwer: https://www.wolterskluwer.com/en/expert-insights/preparing-for-your-joint-commission-visit.
10. Team C. What is an anesthesia technician. 2020. Retrieved from citycollege.edu: https://www.citycollege.edu/what-is-an-anesthesia-technician/

3 Pharmacology of the Most Common Anesthesia Drugs

Nabil A. Shallik, Lamia Tawfik, Muhammad Firas Alhammad, Nada N. Shallik, and Cherif Boutabba

Contents

N. A. Shallik (✉) · L. Tawfik · M. F. Alhammad
Department of Anesthesia, ICU and Perioperative Medicine, Hamad Medical Corporation, Doha, Qatar
e-mail: nshallik@hamad.qa; ltawfik@hamad.qa; MAlhammad@hamad.qa

N. N. Shallik
Faculty of Oral and Dental Medicine, Future University Hospital, New Cairo, Egypt

C. Boutabba
Anesthesia Department, Women's Wellness and Research Center, Doha, Qatar
e-mail: cboutabba@hamad.qa

N. A. Shallik et al. (eds.), *Improving Anesthesia Technical Staff's Skills*,
https://doi.org/10.1007/978-3-030-88849-7_3

3.1 Introduction

This chapter includes a thorough overview of the key knowledge about various anesthetic drugs required for anesthesia technician or technologist's day-to-day workflow.

3.2 Pharmacology

3.2.1 Introducaiton to Types of Anesthesia

General Anesthesia

General anesthesia (GA) is appropriate for most major surgical procedures. A reversible state of Stage III surgical anesthesia is established, including the following goals:

- Hypnosis/unconsciousness.
- Amnesia.
- Analgesia.
- Muscle relaxation or immobility as appropriate for the procedure.
- Autonomic and sensory blockade of responses to noxious surgical stimulation.

Anesthesia or sleeping with general anesthesia occurs in four stages that may not be observed, as they can occur very quickly.

Sage I (Analgesia) The patient experiences analgesia or pain loss but remains conscious that the conversation can continue.

Stage II (Excitement) The patient may have delirium or become violent. Blood pressure decreases and the rate of respiration increases. The administration of barbiturates typically bypasses this stage.

Stage III (Surgical Anesthesia) The skeletal muscles relax during this stage, and the patient's breathing becomes regular, eye movements slow then stop, and surgery can begin.

Stage IV (Medullary Paralysis) This stage happens when the respiratory centers in the brain's medulla oblongata, which regulate the breathing and other vital functions, cease to operate. Death can result if the patient is not quick to be revived. We should never reach this stage. Careful control of the anesthetic amounts administered prevents this occurrence.

GA has three distinct phases: induction, maintenance, and emergence, as described below.

Induction

GA induction may be done with intravenous (IV) and/or inhalation agents. Administration of a sedative-hypnotic agent (e.g. Propofol, Etomidate, and Ketamine) and one or more adjuvant IV agents (e.g. opioids and/or benzodiazepine, commonly used Midazolam) as well as a neuromuscular blocking agent (NMBA) when planning for endotracheal intubation.

Maintenance

Additional agents are required immediately after GA induction to sustain the anesthetic state. Anesthesia is often sustained through the use of a primary inhalation technique. Total Intravenous Anesthesia (TIVA) is an alternative technique. Most commonly, inhalation and/or IV anesthetic combinations are administered to maintain GA, with the aim of reducing the total dose of any one agent.

If muscle relaxation or complete paralysis is required to facilitate surgery, then an NMBA is used.

Emergence

GA emergence is the return of consciousness and movement at the end of the surgical procedure, after discontinuing anesthetic and adjuvant administration and reversing residual NMBA effects. The trachea may be extubated without assistance when the patient has sufficient spontaneous ventilation.

3.2.2 Main Types of Medication in Anesthesia Practice

Main types of medications used in general anesthesia are as follows:

- *Induction* medications to produce and maintain unconsciousness including intravenous and volatile agents.
- *Analgesics* to provide pain relief.
- *Muscle relaxants* to induce muscle relaxation.

Other medications which are used frequently in anesthesia field include the following:

- medications that produce short-term memory loss or amnesia;
- medications that minimize nausea and vomiting (*antiemetics*);
- medications that counteract the effect of other medications (*antagonists*);
- and medications that suppress or stimulate certain nervous reflexes i.e. medications modulate sympathetic and parasympathetic response.

Essential Introduction to Pharmacology

The difference between pharmacokinetics and pharmacodynamics:

Before we go into further detail, let us differentiate between pharmacokinetics and pharmacodynamics. The difference between pharmacokinetics (PK) and pharmacodynamics (PD) can be summed up pretty simply. *Pharmacokinetics* is the study of what the body does to the drug and *Pharmacodynamics* is the study of what the drug does to the body.

Pharmacokinetics:

It is defined simply by how the body is acting towards the drug. It is divided to four stages: absorption, distribution, metabolism, and excretion.

Absorption It is related to the route of administration which can be oral, transdermal, rectal, sublingual, inhalational, intramuscular, intrathecal, and intravenous.

Distribution It is related to lipid solubility, protein binding, drug ionization, and molecular weight.

Metabolism Most of the drugs metabolized in liver through two phases as follows.

Phase 1: It is also known as non-synthetic phase. It includes oxidation, reduction, and hydrolysis.

Phase 2: It is also known as synthetic phase. It includes glucuronidation, sulfation acetylation, methylation, and glycination. The main aim of this phase is to increase the solubility of the metabolized drug.

Excretion It is simply removal of the medication out the body. "It differs from elimination which is removal of the medication out the plasma." Most of the drugs excreted by bile and urine however other possible excretion routs are breast milk and tears.

Pharmacodynamics:

It is defined as the effect of drug on the body, it is simply the mechanism of action of a drug. In fact, there are three ways that drug can act in our bodies, these are:

1. depending on the physiochemical properties of the medication,
2. binding specific receptors to produce a certain effect,
3. binding specific enzymes in order to inhibit/decrease its activity.

3.2.3 Induction Medications

Generally speaking, induction agents could be intravenous drugs or inhalation agents.

Intravenous drugs include but not limited to thiopentone, etomidate, ketamine, and propofol. These drugs easily make patients unconscious when given by intravenous injection. This rapid loss of consciousness makes anesthesia induction much more pleasant than before when patients were forced to breathe Ether or Chloroform and necessarily avoiding stage 2 excitement stage as well.

3.2.3.1 Intravenous Anesthetics

Thiopentone sodium

Generic name: Thiopental sodium (Thiopental) Fig. 3.1a:

Form: Injection (powder for solution for injection) 0.5-g and 1-g vials.

Uses: induction of anesthesia prior to administration of inhalational anesthetic; anesthesia of short duration.

Contraindications: inability to maintain airway, cardiovascular disease, dyspnoea or obstructive respiratory disease; hypersensitivity to barbiturates "porphyria."

Precautions: local extravasation can result in extensive tissue necrosis and sloughing; intra-arterial injection causes intense pain and may result in artery spasm; hepatic impairment.

Dosage: Induction, by intravenous injection as a 2.5% (25 mg/mL) solution over 10–15 s, adult 100–150 mg (reduced in elderly or debilitated patients), followed by a further 100–150 mg if necessary according to the response after 60 s or up to 4 mg/kg; child 2–7 mg/kg repeated if necessary according to the response after 60 s.

Preparation: Solutions containing 25 mg/mL should be freshly prepared by mixing 20 mL of water for injections with the contents of the 0.5-g vial or 40 mL with the 1-g vial. Any solution made up over 24 h previously or in which cloudiness, precipitation or crystallization is evident should be discarded

Adverse effects: rapid injection may result in severe hypotension and hiccup; cough, laryngeal spasm, allergic reactions.

Ketamine

Generic name: ketamine (Fig. 3.1b)

Form: Solution for injection 50 mg/mL, 10 mL or 10 mg/mL vials.

Uses: induction and maintenance of general anesthesia either alone or in combination with other medications; analgesia for painful procedures of short duration.

Contraindications: thyrotoxicosis; hypertension (including pre-eclampsia); the history of cerebrovascular accident, cerebral trauma, intracerebral mass or hemorrhage, or other cause of raised intracranial pressure; eye injury and increased intraocular pressure; psychiatric disorders particularly hallucinations

Precautions: Supplementary analgesia, which is frequently needed during recovery in surgical procedures involving acute pain, patients must remain undisturbed while under observation.

Dosage:

Induction by intramuscular injection: Adult and child 6.5–13 mg/kg (10 mg/kg usually produces 12–25 min of anesthesia). Induction, by intravenous injection over at least 1 min, adult and child 1–4.5 mg/kg (2 mg/kg usually produces 5–10 min of anesthesia).

Induction by intravenous infusion: of a solution containing 1 mg/mL, adult and child total induction dose 0.5–2 mg/kg; maintenance (using

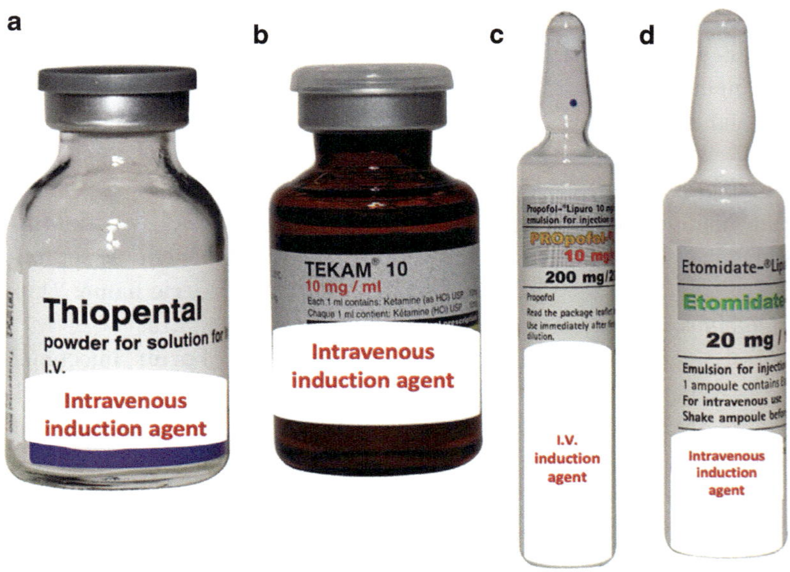

Fig. 3.1 Intravenous induction agents: (**a**) Thioptntal, (**b**) Ketamine(Tekam), (**c**) Propofol, (**d**) Etomidate

micro drip infusion), 10–45 mg/kg/min, rate adjusted according to response.

Analgesia: by intramuscular injection, adult and pediatric initially 4 mg/kg.

Adverse effects: Hallucinations and other emergence reactions (during recovery are accompanied by behavioral changes and these effects are rarely persist for more than a few hours). Transient elevation of heart rate and blood pressure are common; arrhythmias, occasional hypotension, and bradycardia have occurred.

Propofol

Generic name: Propofol Fig. 3.1c

Forms: injectable solutions 10 mg/mL 20 mL vials and 50 mL PFS.

Uses: Induction and maintenance of general anesthesia, sedation for short procedures, combined sedation and regional anesthesia, and in ICU sedation of intubated and mechanically ventilated patients.

Contraindications: Hypersensitivity (documented), egg, and soybean allergy.

Precautions: Do not use quick bolus because it increases the likelihood of unwanted cardiorespiratory depression, hypotension, apnea, and/or oxygen desaturation.

Doses:

Induction: by intravenous injection, adults (2–2.5 mg/kg) and child 2.5–3.5 mg/kg.

Maintenance: by intravenous infusion, adults (0.1–0.2 mg/kg/min) and child (0.125–0.3 mg/kg/min).

Adverse effects: Hypotension, Apnea which may last for 30–60 s, injection site burning/pain which may be decreased by administering IV lidocaine before propofol bolus, rash, itching, arrhythmia (irregular heart rate), bradycardia or tachycardia.

Etomidate

Generic Name: Etomidate Fig. 3.1d:

Form: injectable solution, 2 mg/mL, 10 mL vial.

Uses: Induction of general anesthesia and rapid sequence intubation, also can be used for the maintenance of GA and sedation. It is an ideal choice for shock trauma, hypovolemic patients, or patients with significant cardiovascular disease.

Contraindications In any patient with a known hypersensitivity reaction, etomidate is contraindicated. It is commonly used in intubation with rapid sequence (RSI). Septic patients have an increased risk of developing adrenal suppression which in some research has been associated with increased mortality. Lower doses may be used with caution in liver disease and renal impairment, as it is metabolized in the liver and excreted by the kidneys.

Dose: An induction dose of etomidate at 0.2–0.3 mg/kg, injected over 30–60 s for adults, not recommended for children below 10 years. Etomidate is no longer administered by continuous infusion because of the risks of sustained suppression of endogenous cortisol and aldosterone production.

3.2.3.2 Volatile Anesthetics

Inhalational Anesthetics

Those medications render patient unconscious during surgery and might be used for inhalational induction particularly in infants, however, because the second stage is remarkably prolonging when using these medications, the main use is to maintain anesthesia and not to induct it. These medications are called inhalational agents as they are inhaled by patients. Halothane was introduced in the 1950s and replaced the older agents like Ether. Halothane has now largely been substituted and the commonly used agents nowadays include enflurane, isoflurane, sevoflurane, and desflurane.

- ***Non-volatile gases:*** nitrous oxide (N_2O), xenon "the only two available in gas form."
- ***Volatile gases:*** halothane, isoflurane, desflurane, and sevoflurane.

Halothane Volatile Liquid

Uses: induction, maintenance of anesthesia, and adjunctive anesthesia maintenance to intravenous (IV) anesthetic agents (i.e., midazolam and propofol).

Contraindications: History of unexplained liver dysfunction or pyrexia following previous exposure to halothane; family history of malignant hyperthermia; reduced ejection fraction heart failure, pheochromocytoma.

Precautions: Anesthetic history should be taken carefully to determine previous exposure and reactions to halothane (at least 3 months should be allowed to elapse between each re-exposure, arrhythmias, pregnancy, and breastfeeding.

Dosage:

Induction: Using a specifically calibrated vaporizer, gradually increase inspired gas concentration to 2–4% adult or 1.5–2% pediatric in oxygen or nitrous oxide/oxygen.

Maintenance: adult and pediatric 0.5–2%.

Adverse effects: Arrhythmias; bradycardia; respiratory depression; hepatic damage.

Malignant hyperthermia, halothane was the most common agent which caused this reaction when used with depolarizing neuromuscular blocker (succinylcholine).

Isoflurane Volatile Liquid

Uses: It is a non-flammable volatile anesthetic, but it has a strong pungent odor which makes it difficult to use it for induction of inhalational general anesthesia.

Contraindications: All halogenated volatile anesthetics, including isoflurane, in susceptible patients, are known to trigger malignant hyperthermia. Any patient with a confirmed or suspected history of malignant hyperthermia should be considered at elevated risk for malignant hyperthermia; relative contraindication in patients with severe asthma or active bronchospasm due to the pungency of the agent.

Precautions: Isoflurane is rarely used for induction of anesthesia, but instead, IV anesthetic agent can be used for induction of anesthesia.

Dosage: MAC of isoflurane is 1.2%.

Adverse effects: Isoflurane should be carefully titrated to the patient as it can cause a drop in blood pressure due to dose-dependent peripheral vasodilation.

Desflurane Volatile Liquid: (Fig. 3.2a)

Uses: induction or maintenance of anesthesia in adults. It may also be used for maintenance of anesthesia in pediatric patients following induction with agents other than desflurane.

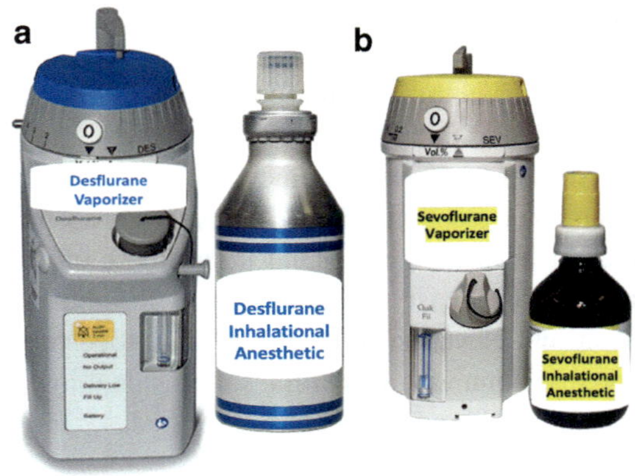

Fig. 3.2 (**a**) Desflurane & Vaporizer (**b**) Sevoflurane & Vaporizer

Contraindications:

- induction of anesthesia in pediatric patients because of a high incidence of moderate to severe upper airway adverse reaction as laryngospasm.
- in patients with known or suspected susceptibility to malignant hyperthermia.
- history of moderate to severe hepatic impairment following general anesthesia with desflurane.
- Increased intracranial pressure.
- relative contraindication in patients with severe asthma or active bronchospasm due to the pungency of the agent.

Precautions: It has a non-pungent odor, making it suitable to use for the induction of general anesthesia. It is used most commonly for maintenance of general anesthesia after induction with an IV or another inhalational agent.

Dosage: (MAC) of desflurane is 6.0%.

Adverse effects: It is a potent vasodilator and can cause a decrease in blood pressure by decreasing systemic vascular resistance (SVR) which may lead to an increase in heart rate. It enhances the effects of rocuronium, greater than either sevoflurane, isoflurane or intravenous anesthetics.

Sevoflurane Volatile Liquid (Fig. 3.2b)

Uses: Inhalational induction of general anesthesia in neonatal and pediatric patients in absence of pre-induction intravenous access.

Inhalational induction of general anesthesia in adult patients whose clinical condition requires spontaneous respirations during induction.

May be used for complete maintenance of general anesthesia or concurrently with intravenous anesthetics to maintain general anesthesia in adult and pediatric patients.

Contraindications:

- Hypersensitivity to sevoflurane or any other halogenated anesthetics.
- Patient with known or suspected susceptibility to malignant hyperthermia.
- relative contraindication in patients presenting with renal dysfunction undergoing extensive surgical procedures.

Precautions: It has a non-pungent odor, making suitable it difficult to use for the induction of general anesthesia. It is used most commonly for maintenance of general anesthesia after induction with an IV or another inhalational agent.

Dosage: *Adults MAC Values for Surgical Levels of Anesthesia*

- Age 25 years: Sevoflurane in oxygen: 2.6%.
- Age 40 years: Sevoflurane in oxygen: 2.1%.
- Age 60 years: Sevoflurane in oxygen: 1.7%.
- Age 80 years: Sevoflurane in oxygen: 1.4%.

Pediatric MAC Values for Surgical Levels of Anesthesia

- Newborn to 1-month-old full-term neonates: Sevoflurane in oxygen: 3.3%.
- One to younger than 6 months: Sevoflurane in oxygen: 3%.
- Six months to younger than 1 year: Sevoflurane in oxygen: 2.8%.
- One to younger than 3 years: Sevoflurane in oxygen: 2.8%.

Adverse effects:

- Hypotension, hypertension, tachycardia, bradycardia.
- Emergence delirium and agitation.
- Postoperative nausea and vomiting.
- Respiratory: Laryngospasm (2–8%), breath-holding, apnea.
- Anaphylaxis, anaphylactoid reaction, cardiac arrhythmias, QT prolongation, increased intracranial pressure, hepatotoxicity, electrolyte disturbances, and malignant hyperthermia.

Nitrous Oxide Inhalation Gas

Odorless, colorless, and non-flammable gas

Uses: Maintenance of anesthesia in combination with other anesthetic agents (volatile or intravenous agents) and muscle relaxants. Analgesia for obstetric practice is 50% mixture with oxygen.

Contraindications:

- Critically ill patients: Nitrous oxide inactivates methionine synthase by cobalt oxidation in vitamin B12 and can cause megaloblastic anemia. This enzyme is important for the metabolism of vitamin B12 and folate and plays a role in other substances' synthesis and synthesis of DNA and RNA.
- Severe cardiac disease: Methionine synthase is also needed to convert homocysteine to methionine, and high levels of serum homocysteine are associated with an increased risk of adverse coronary events. The clinician should avoid using nitrous oxide in the setting of severe cardiac disease.
- The first trimester of pregnancy: Due to the above-referenced impact on B12 and folate metabolism, nitrous use is not recommended in the first trimester of pregnancy.
- Venous or arterial air embolism.
- Since nitrous oxide is 30 times more soluble than oxygen, so, it is not used in the following conditions: pneumothorax, small bowel obstruction, middle ear surgery, retinal surgery, and head and neck procedures. It diffuses faster into closed spaces than nitrogen resulting in increased volume and pressure of the gas within closed spaces. It may accumulate in the pneumoperitoneum in laparoscopic cases.
- Pulmonary hypertension: Nitrous oxide can increase pulmonary artery pressures.

Precautions: minimize exposure of staff, pregnancy.

Dosage:

Anesthesia: adult and pediatric nitrous oxide mixed with 25–30% oxygen.

Analgesia: 50% nitrous oxide mixed with 50% oxygen.

Adverse effects: Nausea and vomiting. Megaloblastic anemia after prolonged administration due to depressed white cell formation. Peripheral neuropathy.

Oxygen: In fact, this gas in essential in anesthesia practice. The air we inhale contains roughly 21% of oxygen gas.

Uses: To maintain an adequate oxygen tension during inhalational anesthesia.

Dosage: The concentration of oxygen in inspired anesthetic gases should never be less than 21%.

Adverse effects: Concentrations above 80% have a toxic effect on the lungs that leads to pulmonary congestion, exudation, and atelectasis.

3.2.4 Analgesics

Analgesia medication are varies in their mechanism of action to produce reducing or elimination the unpleasant feeling of pain. Opiates or narcotics are well known painkillers, they are either extracted from opium (such as morphine) or synthesized in a laboratory (such as pethidine or meperidine, fentanyl, alfentanil, sufentanil, and remifentanil). In modern practice the concept of multimodal analgesia is evolving and many recommends sharing opioids with other subtypes of medications. Other main targets for analgesia medications include cyclooxygenase 1 & cyclooxygenase 2, and *N*-Methyl-D-aspartic acid or *N*-Methyl-D-aspartate (NMDA) (ketamine).

3.3 Analgesics and Opioid Antagonists

Opioid analgesics, such as morphine, fentanyl, and remifentanil, may be used to supplement general anesthesia. Repeated doses of intraoperative analgesics should be given with care, since respiratory depression may persist into the postoperative period.

Morphine: (Fig. 3.3a)
Form: Its administration is most often via the following routes: orally (PO), intravenously (IV), intramuscular (IM), subcutaneous (SC), epidural, and intrathecal.

Uses: adjunct during major surgery; postoperative analgesia; pain, myocardial infarction, acute pulmonary edema.

Contraindications: acute respiratory depression; increased intracranial pressure, head injury or brain tumor; severe hepatic impairment; hypothyroidism; convulsive disorders; acute alcoholism, spastic conditions of colon; recent surgery on biliary tract; diarrhea due to toxins.

Precautions: asthma, heart failure secondary to chronic lung disease; inability to maintain airway; renal impairment.

Dosage:

Premedication: by subcutaneous or intramuscular injection 1 h before surgery, adult 150–200 mcg/kg; by intramuscular injection 1 h before surgery, pediatric 50–100 mcg/kg.

Intraoperative analgesia: by intravenous injection, adult and pediatric 100 mcg/kg, repeated every 40–60 min as required.

Postoperative analgesia: by intramuscular injection, adult 150–200 mcg/kg every 4 h, pediatric 100–200 mcg/kg; or by intravenous infusion adult 8–10 mg over 30 min, then 2–2.5 mg/h

Adverse effects: respiratory depression; anorexia, nausea, vomiting, constipation; euphoria, dizziness, drowsiness, confusion, headache; dry mouth; spasm of urinary and biliary tract; circulatory depression, hypotension, bradycardia, palpitations; miosis; allergic reactions; physical dependence.

Fentanyl: (Fig. 3.3b)
Form: Its administration is most often via the following routes: orally (PO), intravenously (IV), intramuscular (IM), subcutaneous (SC), transdermal as skin patches (TD), intranasally (IN) in the form of a volatile nasal spray, transmucosal, epidural, and intrathecal.

Uses: 50–100 times more potent than morphine, used as adjunct during minor or major surgery; postoperative analgesia; pain management, myocardial infarction, acute pulmonary edema.

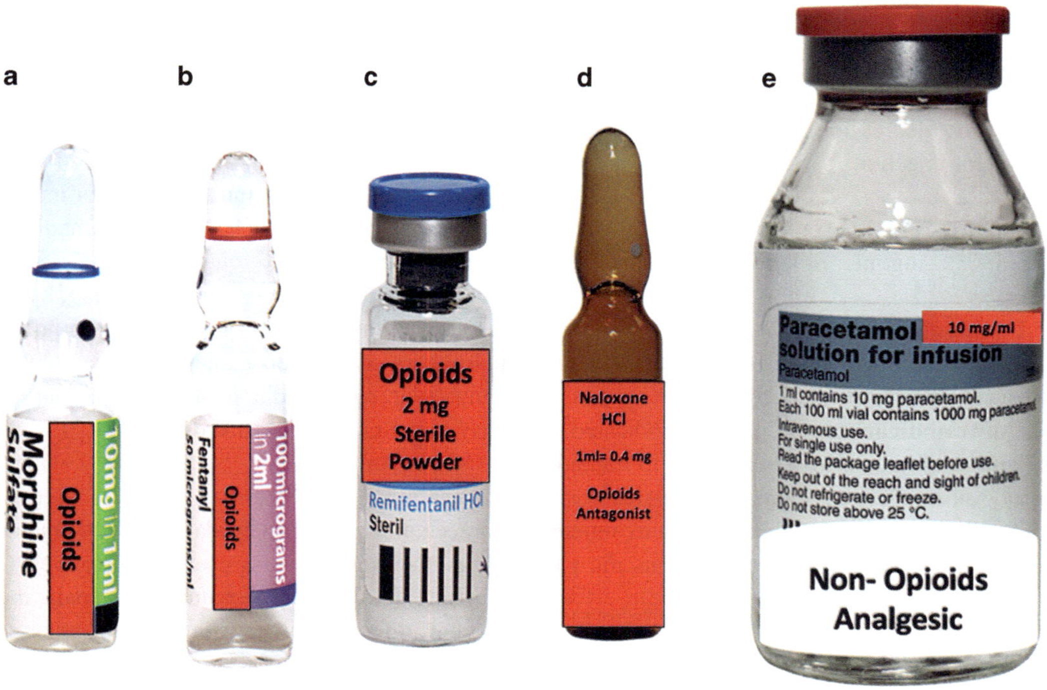

Fig. 3.3 (**a**) Morphine; (**b**) Fentanyl; (**c**) Remifentanil, (**d**) Naloxone, (**e**) Paracetamol

Contraindications: Fentanyl is relatively contraindicated or can be given with some precautions in the following conditions: postoperative in biliary tract surgeries, respiratory depression or obstructive airway diseases (i.e., asthma, COPD, obstructive sleep apnea OSA, obesity, liver failure, hypersensitivity (i.e., anaphylaxis).

Precautions: asthma, heart failure secondary to chronic lung disease; inability to maintain airway; renal impairment.

Dosage:

Premedication: 50–100 mcg IM or slow IV 30–60 min prior to the surgery.

Adjunct to general anesthesia: 1–2/kg mcg IV.

Adjunct to regional anesthesia: 25 mcg IT.

Patient-controlled anesthesia (PCA): 10 mcg/mL IV infusion, usual concentration 20 mcg demand dose with 5–10 min lockout time interval and base rate of ≤50 mcg/h.

Adverse effects: euphoria, confusion, respiratory depression (which, if extensive and untreated, may lead to arrest), drowsiness, nausea, visual disturbances, dyskinesia, hallucinations, delirium, constipation, narcotic ileus, muscle rigidity, constipation, addiction, loss of consciousness, hypotension, coma, and even death.

Remifentanil: (Fig. 3.3c)
Form: 2 mg or 5 mg powder concentrate for solution for injection or infusion.

Uses: Induction and maintenance of anesthesia, administration by Target-Controlled Infusion (TCI).

Contraindications: Remifentanil is contraindicated for epidural and intrathecal use in patients with known hypersensitivity to remifentanil and other fentanyl components of the remifentanil and for use as the sole agent for induction of anesthesia.

Precautions: Use with caution in patients with hypovolemia, cardiovascular disease (including acute MI), or drugs which may exaggerate hypotensive effects, bradycardia, and respiratory depression.

Dosage: Induction of anesthesia: 0.5–1 mcg/kg/min.

Maintenance of anesthesia: 0.05–2 mcg/kg/min.

Adverse Effects: Hypotension, bradycardia, headache, nausea and vomiting muscle rigidity, respiratory depression, apnea, pruritus, pain at the site of injection.

Tramadol: (Fig. 3.3d)
Form: 50 mg/mL Solution for Injection or Infusion.

Uses:

For the treatment and prevention of moderate to severe pain.

Contraindications: It is contraindicated in patients with known hypersensitivity to tramadol or any other of its components; in patients with epilepsy not adequately controlled by treatment.

Precautions: Intravenous injections must be given slowly over 2–3 min.

Dosage:

50 mg or 100 mg every 4 to 6 hours by either injection IM or IV routes. The dose should be adjusted according to the severity of the pain and the response.

For postoperative pain: An initial bolus of 100 mg is given. During the 60 min following the initial bolus, further doses of 50 mg may be given every 10–20 min, up to a total dose of 250 mg including the initial bolus. Subsequent doses should be 50 mg or 100 mg 4–6 hourly up to a total daily dose of 400 mg.

Adverse effects

Nausea, dizziness, constipation, vomiting, somnolence, and headache usually occur during the initial treatment rather than maintenance doses of the drug.

Significant side effects include respiratory depression that can lead to death.

3.3.1 Opioid Antagonists

Naloxone Hydrochloride (Fig. 3.3d)
Form: solution for injection, 400 mcg/mL.

Uses: to counteract respiratory depression induced by opioids during anesthesia and opioids overdose.

Precautions: dependence on opioids; cardiovascular disease.

Dosage: Opioid-induced respiratory depression, by intravenous injection, adult 100–200 mcg, repeated every 2–3 min to obtain required response; pediatric initially 10 mcg/kg, if no response followed by 100 mcg/kg.

Opioid-induced respiratory depression at birth, by subcutaneous, intramuscular, or intravenous injection, neonate 10 mcg/kg immediately after delivery.

Adverse effects: nausea and vomiting, hypertension and hypotension, left ventricular failure, pulmonary edema, seizures; arrhythmias such as ventricular tachycardia or fibrillation, particularly in pre-existing cardiac disease.

Paracetamol (Fig. 3.3e)
Paracetamol and nonsteroidal anti-inflammatory drugs (NSAD) may be useful alternatives (or adjuncts) for the relief of postoperative pain; they do not affect respiration and gastrointestinal motility.

Form: solution for injection one 100 mL vial contains 1000 mg paracetamol.

Uses: for the short-term treatment of moderate pain, especially following surgery and for the short-term treatment of fever.

Contraindications:

In patients with hypersensitivity to paracetamol or to propacetamol hydrochloride (prodrug of paracetamol).

In cases of severe hepatocellular insufficiency.

Precautions:

Hepatocellular insufficiency, severe renal insufficiency, chronic alcoholism, and dehydration.

Dosage:

15 mg/kg, the maximum daily dose must not exceed 3 g.

Adverse effects:

Malaise, hypotension, hypersensitivity reactions very rarely.

3.3.2 Muscle Relaxants

These medications work specifically to weaken or relax skeletal muscles of the body (voluntary and involuntary skeletal muscles will be relaxed as well i.e. upper part of esophagus). However, they do not affect the muscles of the heart, nor smooth muscles (i.e., intestines or bronchial tree). Muscle relaxants include two family groups: depolarizing, i.e., suxamethonium (succinylcholine) and non-depolarizing (pancuronium, atracurium, cisatracurium, vecuronium, and rocuronium).

3.4 Muscle Relaxants and Cholinesterase Inhibitors

Skeletal muscle relaxants are divided into two groups according to their mode of action:

A. Depolarizing muscle relaxants (e.g., succinylcholine).
B. Non-depolarizing muscle relaxants (e.g. vecuronium, pancuronium, rocuronium, mivacurium, atracurium, and cisatracurium).

Succinylcholine (Suxamethonium) (Fig. 3.4a)
Indications:

It is the only widely used muscle-relaxing depolarizer. It causes sudden, complete paralysis, which is very short-acting and has particular importance for laryngoscopy and rapid sequence intubation and emergency cases.

Electroconvulsive therapy (ECT) to control muscle contractions induced as a result of the electrical impulses delivered during the procedure.

Adverse effects and contraindications

Hyperkalemia, increased intracranial and intraocular pressure, malignant hyperthermia, bradycardia, massive tissue trauma, myopathies, and burn injuries.

Dose:

1–1.5 mg/kg, average (1 mg/kg).

Vecuronium bromide

It is a non-depolarizing muscle relaxant.

Form: Powder for solution for injection 10 mg vial.

Uses: For intubation and muscle relaxation during surgery.

Contraindications: Pulmonary diseases; dehydrated or severely ill patients, myasthenia gravis, or other neuromuscular disorders.

Precautions: renal impairment, hepatic impairment; possibly increase the dose in patients with burn injury; electrolyte disturbances, history of asthma, severe obesity, pregnancy, and breastfeeding.

Dosage: for intubation by intravenous injection.

Intubating dose: adults and pediatrics for more than 5 months (80–100 mg/kg).

Maintenance: 20–30 mg/kg.

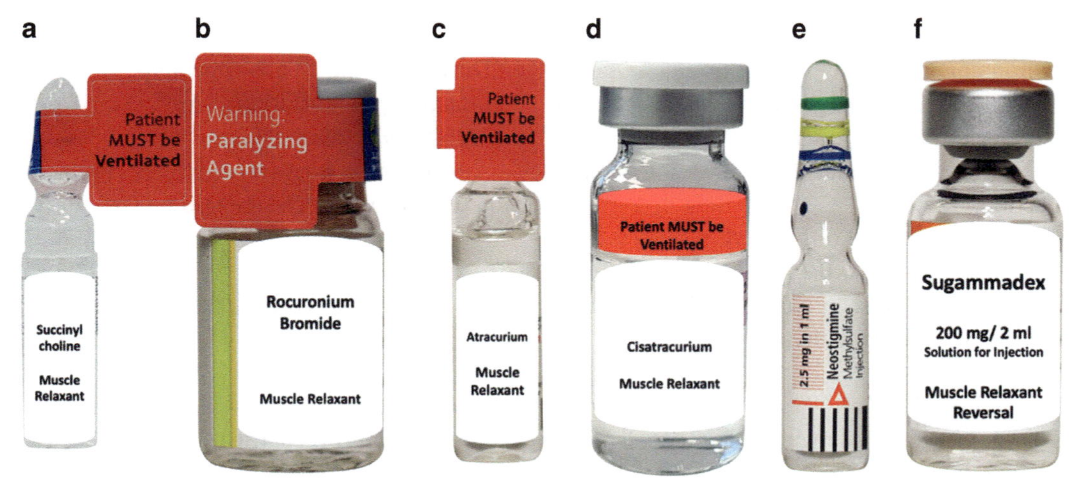

Fig. 3.4 (**a**): Suxamethonium (Succinyl-choline). (**b**): Rocuronium (**c**): Atracurium (**d**): Cisatracurium (**e**): Neostigmine (**f**): Sugammadex

Adverse effects: the minimal release of histamine (rarely hypersensitivity reactions including bronchospasm, hypotension, tachycardia, edema, erythema, and pruritus).

Pancuronium Bromide
It is a long-acting non-depolarizing muscle relaxant.

Form: 2 mg/mL solution for injection.

Uses: intubation and muscle relaxation during surgery.

Contraindications: hypersensitivity to pancuronium.

Precautions: renal and/or hepatic impairment.

Dosage: for intubation by intravenous injection.

Intubating dose: 0.1 mg/kg.

Maintenance dose: 0.02 mg/kg.

Adverse effects: prolonged neuromuscular blockade in patients with renal impairment.

Rocuronium Bromide (Fig. 3.4b)
It is an intermediate-acting non-depolarizing muscle relaxant.

Form: 10 mg/mL solution for injection/infusion.

Uses: for rapid sequence intubation because it has a faster onset than other non-depolarizing muscle relaxants and routine tracheal intubation and to provide muscle relaxation during surgery or mechanical ventilation.

Contraindications: hypersensitivity to rocuronium.

Precautions: renal and/or hepatic impairment, neuromuscular diseases.

Dosage: for Intubation by intravenous injection.

Intubating dose: 0.6–1.2 mg/kg.

Maintenance dose: 0.15 mg/kg.

Adverse effects: prolonged neuromuscular blockade in patients with renal impairment.

Atracurium (Fig. 3.4c)
It is an intermediate-acting non-depolarizing muscle relaxant.

Form: 10 mg/mL solution for injection or infusion.

Uses: for routine tracheal intubation, and to provide muscle relaxation during surgery or mechanical ventilation. It is metabolized by non-enzymatic degradation (Hofmann elimination), it can be used in patients with renal and liver diseases.

Contraindications: hypersensitivity to atracurium or cisatracurium.

Precautions: bronchial asthma, neuromuscular diseases.

Dosage: for Intubation by intravenous injection.

Intubating dose: 0.5 mg/kg.

Maintenance dose: 0.1 mg/kg.

Adverse effects: increases plasma histamine levels, causing skin flushing, hypotension, and tachycardia.

Cisatracurium (Fig. 3.4d)
It is an intermediate-acting non-depolarizing muscle relaxant.

Form: 2 mg/mL solution for injection or infusion.

Uses: for routine tracheal intubation, and to provide muscle relaxation during surgery or mechanical ventilation. It is metabolized by non-enzymatic degradation (Hofmann elimination), it can be used in patients with renal and liver diseases.

Contraindications: hypersensitivity to atracurium or cisatracurium.

Precautions: bronchial asthma, neuromuscular diseases.

Dosage: by intravenous injection.

Intubating dose: 0.15 mg/kg.

Maintenance dose: 0.03 mg/kg.

Adverse effects: Adverse effects are uncommon with the use of cisatracurium.

3.4.1 Reversal of Neuromuscular Block

Cholinesterase Inhibitor—Neostigmine Methylsulfate: (Fig. 3.4e)
Form: solution for injection, neostigmine 500 mcg/mL, 1-mL ampoule; 2.5 mg/mL, 1-mL ampoule.

Uses: counteract effect of non-depolarizing muscle relaxants administered during surgery; postoperative non-obstructive urinary retention; myasthenia gravis.

Contraindications: recent intestinal or bladder surgery; mechanical intestinal or urinary tract obstruction; after suxamethonium; pneumonia; peritonitis.

Precautions: asthma; urinary tract infections; cardiovascular disease, including arrhythmias (especially bradycardia or atrioventricular block); hypotension; peptic ulcer; epilepsy; parkinsonism; hyperthyroidism.

Dosage: Reversal of non-depolarizing block, by intravenous injection over 1 min.

Adult: 2.5 mg, followed if necessary, by supplements of 500 mcg to maximum total dose of 5 mg;

Pediatric: 40 mcg/kg (titrated using peripheral nerve stimulator).

Note. To reduce muscarinic effects atropine sulfate by intravenous injection (adult: 0.6–1.2 mg, pediatric: 20 mcg/kg) with or before neostigmine administration.

Adverse effects: increased salivation and bronchial secretions, nausea and vomiting, abdominal cramps, diarrhea; allergic reactions, and hypotension.

Sugammadex (Fig. 3.4f)
Form: 100 mg/mL solution for injection.

Uses: it is a novel agent that binds with molecules of rocuronium and other steroidal neuromuscular blocking agents (e.g., vecuronium and pancuronium), thereby rapidly reversing their neuromuscular blocking effects.

Contraindications:

Patients who have a known hypersensitivity, which ranges from isolated skin reactions to anaphylaxis.

Advanced renal disease and renal failure.

Precautions: marked bradycardia may occur after administration of sugammadex. Although rare, anaphylaxis within minutes after sugammadex administration has occurred.

Dosage: Reversal of rocuronium and steroidal non-depolarizing block, by intravenous injection 2–16 mg/kg.

Adverse effects: bradycardia, recurrence of neuromuscular blockade is possible with an insufficient reversal with sugammadex, bronchospasm, allergic reactions.

3.4.2 Other Medications

Atropine: (Fig. 3.5a)
Atropine is prepared as a Racemic mixture to use, however, only l-atropine is active in the body, it is as follows.

Chemical structure: It is Atropine sulfate.

Route of administration: oral, intramuscular, and intravenous.

Metabolism: atropine is metabolized by liver esterase then excreted with urine very small amount excreted unchanged.

Dose: adults' dose: 0.2–0.6 mg, pediatric dose: 20 mcg/kg.

Uses:

Atropine is used widely in anesthesia field as a treatment for bradycardia and as antisialuge in premedication and intraoperative, in addition, it can be used as antidote. In case of anticholinesterase toxicity, even though it has antiemetic properties currently it is not labeled as antiemetic medication because it is cardiovascular side effects, indicated in special scenario in advanced life support (asystole/PEA).

Atropine is naturally occurring tertiary amines extracted from plants of the deadly nightshade.

family.

Mechanism of action: Competitive antagonist at muscarinic receptors, vagolytic.

Side Effects: Antiparkinsonian effects, mouth dryness, urinary retention, and blurred vision.

Effects

Central nervous system: atropine is tertiary amine that can cross blood–brain barrier and can cause a central sedation and cholinergic crisis, however, it is unlikely.

Cardiovascular: antimuscarinic properties cause significant tachycardia it on other wise atropine in small doses intravenously may cause bradycardia initially this bradycardia explained by the effect of atropine on vagal nucleus centrally or by partial agonist effect peripherally.

Respiratory system: atropine works as a bronchial dilator as it is antagonizing muscarinic receptors in bronchial smooth muscles, it has anti-sialagogue effect by reducing the secretions from respiratory glands.**Gut:** reduce lower esophageal sphincter tone and gastric acid secretions.

Miscellaneous: may induce hyperthermia especially in pediatric population as it inhibits sweat glands secretions, caution when used in glaucoma patients as atropine may increase intraocular pressure.

Glycopyrolate: (Fig. 3.5b)
Mechanism of action: Competitive antagonist at muscarinic receptors, vagolytic.

Quaternary amine not able to cross blood–brain barrier which prevent central nervous system side effects.

Dose: adult: 0.2–0.4 mg IV or IM, pediatric: 4–10 μg/kg.

Metabolization: only 20% metabolized in liver and the remaining excreted unchanged with urine.

Poorly absorbed by intestine so the oral bioavailability is less than 5%.

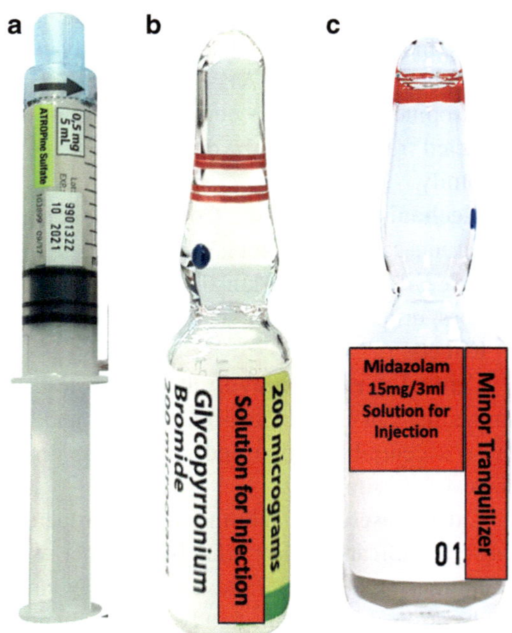

Fig. 3.5 (**a**) Atropine, (**b**) Glycopyronium (Glycopyrrolate), (**c**) Midazolam

Uses:
- anti-sialagogues as a premedication treatment of bradycardia.
- To attenuate effects of Anticholinesterases, commonly mixed with neostigmine in reversing non-depolarizing neuromuscular medications.
- Hyperhidrosis.

Systemic Effects:
Cardiovascular system
- Tachycardia the duration of action can last up to 2–3 h.

Respiratory system
- Bronchodilation.

Central nervous system
- Does not cross BBB, however, can causes headache and sedation.

Gastrointestinal:
- Ant sialagogue as it reduces oral secretions.

Miscellaneous
- reduce sweating secretion.
  Antimuscarinic effects
  like antimuscarinic effect of Atropine

- Tachycardia, dry mouth, urinary retention, and blurred vision.

Midazolam Fig. 3.5c
Introduction:

It belongs to imidazolbenzodiazepine, benzodiazepine family. Supplies are clear colorless solution. Midazolam has two different form depending on the surrounding PH in it is preparation the PH is 4 the midazolam is ionized in solution (open structure).

When enter the body at physiological pH 7.4 it changed its structure rendering to lipid soluble agent (closed structure) which allow it to cross blood–brain barrier.

Dose not cause pain on injection.

Uses:
- reduce the risk of awareness intraoperative even with small doses 2 mg.

- adjunct to anesthetic agents (propofol) which reduces the dose of propofol to reach the targeted effect.
- Sedation in minor procedures.
- Anterograde amnesia effect.
- Sedation at intensive care unit.
- Anxiolytic.

Rout of administration: Orally with 40% bioavailability, intranasally, intramuscularly, rectally, intrathecally, and epidurally.

Dose:
- Oral: 0.5 mg/kg (maximum dos should not exceed 20 mg).
- IV: 0.02–0.1 mg/kg for sedation, titrate to effect.
- Spinal: 0.3–2 mg.
- Epidural: 0.1–0.2 mg/kg.

Metabolism: midazolam is hydroxylaized to active compound 1-hydroxymidazolam then conjugated with glucuronic acid before excreted with urine.

Systemic effect:
Cardiovascular system
- reduce systemic vascular resistance by one-third.
- increase heart rate.
- Obtunds response to laryngoscopy when combined with opioid.

Respiratory system:
- respiratory rate.
- tidal volume.
- No significant change in minute ventilation.
- can cause apnea.
- Blunts the normal response of respiratory center to pCO_2.

Cervical nervous system:
- Hypnosis, sedation, anxiolysis, and amnesia (anterograde).

Gastroenterology system:
- decrease hepatic blood flow.

Genitourinary system:
- decrease Renal blood flow.

Antidote: flumazenil is the drug of choice to reverse midazolam effect, it antagonize the midazolam at the benzodiazepine site.

Miscellaneous

Midazolam is metabolized by the same hepatic P450 isoenzyme (3A3/4) which metabolize alfentanil this might prolong the effect of alfentanil when used in conjunction with midazolam.

Dexmedetomidine

It belongs to the Medetomidine family which is an alpha-agonist, has been used widely in animals for it sedation and analgesia effect.

It is becoming more popular in clinical practice in the last few years.

Mechanism of action

Full agonist, similar to clonidine act by binding a-2 receptors, it is much more potent than clonidine and has a higher affinity for a-2 receptors.

	Clonidine	Dexmedetomidine
Alpha 1 affinity/ alpha2	1/200	1/1600

Rout of administration

Intravenously (bolus/infusion) intranasally.

Kinetics: It's oral absorption is unpredictable but does avoid the initial hypertension that parenteral administration produces. It has an elimination half-life of 2 h.

Uses: Dexmedetomidine can be used for different purposes knowing that not all of them approved by FDA.

- Anxiolysis.
- Sedation.
- Analgesia.
- Adjunctive to anesthesia.
- Anti-shiviring.
- Neurosurgical procedures, airway procedures.

Doses:

Different regimen doses have been recommended by FDA and Europe.

Not approved yet to be used in pediatric; however, it has been used in pediatric population for the last 10 years.

The adult dose regimen includes loading dose 0.5–1 mcg/kg within 10 min then infusion 0.5–1 mcg/kg/h.

Side Effects: Hypotension

Bradycardia/bradyarrhythmia

Tachycardia might happen (initially after injection)

Antidote: Atipamezole can reverse the effect of dexmedetomidine.

3.4.3 Others Medications

The anesthetist may use other drugs to minimize the risk of recalling something happening in the Operating Room (OR). These drugs belong to a family class of drugs called benzodiazepines. Diazepam and midazolam are examples of these medications that used frequently in operating theater.

- Reversal drugs or antidotes drugs are medications that usually given to counteract the effects of other drugs. Some examples include the following:
  - naloxone, to counter the effects of an opiate or narcotic;
  - flumazenil, to counter the effects of a benzodiazepine;
  - neostigmine/sugammadex, to reverse the actions of ammonio steroids types of non-depolarizing muscle relaxants (i.e. rocuronium, vecuronium, and pancuronium).
- Sympathetic and parasympathetic medications are used widely for different purposes will not covered here, for instance, to act on heart rate include atropine (to increase it) and esmolol (to decrease it).
- Antiemetic: these medications help reduce nausea and vomiting and so are termed anti-nauseates or antiemetics. They classified depending on receptors to dopamine antagonists, 5HT3 antagonists, anti-cholinergic, anti-histamines, and other classes with unknown mechanism.
- Vasopressors and vasodilation drugs medications used to maintain hemodynamic stability some drugs can raise blood pressure (epinephrine or adrenaline) and others can lower it (nitroprusside) (Refer to the last part of the chapter).

3.4.4 Local Anesthetics

A local anesthetic injection around a nerve or a group of nerves temporarily blocks the transmission of electrical impulses in the nerve. Lack of transmission causes the nerve-supplied area of the body to become numb. This is also known as a “sensory block” which, depending on the concentration and dose of the local anesthetic used, may progress to muscle weakness.

Drugs used for conduction anesthesia (also called local or regional anesthesia) act by causing a reversible block to conduction along nerve fibers. Local anesthetics are widely used in dental practice, for brief and superficial interventions, for obstetric procedures, and for specialized regional anesthesia techniques requiring highly developed skills. As patient cooperation is required, the patient needs to be prepared psychologically to accept the proposed procedure. The resuscitation services and equipment should be readily accessible at all times. To detect inadvertent intravascular injection, local anesthetic injections should be given slowly.

Classification

Commonly used local anesthetics in clinical practice include the following:

Amino Amides

- Mepivacaine.
- Lidocaine.
- Etidocaine.
- Bupivacaine.
- Levobupivacaine.
- Ropivacaine.

Amino Esters

- Procaine.
- Cocaine.
- Chloroprocaine.
- Tetracaine.
- Benzocaine.

Local anesthetics are classified by where the metabolism occurs. The amino amides are hydrolyzed in the liver and the amino esters are metabolized by plasma cholinesterases.

Local anesthetics work in the nonionic form. The ionized form is dominant in the presence of a low pH, and this may prolong the initiation of action; this also explains why local anesthetics are not successful at inflammatory sites, where an acidic environment is normal. Thus, many clinicians are adding sodium bicarbonate to overcome the acidity and increase local anesthetic efficacy.

Epinephrine is often added to a local anesthetic solution which enables the clinician to use a lower anesthetic dose and improve safety. Furthermore, epinephrine acts as a vasoconstrictor and delays absorption of the anesthetic, thus increasing the duration of action. The addition of epinephrine can also improve hemostasis by inducing vasoconstriction in the surgical field.

Lidocaine: (Fig. 3.6a–c)

Indications and Administration

Different routes of administration utilize various lidocaine preparations.

- Diluted concentrations of 0.05–0.1% may be subcutaneously infiltrated in large volumes to provide tumescent local anesthesia, resulting in site swelling and firmness that may be beneficial for certain surgical procedures (liposuction).
- Dilute solutions of 0.25–0.5% are used for intravenous regional anesthesia (Bier's block) or infiltration into subcutaneous tissue.
- Solutions of 1–2% are used for regional nerve blocks including epidural anesthesia and are

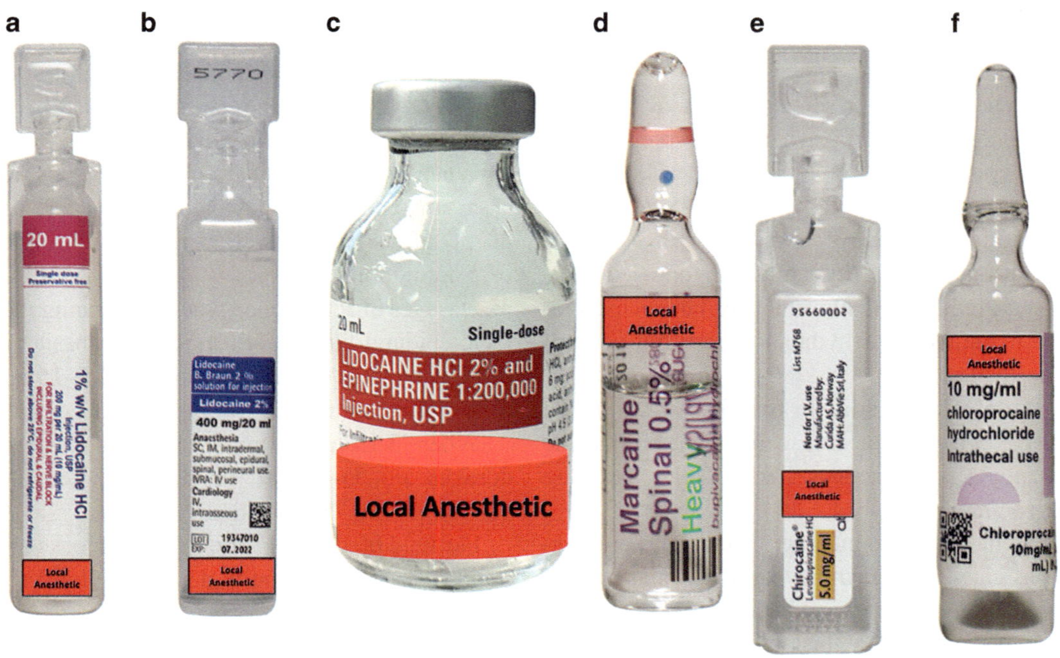

Fig. 3.6 (**a**): Lidocaine 1% (**b**): Lidocaine 2% (**c**) Lidocaine 2% and Epinephrine 1:200,000, (**d**): Levobupivacaine 0.5 Spinal (**e**): Levobupivacaine (**f**): Choloroprocaine

also available in intravenous preparations for antiarrhythmic use.

- Aqueous gels of 1 –2% containing antiseptic (chlorhexidine) are used to topicalize and lubricate urethra prior to catheterization with Foley's catheter.
- A solution of 4% is used for topical anesthesia of the mucous membranes of the airway, including the mouth, pharynx, and respiratory tract, either by gargling, spraying or using an atomizer.
- Ointment of 5% mixed with hydrocortisone is employed topically on other mucous membranes such as the skin or in the rectum.
- A solution of 10% is also used topically for airway anesthesia by spraying from a metered-dose atomizer.

The aqueous preparations from 0.5% to 2% are available in either plain forms or with 1 per 200,000 epinephrine (dentistry sometimes uses versions with 1 per 100,000 epinephrine or more) and are available with or without preservatives. Premixed lidocaine and prilocaine are available in a eutectic 5% cream (containing 2.5%) which is often used to anesthetize small areas of skin prior to procedures.

Doses: Maximum safe dose by body weight is 3 mg/kg or 7 mg/kg when using preparations with epinephrine in regional anesthesia.

The dose is 1–2 mg/kg given 2–5 min before intubation to suppress airway reflexes.

For cardiac dysrhythmias, the initial dose is 1–1.5 mg/kg given intravenously, but not used for the treatment of arrhythmias as a result of local anesthetic toxicity.

Contraindications In patients with a known severe adverse reaction to lidocaine. Lidocaine anaphylactic reactions are likely but are uncommon.

Epinephrine-containing lidocaine preparations cause demonstrable cardiovascular effects, even if only given in small quantities especially if the patient has a history of cardiovascular disease.

Bupivacaine (Fig. 3.6d)
Form: It is available in three different concentrations: 0.25%, 0.5%, and 0.75%.

Indications and administration Used in regional anesthesia (epidural anesthesia and spinal anesthesia) and local infiltration. The administration is by local infiltration (post-surgical analgesia), peripheral nerve blocks for various surgeries, spinal anesthesia for abdominal surgery, orthopedic, urologic surgeries or cesarean delivery, epidural anesthesia/analgesia for labor pain, and caudal block (anesthesia and analgesia below the umbilicus, commonly used for pediatric surgery).

Dose: Maximum safe dose by body weight is 2–2.5 mg/kg

Contraindications: Infection at the injection site, hypersensitivity to the drug or its components, liver and/or renal impairment, impaired cardiac function as heart block, hypovolemia, hypotension, or acutely ill patients.

Levobupivacaine: (Fig. 3.6e)
Levobupivacaine (bupivacaine enantiomer) is approximately equipotent with it, having a shorter duration of surgical anesthesia. Its dose is 2 mg/kg.

Ropivacaine:

It is used in an epidural block for various surgeries, major nerve blocks, and local infiltration and postoperative or labor pain control.

Indications and Administration

When used in lumbar epidural blocks for cesarean section, the doses for ropivacaine are 20–30 mL of 0.5% solution and 15–20 mL of 0.75% solution.

Dosages of ropivacaine when performing thoracic epidural blocks for surgical anesthesia are 5–15% mL dose of 0.5% solution and 5–15 mL of 0.75% solution.

When performing major nerve blocks, the dosages are 35–50 mL of 0.5% solution and 10–40 mL of 0.75% solution.

For field blocks (e.g., minor nerve blocks and infiltration), ropivacaine is dosed at a 1–40 mL dose of 0.5% solution.

When managing postoperative pain, peripheral nerve blocks are continuously infused at a dose of 5–10 mL/h of 0.2% solution. For pain management through lumbar or thoracic epidurals, the continuous infusion dose of ropivacaine is at 6–14 mL/h of 0.2% solution.

Dose: 2–3 mg/kg.

Contraindications: Hypersensitivity to the drug.

Chloroprocaine: (Fig. 3.6f)

Form: It is supplied as both 2% and 3% solutions.

Indications and administration

For neuraxial anesthesia (spinal, epidural, and caudal), as well as peripheral nerve blocks and obstetric anesthesia (pudendal and paracervical nerve blocks).

It is short-acting leads to faster discharge times, lower pain scores, and lower costs than general anesthesia and shorter motor blockade than spinal bupivacaine in ambulatory surgeries.

Dose: The maximum dose is 11 mg/kg not to exceed a maximum total dose of 800 mg; with epinephrine (1:200,000), 14 mg/kg, not to exceed a maximum total dose of 1000 mg.

Contraindications

It should be used with caution in patients with hepatic and renal diseases.

3.5 Vasoconstrictors

Vasoconstrictors medication can act directly or indirectly depending on binding the targeted receptors or increase releasing of a ligand that binds the targeted receptor.

Ephedrine Hydrochloride (Fig. 3.7a)

Form: Solution for injection ephedrine hydrochloride 30 mg/mL 1 mL ampoule.

Uses: Management of hypotension during regional or general anesthesia.

Precautions: Hyperthyroidism, diabetes mellitus, ischemic heart disease, hypertension, and angle-closure glaucoma.

Dosage: To prevent or treat hypotension during anesthesia, by slow intravenous injection of a solution containing 3 mg/mL, 3–6 mg (maximum single dose 9 mg), repeated if necessary, every 3–4 min; maximum dose 30 mg.

Adverse effects: Anorexia, hypersalivation, nausea, vomiting; tachycardia arrhythmias, anginal pain, vasoconstriction with hypertension, headache, dizziness, anxiety, restlessness, confusion, tremors; difficulty in micturition; sweating, flushing; changes in blood glucose level.

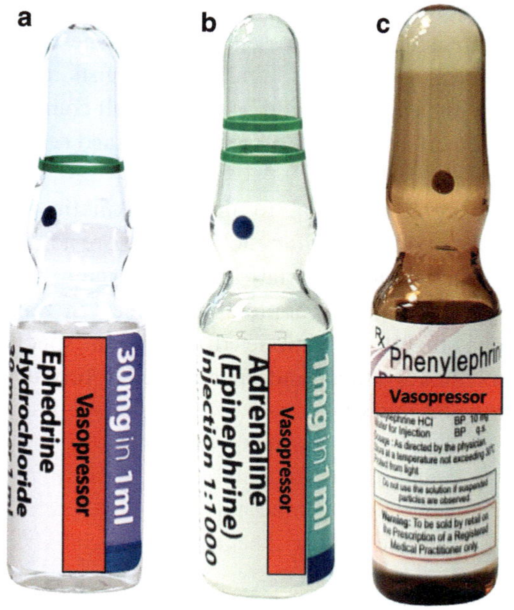

Fig. 3.7 (**a**): Ephedrine, (**b**): Adrenaline, (**c**): Phenylephrine

Epinephrine (Adrenaline) (Fig. 3.7b)

Uses: Anaphylaxis, it is the first and most important treatment.

Vasoconstrictor to decrease systemic absorption of infiltrated local anesthetics.

Contraindications:

Extremities as ring block of digits, penis, or other situations where there is a risk of local ischemia.

Precautions:

Hypertension, ischemic heart disease, heart block; cerebral vascular insufficiency, thyrotoxicosis or diabetes mellitus.

Dosage:

IM route: 0.01 mg/kg (maximum dose of 0.5 mg) per single dose, injected IM into the mid-outer thigh.

IV route: Slow, continuous infusion is preferred.

Adults: infusion at 0.1 mcg/kg/min.

Infants and children: infusion at 0.1–1 mcg/kg/min.

Take-Home Message

Pharmacology is an essential part in anesthesia practice, technicians, and technologists aside with anesthetists should be aware of all common medications used in operating theater and remote area.

Special attention to pharmacokinetic and pharmacodynamic for each drug before administration. Dose variation and variant dose response among people should keep in mind as a result of genetic diversity in special enzymes systems and special genes products between races.

Suggested Reading

Gropper M, Eriksson L, Fleisher L, Wiener-Kronish J, Cohen N, Leslie K, editors. Miller's anesthesia. 9th ed. Elsevier; 2019.

Mahmoud M, et al. Dexmedetomidine: review, update, and future considerations of paediatric perioperative and periprocedural applications and limitations. Br J Anaesth. 2015;115:171–82. https://doi.org/10.1093/bja/aev2.

Peck TE, Hill SA, Williams M. Pharmacology for anaesthesia and intensive care. 3rd ed. Cambridge University Press; 2009. ISBN 978-0-521-70463-2

Stoelting R, Flood P, Rathmell J, Shafer S, editors. Stoelting's handbook of pharmacology and physiology in anesthetic practice. 3rd ed. Wolter S Kluwer; 2014.

Pharmacy, Drugs Labeling, and Storage

4

Nabil A. Shallik, Lamia Tawfik, Muhammad Firas Alhammad, Cherif Boutabba, and Nada N. Shallik

Contents

4.1 Introduction

The drug preparation, handling and use, management of medication errors, and safe handling of high alert medications will be discussed.

N. A. Shallik (✉) · L. Tawfik · M. F. Alhammad
C. Boutabba
Department of Anesthesia, ICU and Perioperative Medicine, Hamad Medical Corporation, Doha, Qatar
e-mail: nshallik@hamad.qa; ltawfik@hamad.qa; MAlhammad@hamad.qa; CBoutabba@hamad.qa

N. N. Shallik
Faculty of Oral and Dental Medicine, Future University Hospital, New Cairo, Egypt

4.2 Anesthesia Drug Preparation

Recently, the pharmacy is enrolled in preparing medications for the operating room has been recognized to help in improving drug safety in anesthesia. This process in a central pharmacy supposed to decrease the incidence of medication error related to drug preparation because in the pharmacy two people check each other's work "double check in preparation, " multiple syringes are prepared for one drug at a time which also should reduce error chance, and the environment is one in which distractions are few, order reigns, and time is available to check and

N. A. Shallik et al. (eds.), *Improving Anesthesia Technical Staff's Skills*,
https://doi.org/10.1007/978-3-030-88849-7_4

recheck away from theater stress. In addition, dispensing accuracy generally improves administration accuracy.

4.3 Drugs Handling

4.3.1 Medication Errors During Anesthesia, Standardization of the Anesthesia Drug Tray System

Medication errors in anesthesia practice is a real concern in fact the accurate prevalence of this problem is not well known however estimation is roughly between 1–5% of administered anesthetic medications this might be due to many of medications error is not noticed and others not reported.

Human error occupies a big part of this error in general the literature is lack of evidence in a clear strategic plan to eliminate administration of wrong anesthetic medication.

Medication errors, which can lead to adverse drug reactions, require clear and unambiguous definitions, so that patients, prescribers, manufacturers, and regulators can all understand each other. The classification of medication errors on the basis of the underlying psychological mechanisms, based on how errors occur, can suggest strategies that help to reduce their occurrence.

Using a multimodal system reduce documentation and drug administration errors in anesthesia, customized at site with well-organized workspaces, prefilled syringes for the most commonly used drugs, large lettered and legible drug labels with standardized color coding in purpose designed drug drawers, a barcode reader linked to a computer, speakers, and touch screen to provide automatic auditory and visual verification of a drug immediately before its administration (Fig. 4.1).

In our days, many healthcare facilities especially in ORs starts using technologies to enable smarter, safer medication management known as the automated drugs cabinet.

All anesthetic drugs are placed in a pharmacologic class or from the more to the less usage order inside separate bins, healthcare worker must have a biometric access as a fingerprint to pull drugs, by entering the patient name, a page will open showing all the ordered drugs write the needed drugs name a specific bin will open and a light blink for guidance. The high alert medications and the narcotics need a second person as a witness for safety reason.

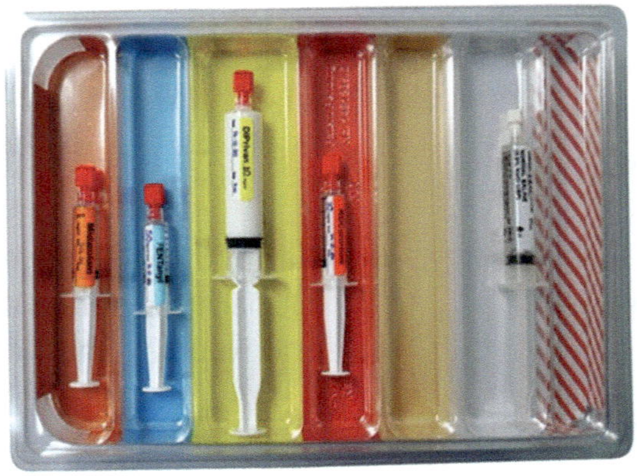

Fig. 4.1 Standardized color coding of prefilled syringes

Once the drugs have been loaded in a labeled color-coded syringe with date, dosage, initial and patient sticker, a specific tray will take a place to regroup all those syringes in clear manner. The used drug's tray must be removed at the end of each case and replaced by a new drug tray, later the used drugs are restocked by pharmacy technician.

Errors usually happen when the intended action intended but could not performed, the reason for this can be divided either due to mistakes (deficiency in planning) or due to slips and lapses.

Fig. 4.2 demonstrates the errors which can be reduced by managing the gaps as follows:

1. knowledge,
2. well-built rules,
3. improve technical supplementation,
4. avoiding lapses and improving memory.

Currently, there are some features to prevent medication errors in anesthetic gases and volatile agents which show significant improvement in safe inhalational drugs delivery to the patient.

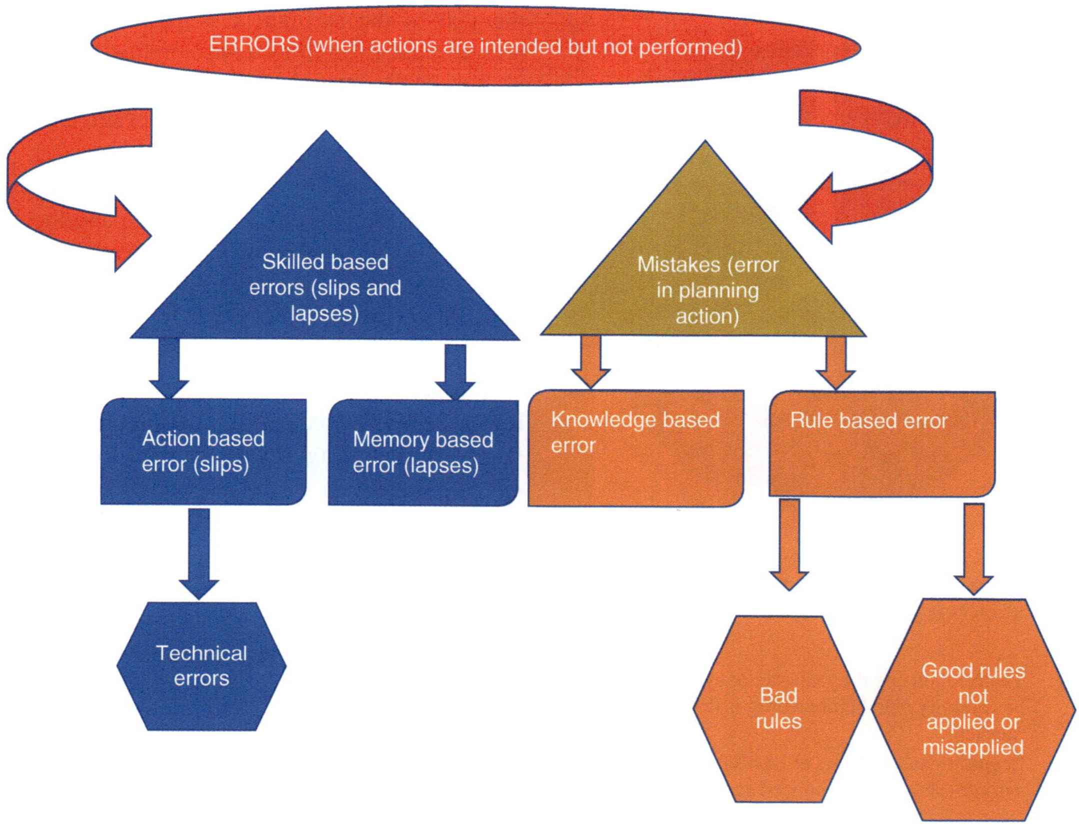

Fig. 4.2 Shows the possibility of errors how they may occur

For example, gas lines and gas cylinders have Diameter-Index Safety Systems and Pin-Index systems, respectively, also anesthetic vaporizers have special keyed fillers, from the other hand till now there is no effective way to prevent administer a wrong intravenous medication to the patient.

Levels of mistake proofing exist along a 4-level hierarchy:

1. Eliminate the error.
2. Detect the error.
3. Detect the defect.
4. Cognitive aids.

Lessons from the design world do suggest certain themes: (1) infrequently used, emergency medications ought to be in a distinctive location; (2) medications that could be easily confused should be separated; (3) a standard layout helps providers create a mental model that makes mistakes less likely; and (4) in team-based practices, a standard setup creates a shared mental model.

Follow up of medication management process in hospitals wards have reduced medication errors significantly an example is illustrated in Fig. 4.3. however, applying this systematic management process in the operating theater is not practical. Because the nature of anesthetic medication which mandate immediate decision making and response.

Recommendations of Anesthesia and Patients Safety Foundation are based on a systematic review of the entire literature on drug administration error in anesthesia and as validated against actual incident reports.

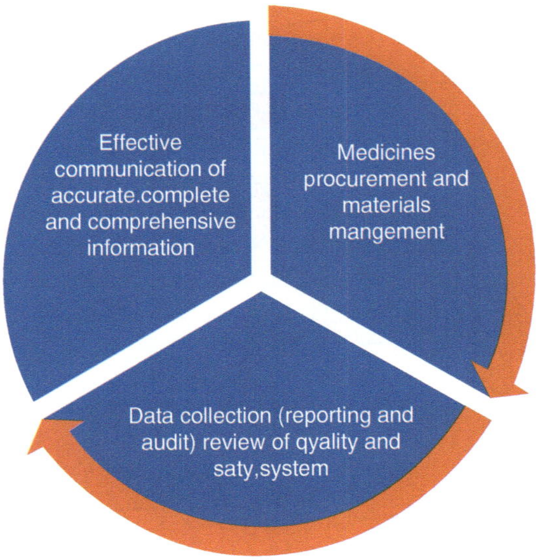

Fig. 4.3 Medication management process to prevent medication errors

1.	The label on any drug ampule or syringe should be carefully read before a drug is drawn up or injected.
2.	Legibility and contents of labels on ampules and syringes should be optimized according to agreed standards in respect to some or all attributes of font, size, color, and the information included.
3.	Syringes should be labeled (always or almost always).
4.	Formal organization of the drug drawers and workspace should be used with attention to tidiness, position of ampules and syringes, separation of similar or dangerous drugs, removal of dangerous drugs from the operating rooms.
5.	Labels should be checked specifically with a second person or a device (such as a barcode reader linked to a computer) before a drug is drawn up or administered.

4.3.2 Standardized Pharmacy Premixed Infusion Bags and Prefilled Syringes and Barcoding Technique (Fig. 4.4)

Many hospitals have begun using prefilled syringes and infusion bags. Those syringe and bags have advantage of removing the necessary work of preparation (transferring the drugs from the vial to the syringe or bag), reduce drugs errors, standardize drugs concentration, and prolong shelf life. The pharmacy and the anesthesiologist can sign an SLA (service level agreement) to develop a standard drug formulary.

Barcoding system and other scanning technique have been introduced wildly in anesthesia practice for tight control of anesthetic medication in addition to the need of second witness before drug administration.

So many prefilled syringes can be prepared by pharmacy in a dedicated IV room or preparation room in aseptic technique to prolog shelf life including but not limited to phenylephrine, oxytocin bags, levobupivacaine epidural bags, and dopamine and dobutamine bags.

4.3.3 High-Risk Medications

Medications involved in a high percentage of errors and/or sentinel events that carry a higher risk for adverse outcomes, as well as medications that carry higher risk for abuse or other adverse outcomes (Table 4.1) (Fig. 4.5).

Chemotherapeutic Agents
Opiates
Insulins
Neuromuscular blocking agents
Antithrombotic
Anesthetics
Epidural and Spinal medications
Concentrated electrolytes
Inotropes and Vasopressors
IV Antiarrhythmics
Oxytocin.

4.3.4 Safe Medication Administration (Right Drug• Right Dose• Right Route• Right Patient• Right Time)

One of the recommendations to reduce medication errors and harm is to use the "five rights": the right patient, the right drug, the right dose, the

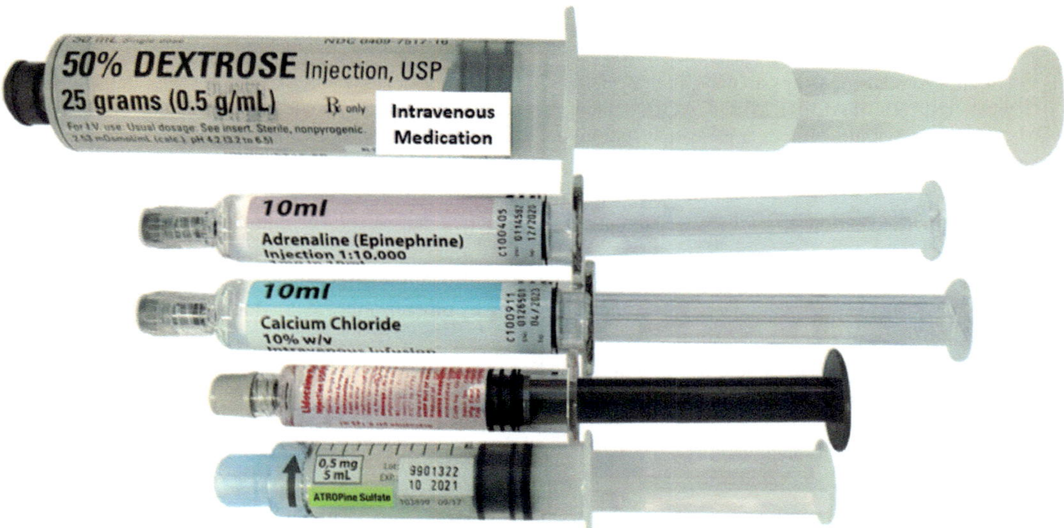

Fig. 4.4 Prefilled syringe

Table 4.1 General safeguard strategies for high alert medications

Procurement	
1	Limit the drug strengths available in the formulary of each healthcare facility
2	Avoid frequent changes of brand or color. Notify the end users whenever there are changes
3	Inform all relevant personnel regarding new High Alert Medications listed in the hospital/clinic formulary
4	Encourage the purchase of equipment and consumables with safety features for safe drug administration
Storage	
1	All personnel must check the High Alert Medication labels carefully before storing to ensure medications are kept at the correct place
2	All High Alert Medications should be kept in individual labeled containers/shelves
3	Whenever possible avoid storing look-alike sound-alike drugs and different strengths of the same drug side by side
4	Use TALL-Man lettering to emphasize differences in medication names (e.g. DOPamine and DOBUTamine)
5	Limit floor stock drugs to the unit/ward requirements
6	Label all containers/shelves containing High Alert Medications with a red label stating in white "HIGH-ALERT MEDICATION"
Prescribing	
1	Do not use abbreviations when prescribing High Alert Medications
2	Do not use trailing zero when prescribing (e.g. 5.0 mg can be mistaken as 50 mg)
3	Specify the concentration, dose, route, and rate of infusion for High Alert Medications prescribed (e.g. IV Dopamine 5 mcg/kg over 1 minute)
4	Prescribe oral liquid medications with the dose specified in weight(w), e.g. gm or weight/volume (w/v)
5	Avoid ordering High Alert Medications verbally. In cases of emergency, phone orders have to be repeated, verified, and documented instantly once possible.
Preparation	
1	All preparations involving High Alert Medications should be independently double checked
2	All diluted medications MUST BE LABELED with the name and strength IMMEDIATELY upon dilution

(continued)

Table 4.1 (continued)

Dispensing/supply	
1	For automated dispensing cabinets, all drawers/cubies that include a High Alert Medication should be labeled with a red "HIGH ALERT MEDICATION" label. In addition, a comment should appear on the machine screen upon withdrawing the medication stating that this is a High Alert Medication
2	Withdrawing a High Alert Medication from automated dispensing cabinets should require another nurse as witness.
3	High Alert Medications to be dispensed directly to patients (e.g. outpatients) should not be labeled as high alert
4	High Alert Medications must be independently double checked before dispensing
5	High Alert Medications should be checked upon receiving by other healthcare providers
Administration	
1	The following particulars should be independently double checked against the order or medication chart at the bedside by two qualified healthcare providers before administration: • Patient's ID using two identifiers • Name and strength of medications • Dosage form • Dose/frequency • Route and rate (pump setting and line placements when necessary) • Expiry date
2	Label the distal ends of all access lines to distinguish IV from epidural lines
3	Wherever possible, smart infusion pumps should be utilized to administer High Alert Medications
4	Wherever available, High Alert Medications should be administered using Bar-Coded Medication Administration
5	Minimize distraction during administration of High Alert Medications to patients.
Monitoring	
1	Closely monitor adverse drug reactions, medication errors, and drug interactions related to High Alert Medications
2	Therapeutic Drug Monitoring should be performed for all narrow-therapeutic-index High Alert Medications
3	Keep antidotes and resuscitation equipment in wards/ units where applicable
Information	
1	High Alert Medications shall be flagged/marked on Cerner or any other Health Information System (HIS)
2	Relevant dilution guidelines should be made available in the wards/units
Education	
1	*Educate patient and family members/caregivers on:* • Medication regimen • Drug–drug/drug–food interactions • Common side effects • Monitoring medication related harm and subsequent management/actions
2	All healthcare providers shall be trained prior to handling of High Alert Medications
3	Staff must be trained to detect potential errors and respond promptly when errors do occur

right route, and the right time. When a medication error does occur during the administration of a medication, we are quick to blame the anesthesia technician and accuse her/him of not completing the five rights. Simply holding healthcare practitioners accountable for giving the right drug to the right patient in the right dose by the right route at the right time to ensure medication safety (Table 4.2).

4.4 Automated Medication Dispensing Machines (Fig. 4.6)

Improving patient safety is always a key focus in the hospital setting, and pharmacists have been exploring a variety of strategies and technologies to achieve this goal. Automated dispensing machines—decentralized medication distribution systems that provide computer-controlled

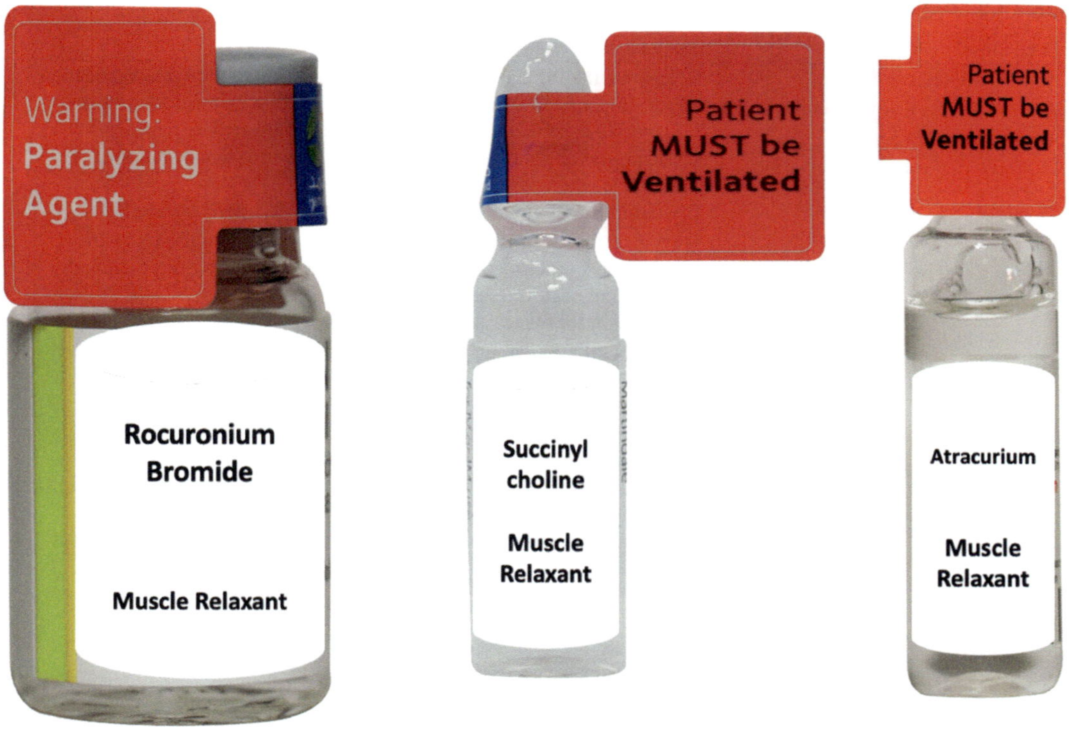

Fig. 4.5 Example of high-risk medications

Table 4.2 Risk reduction strategies for specific high alert medications

Drug class	Risk reduction strategies
Chemotherapeutic agents For example, Cisplatin, 5-flourouracil, Epirubicin, Irinotecan, Paclitaxel, Asparaginase, Trastuzumab, Pembrolizumab, Letrozole, and Tamoxifen	1. Only chemo or specially trained/certified/competent pharmacists are permitted to prepare chemotherapy 2. Only chemo or specially trained/certified/competent nurses are permitted to administer chemotherapy 3. Label these drugs with "Cytotoxic Medication" EXCEPT hormone therapy and non-cytotoxic monoclonal antibodies 4. Extravasation kit should be available where chemotherapy is administered 5. Cytotoxic spill kit should be available where it is necessary 6. Refer to policy: (HMC—CL 6040, CL 7215)
Opiates	1. Naloxone and Oxygen are available 2. PCA protocols are available and used 3. Refer to policy: (HMC—CL 6053)
Insulins	1. Use brand name plus generic name where it is possible 2. Hypoglycemia kit is available where it is necessary 3. Refer to policy: (HMC—CL 6106)
Neuromuscular blocking agents	1. Affix standardized High-Alert and Paralyzing Agent warning labels on all NMBs 2. Segregate storage of NMBs 3. Limit the availability of NMBs outside the Pharmacy to ORs, EDs, and ICUs 4. Refer to NMBs always as "neuromuscular blockers" or "paralyzing agents," NEVER call them "muscle relaxants" 5. Administer NMBs only to patients who are on/to be on ventilator support

(continued)

Table 4.2 (continued)

Drug class	Risk reduction strategies
Anti-thrombotics	1. Separate the storage of different concentrations of the same medication (e.g. Heparin 1000 units/ml and 5000 units/ml) 2. Standardize heparin doses to be prepared and supplied by pharmacy 3. Use premixed solutions and reduce the number of concentrations available where is possible 4. Vitamin K and protamine sulfate are available where are needed
Anesthetics	1. the drug and dose should be verified before administration with the physician's order/medication administration record by two qualified/ competent healthcare providers 2. Education for nurses about the risks 3. Provide appropriate monitoring during the use of anesthetics (e.g. use pulse oximetry) 4. Resuscitation equipment are available where is needed
Epidural and spinal medications	1. Special warning label that the medication is "For Epidural/ Spinal Use Only" on shelves and on the drug before dispensing 2. Independently double check the route of administration before dispensing and administration 3. Epidural/intrathecal can be administered only by privileged physician

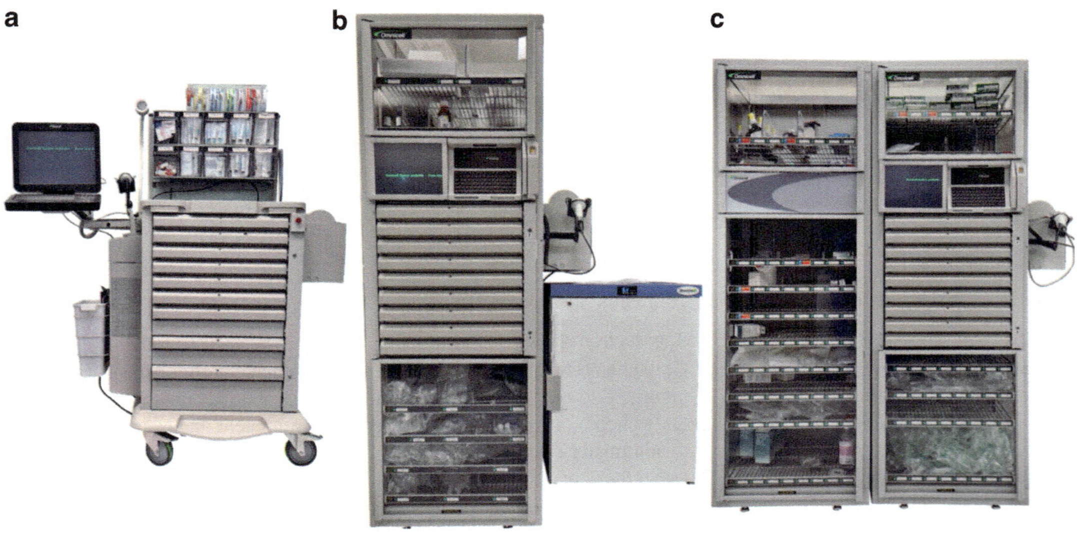

Fig. 4.6 Automated Medication Dispensing Machines (**a**–**c**)

storage, dispensing, and tracking of medications—have been recommended as one potential mechanism to improve efficiency and patient safety, and they are now widely used in many hospitals. Enhance the efficiency of medication distribution, but their ability to reduce medication errors is controversial however they carry many advantages:

- Provide a good balance among security, accessibility, and inventory control of medications, which are all recognized as important characteristics of a safe medication distribution system.
- Automated dispensing machines provide secure medication storage on patient care units, along with electronic tracking of the use of narcotics and other controlled drugs.
- Automated dispensing machines reduce pharmacists' dispensing time, as inventory management is driven by the pre-established minimum and maximum levels and is handled exclusively by pharmacy technicians.

- Automated dispensing machines is the capability to track and proactively monitor drug usage patterns.
- Automated dispensing machines enhance first-dose availability and facilitate the timely administration of medications by increasing their accessibility on patient care units.
- Automated dispensing machines reduce pharmacists' dispensing time, as inventory management is driven by the pre-established minimum and maximum levels and is handled exclusively by pharmacy technicians.

4.5 Infection Control Related to Drugs Use (Aseptic Technique)

Many patients are affected every year by health care associated infection most of these infections related to invasive procedure.

Hence intravenous drug administration is considered as one of the possible sources of infection, aseptic techniques should follow during intravenous medications administrations including in operating theater. Aseptic technique is defined as a process or procedure used to achieve asepsis to prevent the transfer of potentially pathogenic micro-organisms to a susceptible site that may result in the development of infection.

Examples of when to use a medical aseptic technique are as follows:

- Dressing a surgical wound.
- Inserting a peripheral cannula.
- Venipuncture.
- Inserting a urinary catheter.
- Administrating intravenous drugs.

4.5.1 Principles of Aseptic Techniques

The fundamental principle of an aseptic technique/ANTT incorporates protecting key elements of the equipment (usually parts of equipment with contact of internal organs or blood) that should remain free from micro-organisms, contaminating of these parts of equipment will prone the patient to an avoidable infection (Table 4.3).

Table 4.3 Stages of medical aseptic technique

Summary for the Principles of aseptic technique and the rationale behind it	
The Task	Rationale
Hand hygiene	Remove transient micro-organisms from the hands
Safe storage of equipment	Prevent damage to the sterile equipment preserve sterility of the equipment and prevent microbial contamination
Cleaning of the procedure trolley or tray	Reduce microbial contamination
Preparation of equipment	Prevent microbial contamination of sterile equipment
Personnel protective equipment	Aprons provide protection for potential contamination from the health care workers (HCW) uniform and the procedure and also protect HCW from potential contamination from the procedure Non-sterile gloves provide protection the HCW from contamination from blood and body fluid that may contaminated the hands Sterile gloves protect key sites from potential microbial contamination from HCW hands
Preparation of the environment	Reduce microbial contamination during the procedure
Preparation of the patient	Gain informed consent and reduce anxiety
Waste disposal	Prevent contamination of the environment
Documentation	Provide essential communication and meet the standards

It is recommended before intravenous drug injection not to touch any key part of the cannula and using caps and covers, such as the sterile wrapper of a syringe to protect the key part of the syringe before use. To achieve the main goal ideally the health care provider should follow the principles summarized in Table 4.1.

Take-Home Message

Familiarity with simple and serious side effects of used medication is essential and a must.

Minimalizing medications errors is important to avoid any serious harm to the patient, this could be achieved according to hospital policy and resources.

In general, few important aspects to prevent adverse drug event (ADE) which different from adverse drug reaction (ADR) are:

- Attention to medications packaging storing and labeling.
- Attentions to Look alike-sound alike (LASA) drugs.
- Standardized labeling has been developed in the last few decades with color-coded syringes, color-coded labels, and computer-generated labels; however, this should not replace the last step before administering the medication to the patient which is read the label to confirm the appropriate medication and dose.

Suggested Reading

Gropper M, Eriksson L, Fleisher L, Wiener-Kronish J, Cohen N, Leslie K, editors. Miller's anesthesia. 9th ed. Elsevier; 2019.

Mahmoud M, et al. Dexmedetomidine: review, update, and future considerations of paediatric perioperative and periprocedural applications and limitations. Br J Anaesth. 2015;115:171–82. https://doi.org/10.1093/bja/aev2.

Peck TE, Hill SA, Williams M. Pharmacology for anaesthesia and intensive care. 3rd ed. Cambridge University Press; 2009. ISBN 978-0-521-70463-2

Stoelting R, Flood P, Rathmell JP, Shafer S, editors. Stoelting's handbook of pharmacology and physiology in anesthetic practice. 3rd ed. Wolter S Kluwer; 2014.

Checklists: To Get Things Done Right—All the Time

5

Neeraj Kumar, Layla Jasim Mahdi Kily, and Abdul Khader Muhammed

Contents

Abbreviations

AAGBI Association of Anaesthetists of Great Britain and Ireland
AHRQ Agency of Healthcare Research and Quality
APL Adjustable pressure limiting

N. Kumar (✉) · L. J. M. Kily · A. K. Muhammed
Anesthesiology, Intensive care and perioperative Medicine, Hamad General Hospital, Doha, Qatar
e-mail: nkumar@hamad.qa; Lkily@hamad.qa; Amuhammed5@hamad.qa

N. A. Shallik et al. (eds.), *Improving Anesthesia Technical Staff's Skills*,
https://doi.org/10.1007/978-3-030-88849-7_5

ASA	American Society of Anesthesiologist
ASATT	American Society of Anaesthesia Technologists and Technicians.
ETT	Endotracheal tube
FDA	Federation of Drug Administration
HME	Heat Moisture Exchange
LAST	Local anaesthetic systemic toxicity
LMA	Laryngeal Mask Airway
MH	Malignant hyperthermia
OR	Operating Room
POC	Point of care
PPE	Personal Protective equipment
Psig	Pound-force per square inch gauge
RSI	Rapid sequence Induction
WHO	World Health Organization

5.1 Introduction

Operating room (OR) practice is generally reliant on the use of many different checklists that institute as well maintain essential safety standards. To work in an OR without any form of checklist available or non-compliance can be considered unsafe practice that may contribute to errors or patient harm [1].

All OR staff but in particular anaesthesia providers and the technician support staff should be familiar with the array of international standard as well as local hospital checklists within their department. Some may choose to modify the checklist to personalize its use such as the order in which items are checked, which is also acceptable provided no item is omitted.

Checklists contribute to safer work flow, improved communication and facilitation of team work as well as consistency in key steps and availability of functioning equipment [2]. These essential safety checks should be undertaken before, during and after the administration of anaesthesia to the patient and should not be limited to the anaesthesia provider.

This chapter will review the development and importance of regular checklists and give an overview and summary of some existing anaesthesia checklists we are familiar with including the International World Health Organization (WHO) Surgical Safety Checklist, anaesthesia equipment and machine ventilator checklist, room preparation, crisis and emergency checklists, medications and equipment supply. The essential components of these checklists will be discussed.

5.2 History of the Checklist

There is no doubt that practitioners throughout the ages, before administering agents to aid surgical procedures, had their own personal mental checklist to aid the basis of their practice. However, it was not until the analysis of the first death related to anaesthesia which was attributed to the use of Chloroform and published in 1849, that provider safety and practice was questioned and discussed [3]. Since then there have been numerous publications, editorials and discussions on the development of safer anaesthesia practice [1, 3].

The aviation sector has taught anaesthesia many learning points regarding human factors and errors as flying is thought to be comparable to induction during take-off, maintenance during the journey flight and emergence during landing. It is also associated with introducing the anaesthesia world to the all-important checklist to ensure essential steps before each of these processes. This historical introduction of pilot's checklist was founded in 1935 after the analysis of the US Army Air Corps Boeing Model 299 plane crash and despite being flown by highly experienced army pilots, simple pilot errors were established as the cause. Following this, four simple checklists were made to ensure crucial steps were not forgotten during the critical phases of flight; take off, flight, landing and post-landing [4].

In 1985, the Anesthesia Patient Safety Foundation (APSF) was established to ensure "no patient is harmed by anaesthesia" [1]. However, in 1986 The United States Food and Drug Administration (FDA) published the earliest form of anaesthesia checklist which issued a guideline on the generic anaesthesia equipment pre-use check. It recommended checkout to be conducted before anaesthesia and also issued guidelines users were encouraged to modify to accommodate differences in equipment design and variation [5].

Charlton, in his 1990 editorial in the journal *Anaesthesia*, stressed on the importance and development of checklists during anaesthesia practice and their potential cost effectiveness from the reduction in patient harm and litigation. After multiple reported serious accidents with the anaesthesia machine it was suggested to introduce mandatory checklists for the patient's safety, though countries federal bodies that make recommendations using the word "should" are mandatory and not voluntary. Such countries included USA, Australia and Germany [6].

In 2008, the American Society of Anesthesiologists (ASA) Committee on Equipment and Facilities, in conjunction with the AANA and the American Society of Anesthesia Technologists and Technicians (ASATT), started to improve a revised pre-use guideline. These procedures are a guide to other departments for using similar equipment and creating their own checkout procedures [7].

In 2009, the WHO launched their Safe Surgery Saves Lives campaign and published their first guidelines on safety related to checks made at various stages [8]. In 2012 the Association of Anaesthetists of Great Britain and Ireland (AAGBI) developed and published their Checking Anaesthetic Equipment Guideline which is a comprehensive guide to outcomes expected rather than processes [9].

The end of 2019 saw the emergence of a novel Coronavirus SARS-CoV-2, which was declared a pandemic by March 2020. Therefore, to minimize exposure and infection risk to both, staff providing airway management and successive patients, many institutions developed checklist-style guidelines for the assessment, induction and safe airway management of such patients.

5.2.1 Importance of Checklists

A checklist is a cognitive visual aid that serves to remind its user to undertake a specific task or action. With the development and advancement of technology and the need to prevent and minimize errors and unnecessary harm to patients, the checklist has become an integral part of clinical practice.

Human factors are known to contribute to error and patient harm. Simply forgetting and lapses or errors may occur in otherwise competent anaesthesiologists, and the adoption of the checklist has been studied and supported to prevent and reduce such errors [1, 9]. Checklists within the clinical setting have been studied over the years and they not only increase the number of physical safety checks, but also improve efficiency, communication, team work and consistency [1, 10].

Many studies have supported the use of checklists to improve patient outcomes. The use of a checklist to ensure critical infection control and other safety steps caused a reduction in the number of blood borne infections related to their insertion. This also empowered the other staff such as nurses to challenge the doctor if a step was omitted either by accident or deliberately even if it seemed minor as they were now able to raise this concern further [11].

Anaesthesia checklists have been shown not only to improve quality of care but also to reduce perioperative morbidity and mortality especially in intraoperative emergency situations with the use of crisis checklists. However, the acceptance and appreciation of checklists were found in only very junior or experienced providers [1]. In the crisis checklists serve to reduce information that may lead to wrong decision making. They have also been found to improve performance and lower overall mortality.

It is very important when designing a checklist that they are user friendly, adjustable as much as possible to the variable clinical settings and succinct enough to reduce the risk of distraction and rejection; a term called "checklist fatigue" [12]. Another study found that increasing the visibility of the checklist itself by designating a known place within the OR where all staff can see it and assigning a checklist operator, not only increased the number of items completed but also overall performance [13].

5.2.2 Checklist Manifesto

Atul Gawande, public health researcher and surgeon, published a book in 2009, The Checklist Manifesto: How to Get Things Right. In this non-fiction book, the author discussed how the medical profession and the business world could significantly benefit from the implementation of checklists. He stated a distinction between errors of ignorance (mistakes made because we do not know enough) and errors of ineptitude (mistakes made because we do not make proper use of what we know). In his opinion, current practice is due to the latter error. He believed that checklists; literal written guides can walk people through the key steps in any complex procedure [14].

In stressful situations, such as anaesthesia practice, it is not unusual even for experienced physicians to miss steps, questions or fail to implement their plan. Experts also need help and they need to have humility to ask for help. A checklist is one of the tools that experts can use to make sure that they do not miss any important step in their patient care. Dr. Gawande and his research team then developed a safer surgery checklist which is applied around the world and is incorporated within the WHO Surgical Safety Checklist [14].

5.2.3 Cockpit Drill

Anaesthesia induction including airway management and extubation are two very important phases during anaesthesia. Airway complications, once the most common cause of anaesthesia related morbidity and mortality, still is a common concern to patient safety. Most of the airway related complications are preventable and those such as regurgitation and aspiration of gastric contents and difficulty in ventilation and oxygenation can be managed safely with adequate preparation and planning. This includes OR preparation which can be safely accomplished using a checklist to make sure the availability, adequacy and functioning of all necessary equipment. Many anaesthesiologists compare anaesthesia and aviation and suggest that practitioners should check the anaesthetic machines using a "cockpit drill" [15].

5.3 Electronic Checklists

Several strategies for decreasing the possibilities of errors have been suggested along with the checklist. A few examples of these strategies are thorough preparation before anaesthesia, development of meticulous work habits and advanced training methods. As long as humans provide anaesthesia care, the advantage of sensory and reasoning abilities unmatched by any machine will exist, despite the chances of human errors. No amount of training and effort on the part of the individual can eliminate this error. There is, therefore, great potential for decision support tools to aid the specialist and hence reduce the risk of these errors. The electronic checklist can provide more extensive checklists and support information in the form of online "help" to explain checklist points or provide insights for decision making and also reduce the bulk of multiple papers, reducing waste and distraction.

Electronic checklists provide better documentation of clinical work which can be very helpful in medicolegal settings. The handwritten record may be either illegible or an incomplete rendition of events. The use of an electronic checklist can be documented either in print or by an electronic record keeper and takes approximately 5 min. This type of electronic documentation would, therefore, be thorough, reproducible and easily retrieved.

5.4 Anaesthesia Checklists

Numerous different checklists have been developed to ensure consistency in safety checks, patient care, essential monitoring and communication/handover. Various hospitals and international societies have created their own checklists to suit local, environmental and cultural needs. The most popular checklists; the ASA and AAGBI anaesthesia equipment checklist, the

WHO Surgical Safety Checklist, pre-induction checklist and crisis checklists will be discussed further in this section.

The ASA also recommends a standard check-out at the start of the day and additional checks between cases (Table 5.1). Most hospitals have adopted their own checklist which may be a modification of the ASA or AAGBI guidance or a combination of guidelines and checklists from other published sources.

Table 5.1 Summary of ASA anaesthesia checklist items to be conducted daily and between cases

Item	Task to be completed	Daily	Between cases	Responsible Parties
1	Verify auxiliary oxygen cylinder and self-inflating Manual ventilation device available and functioning.	✓		Provider and technician
2.	Verify patient suction is adequate to clear the airway.	✓	✓	Provider and technician
3.	Turn on the anaesthesia delivery system and confirm that AC power is available.	✓		Provider or technician
4.	Verify availability of required monitors, including alarms.	✓	✓	Provider or technician
5.	Verify that pressure is adequate on the spare oxygen cylinder mounted on the anaesthesia machine.	✓		Provider and technician
6.	Verify that the piped gas pressures are ≥50 psig.	✓		Provider and technician
7.	Verify that vaporizers are adequately filled and, if applicable, that the filler ports are tightly closed.	✓	✓	Provider only
8.	Verify that there are no leaks in the gas supply lines between the flowmeters and the common gas outlet.	✓		Provider or technician
9.	Test scavenging system function.	✓		Provider or technician
10.	Calibrate, or verify calibration of, the oxygen monitor and check the low-oxygen alarm.	✓		Provider or technician
11.	Verify carbon dioxide absorbent is not exhausted.	✓	✓	Provider or technician
12.	Perform breathing system pressure and leak testing.	✓	✓	Provider and technician
13.	Verify that gas flows properly through the breathing circuit during both inspiration and exhalation.	✓	✓	Provider and technician
14.	Document completion of checkout procedures.	✓	✓	Provider and technician
15.	Confirm ventilator settings and evaluate readiness to deliver anaesthesia care (anaesthesia time out).	✓	✓	Provider only

Excerpted from (Standards and Guidelines- 2008 ASA Recommendations for Pre-anaesthesia Checkout. www.asahq.org/standards-and-guidelines. Accessed on July 25, 2020) [7]

5.5 Pre-Anaesthesia Checklist in the OR

Anaesthesia equipment which includes the anaesthesia machine as well as all equipment either to be used to provide anaesthesia to the patient or to be used in a potential emergency or crisis situation must be checked [10]. The AAGBI states that the anaesthesiologist has the responsibility to understand the function as well as perform a pre-use safety check [16].

Pre-anaesthesia check may involve either physically checking the equipment and machine themselves or referring to the log book documentation to ensure that the more detailed and comprehensive check has occurred. A basic re-check of airway equipment, machine, monitors, suction, availability of self-inflating bag and medications including emergency medications should always occur before the start of anaesthesia unless there is an urgent lifesaving surgery in which case, the checks that could not be performed due to the urgency of the situation should be clearly documented.

As an anaesthesia team, the first check before starting any case is that of the basic anaesthesia machine check. Anaesthesia equipment failures may contribute to anaesthetic difficulties leading potentially to operative morbidity and mortality. There are many reported guidelines by professional organizations advising anaesthesiologists; pre-use and in-between anaesthesia machine checking. Modern anaesthesia machines incorporate self-checking programmes complemented by personal checking to insure operability of these machines. Recording and authentications can be part of the process to improve operative patient safety.

The anaesthesia machine with its incorporated monitors and computer recording system may also be called the anaesthesia workstation (Fig. 5.1). It is an important component of anaesthesia health and safety and it has many automatic inbuilt monitors included to maintain vigilance over the patient and machine itself. Oxygen concentration and exhaled patient volume monitors may present early warning of hypoxic mixtures, system leaks, or accidental disconnections. This along with integration of other monitors (capnometry, saturation, non-invasive blood pressure) into the anaesthesia system ensures that these monitors should be switched on and functional before using it on any patient or procedure involving gas delivery and improves the management of the workstation and patient safety monitoring.

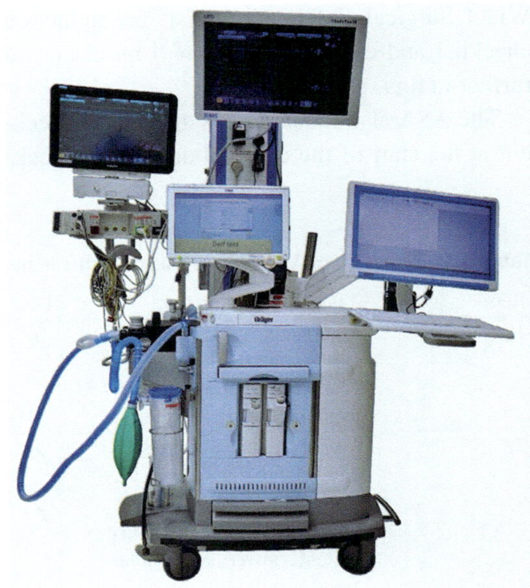

Fig. 5.1 Anaesthesia Workstation. Example of the modern anaesthesia workstation with the incorporation of monitoring and computer system (Drager, Germany)

Some argue that a quick check out at the start of anaesthesia is enough and that any kind of error or malfunction shall be discovered during use and managed intraoperatively. This can be true in some circumstances; nevertheless, modern anaesthetic workstations are generally large and complex. They therefore must be checked carefully to avoid any potential problems. It is just as important to check the older, more "straightforward" machines as they approach the conclusion of their working lives. Many hospitals may have found that it is difficult to replace older machines as a consequence of restraints upon their equipment budgets.

Systematic checkout procedure and the simple documentation usually forms part of the working day and should not be viewed as an additional burden. A general rule known in medicine is "if it isn't written down, it wasn't done". Keeping a record of check out processes performed is important. This may be in the form of either a logbook or simple checkout form kept and stored but performed daily before the start of the day. Higher standards of quality and patient care can be achieved by implementing and auditing these checkout procedures.

5.6 Anaesthesia Machine Checkout Procedure

With advancement of technology, anaesthesia delivery systems have evolved immensely, so much that one checkout procedure may not be applicable to all anaesthesia delivery systems that are currently available. Therefore, the goal of the ASA subcommittee was to provide guidelines applicable to all anaesthesia delivery systems so that individual departments can modify and develop their own pre-anaesthesia checklist that can be performed consistently and quickly even in emergency situations. In addition, they also described the responsible person for each step to carry out such checks so that the time taken to perform the check may be reduced.

In summary the requirements for safe delivery of anaesthetic care include but not limited to the following:

- Reliable delivery of oxygen (from 21 to 100%).
- Reliable means of positive pressure ventilation.
- Availability of functional backup ventilation equipment.
- Anaesthesia vapour delivery.
- Adequate suction.
- Means of standard patient monitoring.

The new ASA guidelines for the pre-anaesthesia checkout procedures consist of 15 items. These items must be performed as part of a complete pre-anaesthesia checkout on a daily basis (Table 5.1). Excerpted from (Standards and Guidelines- 2008 ASA Recommendations for Pre-anaesthesia Checkout. www.asahq.org/standards-and-guidelines. accessed on July 25, 2020) of the ASA. A copy of the full text can be obtained from ASA,1061 American lane schaumbaug, IL 60173–4973 or online at www.asahq.org.

5.6.1 Essential Anaesthesia Workstation Checks

1. Verify auxiliary oxygen cylinders and self-inflating manual ventilation devices are available and functioning.

A major cause of morbidity and mortality related to anaesthesia care is failure to ventilate the patient, one reason may be due to machine equipment failure which can happen at any time. Where the problem cannot be immediately identified or corrected, a manual ventilation device (e.g. AMBU bag Fig. 5.2a) may be required to provide positive pressure ventilation until the problem is resolved. This should be present at every anesthetizing location for every case and should be checked for proper function. An additional source of oxygen such as an oxygen cylinder with a regulator (Fig. 5.2b) as well as cylinder key should be immediately available and checked.

A full E cylinder of oxygen has a pressure of about 2000 pound-force per square inch gauge (psig), which is equivalent to approximately 625 L of oxygen. After checking the oxygen cylinder pressure to ensure adequate supply, the cylinder should be stored with the valve shut off in order to avoid leakage of oxygen.

2. Verify patient suction is adequate to clear the airway.

Safe anaesthetic care requires the immediate availability of adequate suction to clear the airway if needed. A simple gross test of adequate strength is to open the suction on maximum continuous mode and attach the free end to either a finger or palm of hand and once attached, raise the hand to above shoulder height. If the suction tube detaches and falls, this is failure of adequate suction (Fig. 5.3). Suction pressure that is able to hold up 6 feet of tubing with and without glove use on average is −97.7 mmHg [17].

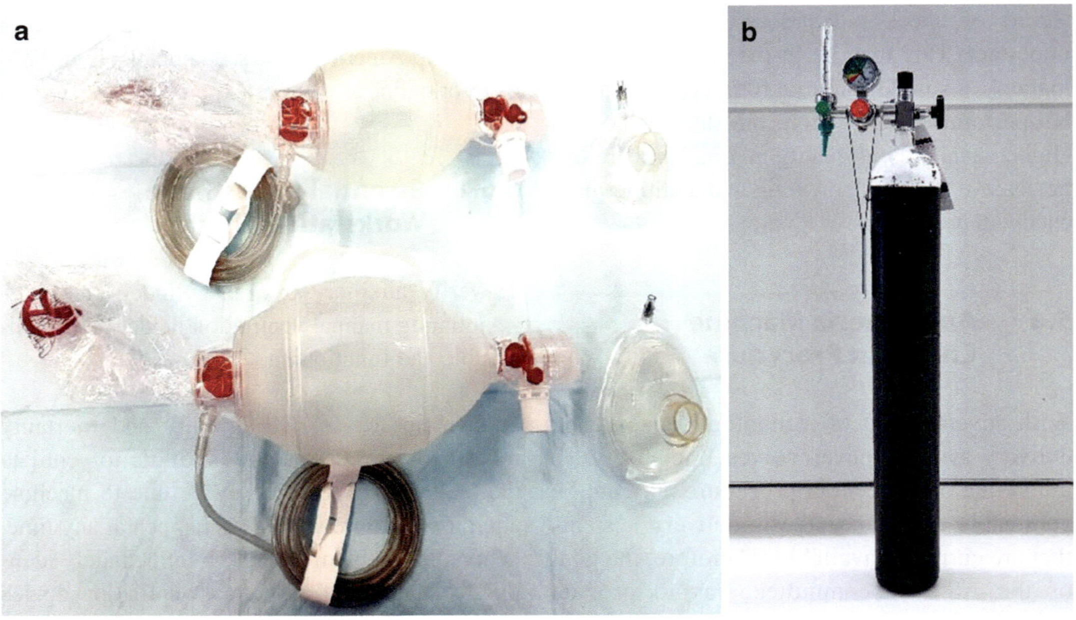

Fig. 5.2 Provisions for emergency ventilation and oxygenation. (**a**). Self-inflating bag plus mask in standard adult and paediatric sizes (**b**) Auxiliary oxygen cylinder

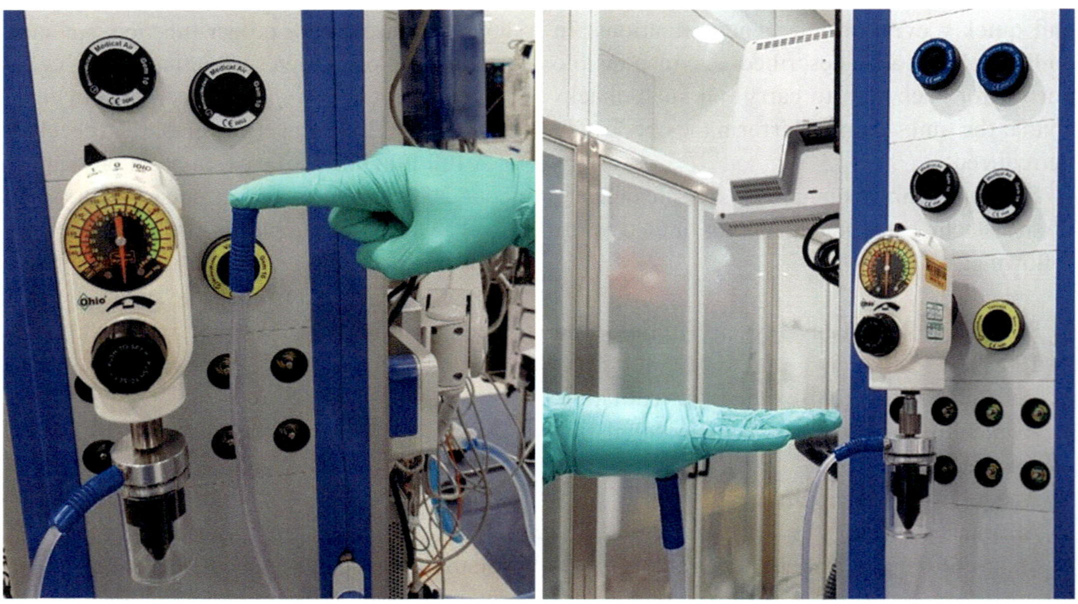

Fig. 5.3 Gross test of adequate suction using either finger or hand held above shoulder height

3. Turn on the anaesthesia delivery system and confirm that AC power is available.

Anaesthesia delivery systems usually operate with backup battery power should AC electrical power fail. Unless the presence of AC power is confirmed, the first obvious sign of power failure could be a complete system shutdown when the batteries can no longer power the machine. Many anaesthesia delivery systems have visual indica-

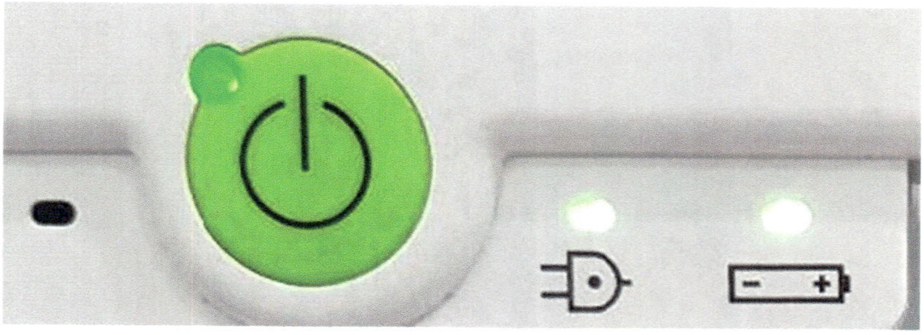

Fig. 5.4 AC electrical and backup battery power indicators to be checked

tors of the power source showing the presence of both AC and battery power (Fig. 5.4). These indicators must be checked and the connection of the power cord to a functional AC electrical power source should be confirmed.

4. Verify availability of required monitors and check alarms.

The standards for patient monitoring are clearly defined during anaesthesia. Before every procedure, the team should visually verify that the minimum mandatory monitoring supplies as recommended by the ASA (BP cuff, oximetry probe, ECG, temperature probe, etc.) are available [18]. They should be turned on and checked whether connected to the power supply. Alarm signal and limits should also be checked and set prior to each case ensuring appropriate limits for adult or paediatric cases (Fig. 5.5). Provided the importance of pulse oximetry and capnography to patient safety, confirming the proper function of these devices prior to anesthetising the patient is vital.

Capnometer function may be checked by physically by exhaling through the breathing circuit or gas sensor to generate a capnogram or by the patient's breathing efforts to generate a capnogram before induction of anaesthesia. Visual and audible alarm signals should be generated when this is discontinued. Pulse oximeter function which emits a variable pitch tone, can be verified by placing the sensor on a finger and observing for a proper recording. The pulse oximeter and alarm can be tested by introducing motion artefacts or removing the sensor. Audible alarms have also been reconfirmed as essential to patient safety by professional societies and accrediting organizations. When pulse oximeter is used, variable pitch pulse tone and the low threshold alarm shall be audible to the anaesthesia provider [18].

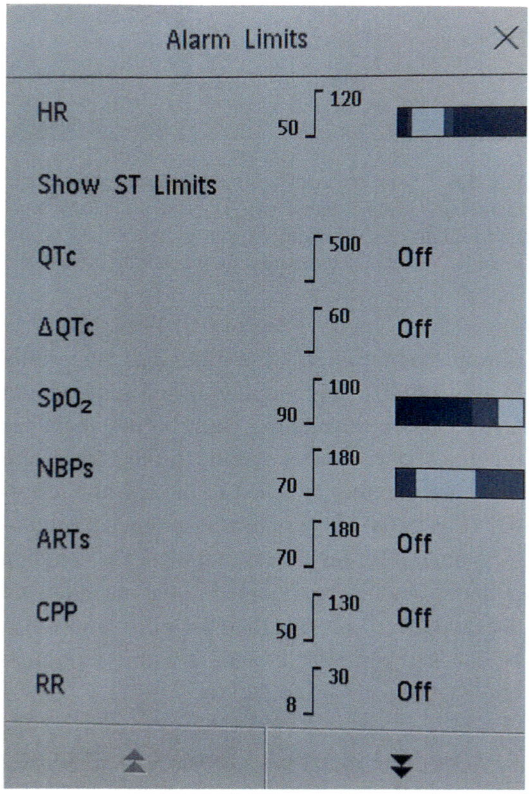

Fig. 5.5 Checking and setting up alarm limits of monitors

5. Verify that pressure is adequate on the spare oxygen cylinder mounted on the anaesthesia machine.

The anaesthesia machine mainly depends on central supply for gases (oxygen, medical air and

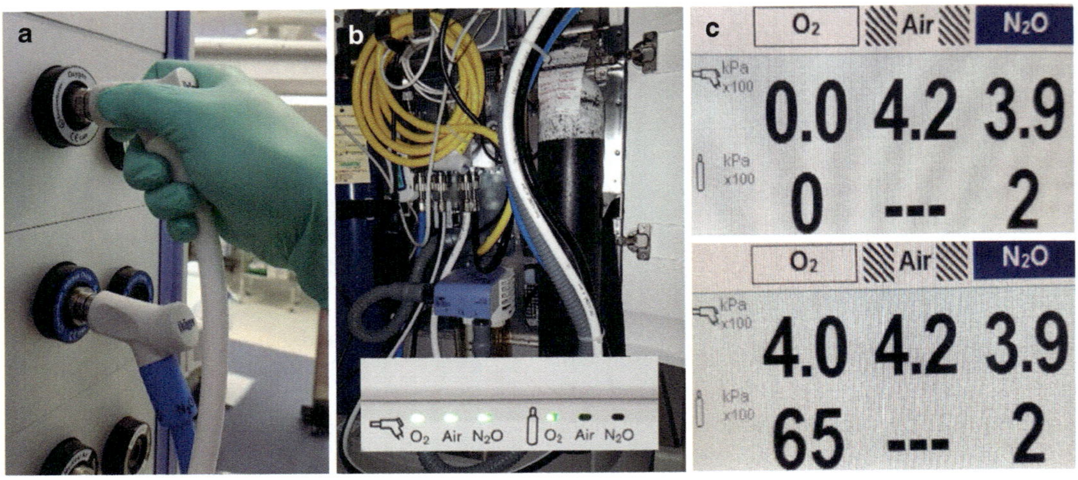

Fig. 5.6 Check of anaesthesia machine oxygen supply including backup cylinder. (**a**) "Tug test" for secure pipeline terminal. (**b**) Backup oxygen cylinder present and mounted within machine (inset indicator light on machine that backup oxygen cylinder present and turned on). (**c**) Oxygen pressure check on main screen of both pipeline and cylinder

nitrous oxide) for its various functions. According to the AAGBI guidelines, this machine should also be checked using the 'tug test'; the main gas pipelines should be manually pulled to ensure there are securely attached to the specific terminal (Fig. 5.6a). Pneumatically-powered ventilators also rely on a gas supply. The oxygen cylinders should be mounted in the machine and checked (Fig. 5.6b) and their pressure should also be checked periodically and be within minimum range ($\geq$50 psig/ $\geq$344.7 kPa).

6. Verify that piped gas pressures are $\geq$50 psig ($\geq$ 344.7 kPa) (Fig. 5.6c).

A minimum gas supply pressure is required for proper function of the anaesthesia delivery system. Gas supplied from a central source can fail for a variety of reasons. Therefore, the pressure in the piped gas supply should be checked at least once daily.

Additionally, flowmeters need to be checked for adequate function and bobbin presence. In non-automated machines the hypoxic guard is an essential check. This checks the presence of a system link between the oxygen flow and Nitrous oxide to ensure the prevention of a hypoxic mixture and hence a minimum oxygen concentration of 21%. This is performed simply by turning up the Nitrous oxide flow without altering the oxygen and observing that the oxygen flow level also rises automatically (Fig. 5.7).

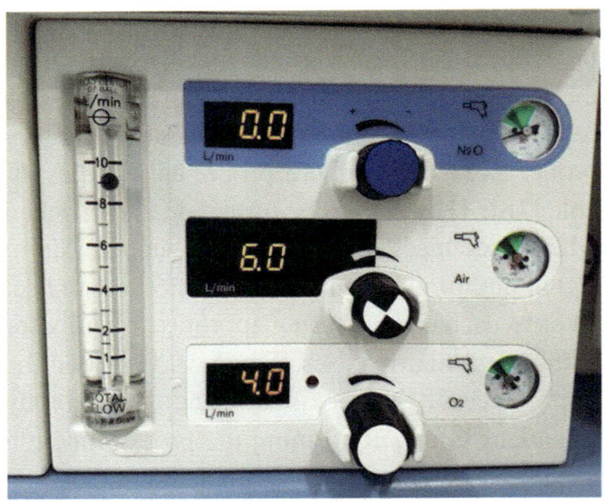

Fig. 5.7 Hypoxic guard proportioning system. The automatic adjustment of oxygen when Nitrous oxide flow is increased to prevent a hypoxic gas mixture

7. Verify that vaporisers are adequately filled and, if applicable, that the filler ports are tightly closed.

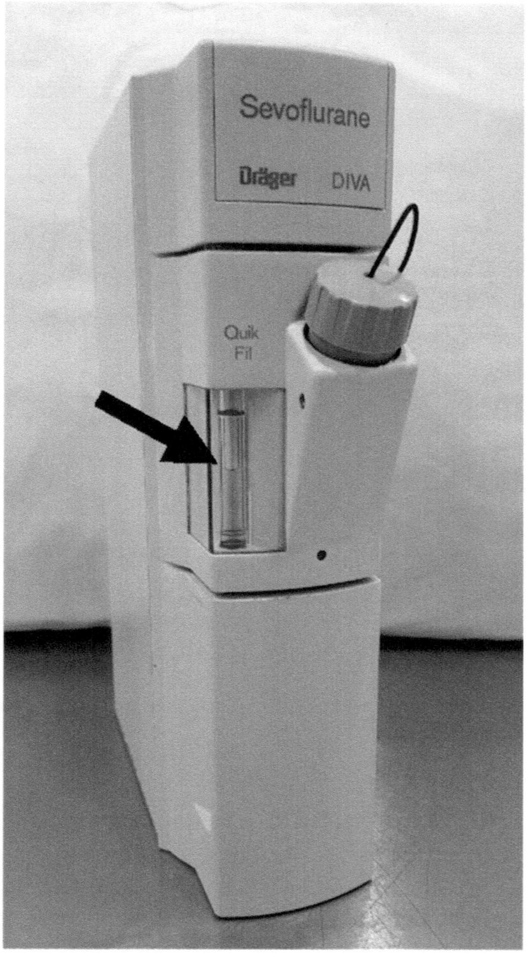

Fig. 5.8 Example of an anaesthesia vaporiser for Sevoflurane. Photo demonstrating an adequate level in the window chamber (arrowed)

All the vaporisers should be adequately filled and tightly closed before the procedure as it may cause light anaesthesia and awareness. This is especially true if an anaesthetic agent monitor with a low agent alarm is not being used (Fig. 5.8).

One of the main reasons for anaesthesia gas vapour leak is improper closure of the filler ports that may not have been noticed or not detected during leak tests. This leak source can be minimized by tightly closing filler ports. Modern vaporiser designs have filling systems that automatically close the filler port. High and low anaesthetic agent alarms are useful to help prevent over or under dosage of anaesthetic vapour. Use of these alarms is encouraged and they should be set to the appropriate limits and enabled.

8. Verify that there are no leaks in the gas supply lines between the flowmeters and the common gas outlet.

The gas supply in this part of the anaesthesia delivery system passes through the anaesthetic vaporiser on most anaesthesia delivery systems. To perform a thorough leak test, each vaporiser must be checked individually. However, in some modern anaesthesia workstations the vaporisers are built-in and the machine itself does the leak tests within the system during the self-test (Fig. 5.9). When using the older anaesthesia machines, which contain automated checkout procedures and include a leak test but may not evaluate leaks at the vaporiser especially if the vaporiser is not turned on during the leak test. When relying upon automated testing to evaluate the system for leaks, the automated leak test would need to be repeated for each vaporiser in place within the machine.

This test should also be completed whenever a vaporizer is changed or refilled. The risk of a leak at the vaporiser depends upon the vaporiser design. Vaporiser designs where the filler port closes automatically after filling can reduce the risk of leaks. Technicians can provide useful assistance to the anaesthesiologist with this aspect of the machine checkout since it can be time-consuming.

In non-automated systems, a simple negative pressure test of the low pressure system of the machine can be performed. This test termed the "bulb squeeze" test is the most sensitive test for leaks as it is independent of flow and can detect as little as 30 ml/min of leakage from common gas outlet [19] (Fig. 5.10).

9. Testing of the scavenging system function.

An adequately working scavenging system prevents room contamination by anaesthetic gases. Proper function depends upon correct con-

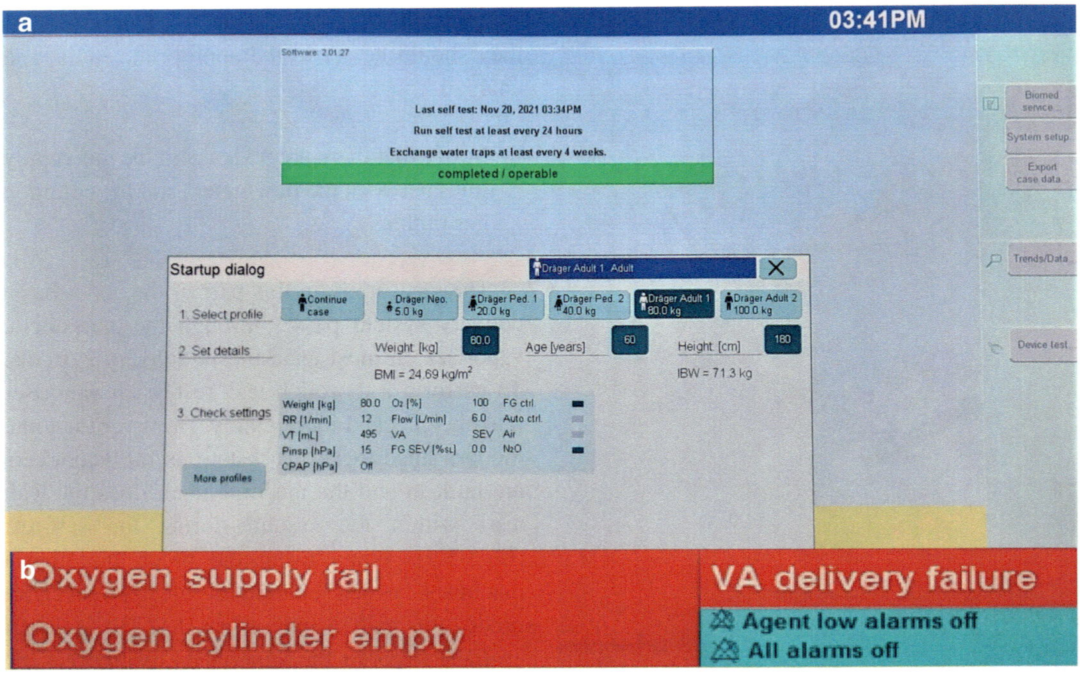

Fig. 5.9 Automated machine screen indicator. (**a**) Self-test screen indicating the individual machine testing points. (**b**) Oxygen failure alarm

nections between the scavenging system and the anaesthesia delivery system within the machine. These connections should be checked daily by a provider or technician. Based upon the scavenging system design, a proper function may also require that the vacuum level is adequate and confirmed daily (Fig. 5.11a). Some scavenging systems have mechanical positive and negative pressure relief valves. Positive and negative pressure relief is important to protect the patient circuit from pressure fluctuations related to the scavenging system. OR ventilation systems should also be checked that they are switched on to ensure continuous OR ventilation to reduce OR staff anaesthetic gas exposure (Fig. 5.11b).

10. Calibrate or verify calibration of the oxygen monitor and check the low oxygen alarm.

Continuous monitoring of oxygen concentration is essential to avoid delivering any hypoxic gas concentration to the patient. These oxygen sensors require calibration once daily, although some workstations have an automated calibrating system of these sensors. For self-calibrating oxygen monitors, they should be verified to read 21% when sampling room air. The sensors which require manual calibrating in older machines can be done by the skilled technical staff to save time. The low oxygen concentration alarm should be checked by setting the alarm above measured oxygen concentration and confirming that an audible alarm signal is generated.

11. Verify carbon dioxide absorbent is not exhausted.

Adequate function of a circle anaesthesia system depends on soda lime adsorbent to remove carbon dioxide from the breathing system. Exhausted soda lime as indicated by the characteristic colour change from white to pinkish purple should be replaced (Fig. 5.12). Some newer absorbents change colour when desiccated but capnography should be utilized for every anaesthetic and when using a circle anaesthesia system.

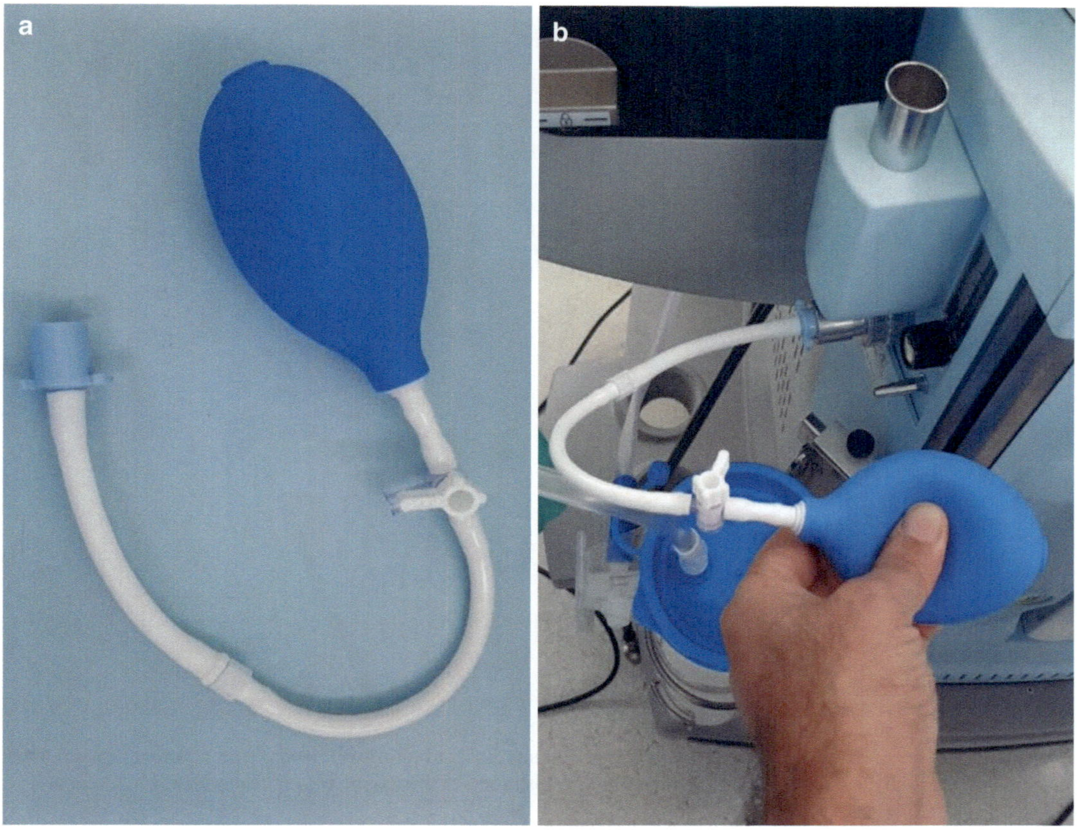

Fig. 5.10 Bulb squeeze test. (**a**) Apparatus used for low pressure testing of leaks which includes simple sphygmomanometer bulb connected to simple tubing and endotracheal tube (ETT) connector. (**b**) Bulb squeezed and when it remains fully collapsed for at least 10 s, this indicates the system is leak free

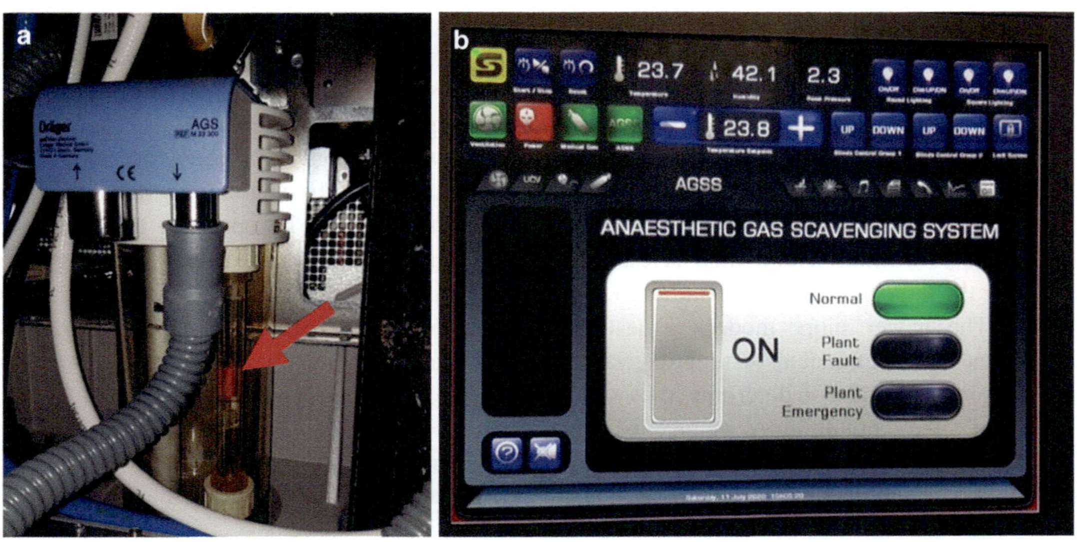

Fig. 5.11 Scavenging system. (**a**) Example of the scavenging interface within a Drager anaesthesia machine. Red bobbin within adequate level (arrowed) (Drager, Germany). (**b**) Main OR scavenging system turned on and functioning normally

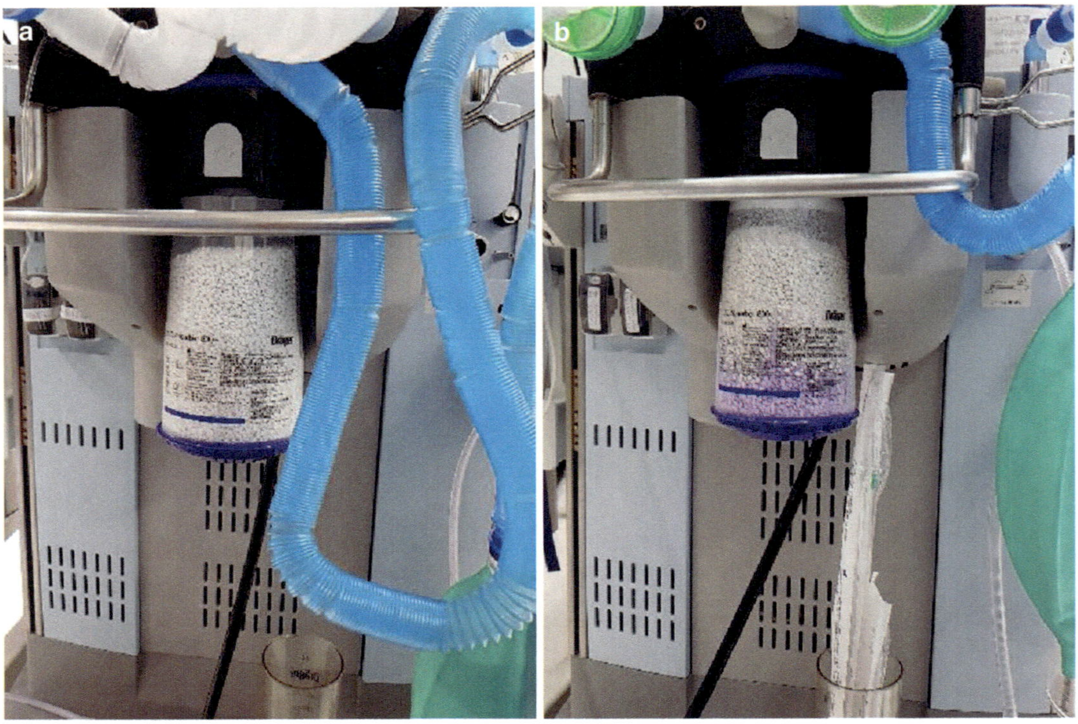

Fig. 5.12 Carbon dioxide soda lime absorbent. (**a**) Example of carbon dioxide soda lime absorbent on a Drager machine. (**b**) Partially exhausted soda lime granules demonstrating characteristic colour change (Drager, Germany)

Rebreathing carbon dioxide as indicated by an inspired carbon dioxide concentration >0 mmHg also indicates exhausted absorbent.

12. Breathing system pressure leak and testing.

The system pressure and leak testing should be performed for the breathing circuit. If any items are replaced such as filters or circuits, the test should be repeated. During the check, pressure can be created in the breathing system during manual ventilation and then released by opening the adjustable pressure limiting (APL) valve. The newer more modern anaesthesia machines have automated testing to evaluate the system leaks and also determine the compliance of the breathing system. Modern Anaesthesia machine automatically adjusts compliance value determined during testing to maintain a constant volume delivery to the patient.

The AAGBI recommends performing the "two-bag" test. This manual test of positive pressure involves the use of a "test lung" reservoir bag attached to the patient end of the circuit (with filter and any angle piece to be used included). The fresh gas flow is set at 5 L/min and the reservoir bag is then manually compressed mimicking manual ventilation. The test lung reservoir bag is felt and observed to be inflating and the whole circuit is also checked for integrity. Both bags are squeezed in turn to test the APL valve. The ventilator is then checked using this test lung by operating the ventilator with minimal to no fresh gas flow, opening each vaporiser in turn and then observing for any loss of volume with the reservoir bag test lung. This contrasts with the negative pressure "bulb squeeze" test (Fig. 5.10).

13. Verify that the gas flows properly through the breathing circuit during inspiration and expiration.

Pressure and leak tests do not rule out all obstruction in the breathing circuit and neither do they confirm the function of inspiratory and expiratory unidirectional valves. A test lung or reservoir bag can be used to confirm the flow of the circuit is unimpeded. This is called a flow test. The inspiratory valve should open, and the expiratory valve should close during inspiration and vice versa on expiration. Automated machine checks may not assess for obstruction to flow within the breathing circuit. Several complications and near misses involving an obstructed breathing circuit have been reported despite the performance of the automated circuit check. A trained person can perform regular valve competence tests.

14. Document completion of checkout procedures.

Everyone in anaesthesia is responsible for the completion of the documentation procedures. Documentations give credit for completion of the task and if any errors can also be traced.

15. Confirm ventilator settings and evaluate readiness to deliver anaesthesia care. (Anaesthesia time out).

The goal is to confirm that appropriate checks have been completed and the essential equipment is available in order to avoid errors. It is essential that the patient specific settings such as weight and age are adjusted on the ventilator to avoid patient harm (Fig. 5.13).

5.7 Airway Equipment Check

This check is an absolute essential part of the pre-anaesthesia check and includes Heat Moisture Exchange (HME) filters, catheter mounts, connectors, ETT's, laryngeal mask airways (LMA), laryngoscopes, suction catheters, plasters, etc. These should be available in a variety of sizes and ideally those of the appropriate size plus half size larger and smaller of each item present and

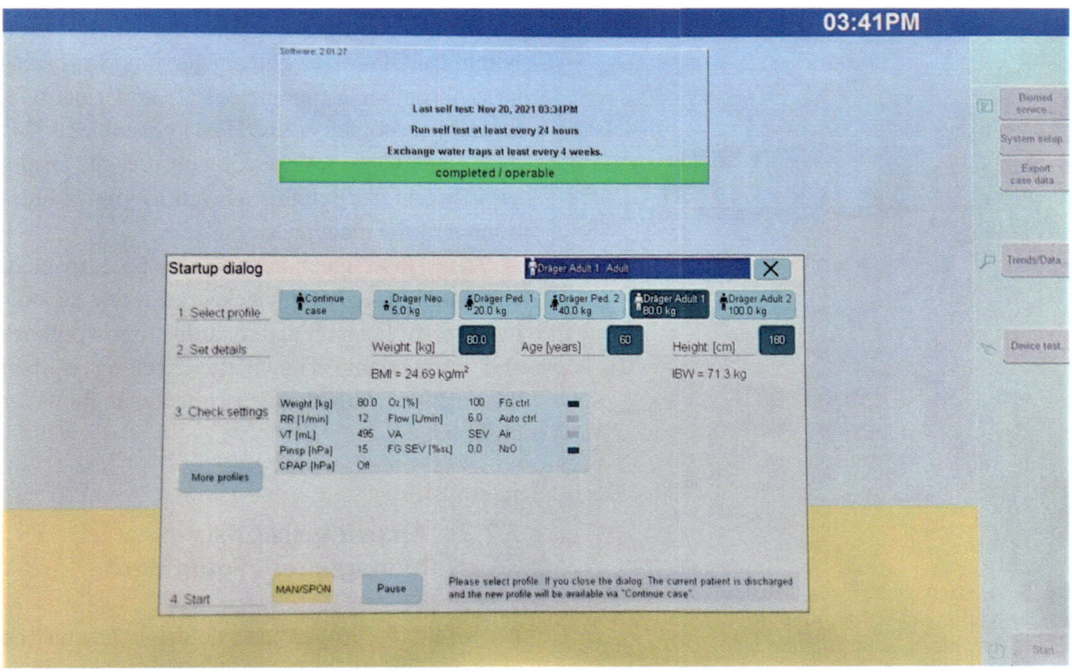

Fig. 5.13 Set up of patient ventilator settings. Example of adult patient detail settings on a Drager anaesthesia machine (Drager, Germany)

checked for patency. A new, single-use antibacterial filter and angle piece must be used for each patient.

The appropriate size laryngoscopes should be available and checked for extension and locking of the blade and adequately functioning light. Equipment for the management of an anticipated or unexpected difficult airway must be available and checked regularly in accordance with departmental policies. Many hospitals have a designated "Difficult Airway Trolley" which is placed in a known labelled location like the emergency (E-cart) resuscitation trolley (Fig. 5.14).

Another important check is that of the patient's trolley, bed or operating table, can be tilted head down rapidly. This is important in cases of unexpected vomiting or suspected aspiration in an anesthetised patient.

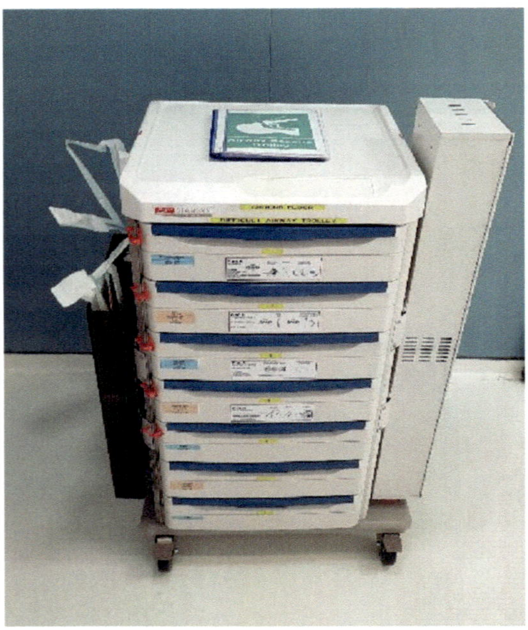

Fig. 5.14 Example of a designated difficult airway trolley. Demonstration of organized trolley with selection of airway equipment and adjuncts and labelled in pre-identified sections on the trolley

5.7.1 Regional Anaesthesia Equipment Area

Equipment needed for regional anaesthesia such as spinal needles, epidural kits, sonographic nerve block needles and sterile drapes, should be placed in a clearly assigned location such as a regional anaesthesia trolley which is easily accessible containing all the essential equipments. On a daily basis and between cases when items are used, these should be refilled against the regional anaesthesia equipment checklist. The location for Intralipid should also be known and ideally labelled.

5.7.2 Point of Care Equipment

The point of care (POC) equipment checklists are also a vital checklist in anaesthesia. POC diagnostic tests of the patient are performed instead of sending a formal sample to the lab which saves time and resources from designated clinical laboratories and is highly valuable in urgent and emergency situations.

Some of the POC machines that can be found within the OR are the glucometer, blood gas analyser, thromboelastogram (TEG) and rotational thromboelastometry (ROTEM) machines. This daily quality control checking ensures the results are efficient and reliable as well as proper functioning of the machines.

These POC machines are usually inspected, calibrated, tested and checked each day according to local hospital and manufacturer's policies and instructions. This daily checking is then documented with the departmental logbook or checklist.

5.7.3 Anaesthesia Crisis Management Equipment

A resuscitation trolley and defibrillator must be available in all locations where anaesthesia is

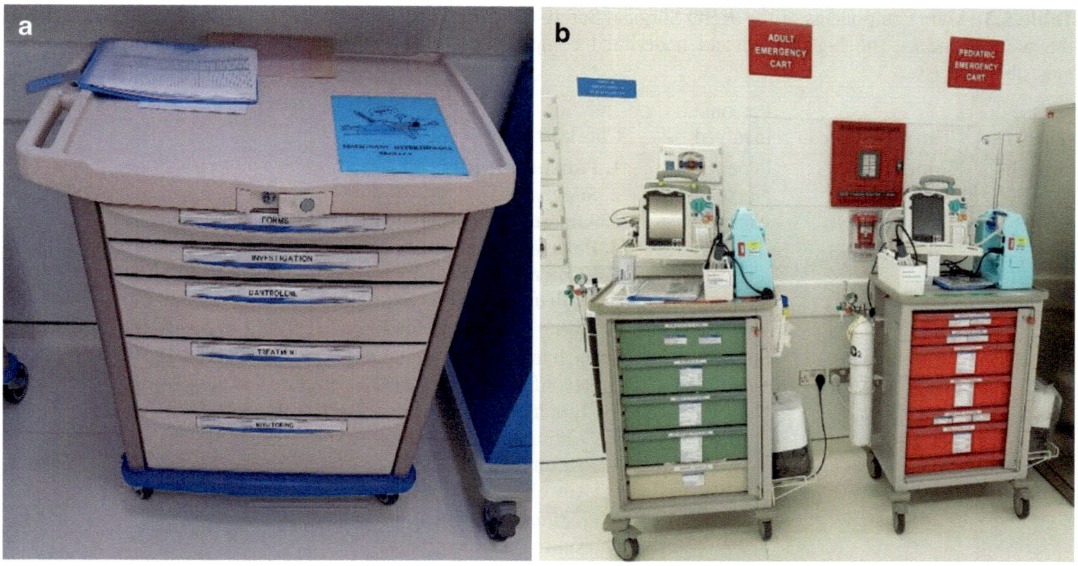

Fig. 5.15 Designated emergency crisis trolleys. (**a**) Example of a malignant hyperthermia trolley where Dantrolene is kept. (**b**) Example of emergency adult and paediatric resuscitation trolleys that contain all emergency medications, defibrillator and portable suction

Table 5.2 List of popular crisis checklists available in most ORs and the pre-arranged trolley and allocated equipment set up for such crises

Crisis Checklist	Trolley/equipment needed
Cardiac arrest	E-cart
Arrhythmias	E-cart
Anaphylaxis	E-cart
Local anaesthetic systemic toxicity (LAST)	LAST trolley/availability and location of Intralipid
Malignant hyperthermia (MH)	MH trolley/availability and location of Dantrolene
Difficult airway	Difficult airway trolley/ video laryngoscopes including fibreoptic videoscope, airway adjuncts, front of neck access.
Paediatric emergency - Cardiac arrest. - Venous air embolism.	Paediatric E-cart
Obstetric emergency - Post-partum haemorrhage. - Pre-eclampsia.	Massive transfusion protocol
Major haemorrhage	Massive transfusion protocol

given and checked regularly in accordance with local policies. Equipment and drugs for rarely encountered emergencies, such as malignant hyperthermia, local anaesthetic systemic toxicity (LAST) and latex allergy must be available and checked regularly in accordance with departmental policies (Fig. 5.15 and Table 5.2).

5.8 Anaesthesia Crisis Checklists

When a patient has an acute event in the perioperative setting, health care practitioners aim to manage the situation according to best practices and to minimize morbidity and mortality. Unfortunately, during the stress of a critical event, most clinicians do not implement all known best practices and lapses may occur.

The choice of having checklists can help minimize or prevent the occurrence of untoward incidents and facilitate appropriate management of intraoperative problems. Errors made in dealing with such problems are sometimes due to fixation on a particular (wrong) diagnosis, omission of

Table 5.3 Main components of the WHO Surgical Safety Checklist. Though the anaesthetist is expected to partake in the whole process, the highlighted and underlined components are those of direct involvement expected of the anaesthesiologist

Phase of checklist	Time conducted	Personnel involved	Checklist component
Sign in	Prior to induction Of anaesthesia	Patient Nurse Anaesthetist	**1. Patients identity confirmed.** 2. Site marked? **3. Anaesthesia machine and medication checked?** **4. Pulse oximeter applied and working?** **5. Known allergies?** **6. Difficult airway aspiration risk?** **7. Risk of > 500 ml blood loss? (7 ml/kg in paediatric patients)?**
Time out	Prior to skin incision	Surgeon Anaesthetist Nurse	8. Each team member role and introduction. 9. Reconfirm patients name, procedure and surgical site. 10. Prophylactic antibiotics given within last 60 minutes? 11. Anticipated critical events 12. To surgeon: (a) Any critical/non-routine steps? (b) Estimated length of procedure? (c) Anticipated blood loss? **13. To Anaesthetist:** (a) **Patient concerns?** 14. To nurse: (a) Sterility of instruments confirmed? (b) Equipment issues/concerns? 14. Any essential radiology displayed?
Sign out	Prior to patients exit from the OR	Surgeon Nurse Anaesthetist	15: Confirms name of procedure 16: Needle, sponge, instrument count complete? 17: Any specimens? And labelled? 18: Any equipment problems? **19: Key concerns for recovery and management of patient (including location, e.g. ICU, PACU, day care)**

important steps in diagnosis or treatment and particularly while dealing with rare events. The crisis checklist can serve in this case as a memory aid and a mechanism for ensuring that all possibilities are considered.

Over the decades in response to unfortunate emergency crisis situations within the perioperative period, many crisis checklists have been formulated and have been shown to reduce morbidity and mortality [1].

There are a number of known and published crisis checklists and algorithms available (Table 5.2).

5.9 WHO Surgical Safety Checklist

The WHO Surgical Safety Checklist is most popular and internationally recognized checklist [20]. It consists of a 19-item list divided into three important phases named Sign In, Time Out and Sign Out. These phases correspond to three identified time critical checkpoints within a patient's journey through the OR (Table 5.3). Several countries have made this checklist mandatory practice. In addition, the administration of antibiotics is considered a key performance Indicator (KPI) for anaesthetists.

During anaesthesia and life support training it is common to learn the mnemonic ABCDE to guide the order of clinical assessment of the patient. During the anaesthesia safety check this mnemonic may also serve as an aid to remember the minimum pre-induction safety checks: A: airway examination, B: breathing system (anaesthesia machine including oxygen; volatile agents and availability of self-inflating bag); C: suction of adequate strength and availability of attached suction catheter; D: Drugs including E: emergency medications and all equipment including a functional pulse oximetry. Though not formally part of

BEFORE PATIENT ARRIVES		INSIDE THEATRE (WEAR PPE)	
PREPARE	**PLAN**	**INTUBATION**	**EXTUBATION**
❑ **Anaesthetic Pre-op Assessment** **Prepare Airway Equipment** ❑ Check Machine ❑ Working Laryngoscope (VL *if available)* ❑ ET Tubes, Syringe, Stylet, Tie/Tape ❑ Adjuncts e.g. Bougie, LMA, Oral airway ❑ Working Suction + Suction Catheter ❑ Breathing Circuit + Viral filter + Facemask ❑ Consider Tube Clamp & Aerosol Barrier **Prepare Drugs** ❑ Induction Agent ❑ NM Blockade (+ Reversal +/– Stimulator) ❑ Emergency drugs e.g. Atropine, Adrenaline ❑ Analgesics / Antiemetics ❑ Antibiotics ❑ Other drugs as relevant ❑ IV Cannulas, Fuids (+ Pumps), Blood ❑ **Additional Items** e.g. Pen/documents, Dedicated waste bag	**Anaesthesia Team Briefing** ❑ Confirm team roles ❑ Discuss & confirm need for intubation and anaesthetic plan **Intubation Plan** Plan A: RSI or Modified RSI Plan B/C: Mask ventilation or LMA LMA/ Supraglottic Airway (2nd generation *if available*) Facemask ▪ 2-Person ▪ 2-Handed ▪ Adjuncts ▪ Low Flow ▪ Low Pressure Plan D: Rescue - FONA ❑ **Team members apply PPE** ▪ Gown, Hat, Eye Protection, N95/FFP mask, gloves (anaesthesia provider double glove for airway management) ❑ **Non-essential personnel leave** ❑ **Patient transferred to theatre wearing surgical mask**	❑ **Essential personnel only** ❑ **Apply patient monitoring** ❑ **Optimise patient position** ❑ **Optimise patient condition** ❑ **Set-up any barrier methods** ❑ **Team confirm anaesthetic plan** ❑ **Pre-oxygenate >3 mins, low flows** ❑ **Proceed with RSI / Modified RSI** ❑ **Minimise Aerosolization** ▪ Avoid BVM ventilation during apnoeic period unless hypoxia ▪ Inflate cuff before ventila:ing ▪ Secure tube & all connections ▪ Avoid unnecessary dis connections ▪ Consider clamping ETT after insertion until ventilator attached ❑ **Confirm ETT placement with Capnography (*if available*) or resource appropriate methods** ❑ **Ensure patient condition stable** ❑ **Proceed with surgery**	❑ **Essure patient condition stable** ❑ **No non-essential personnel in OR** ❑ **Perform suction prior to extubation** ▪ Avoid excessive or over-suctioring ▪ Consider in-line suction *if available* ❑ **Extubate on OR table** ▪ Avoid unnecessary disconnections ▪ Keep any aerosol barrier in place ❑ **Extubate whene indicated** ▪ Minimize coughing at extubation ▪ Apply oxygen mask or facemask when extubated ❑ **Arrange transfer when indicated** ❑ **No entry to OR without PPE until designated time post-extubation (according to OR ventilation)** ❑ **Remove PPE in designated area**

Fig. 5.16 Example of a checklist for the intubation of suspected or positive COVID-19 patients

the WHO checklist but increasingly adopted within the Time Out is the addition of a confirmation of any thromboembolic prophylaxis.

5.10 COVID-19 Checklist

The recent COVID-19 pandemic and the high-risk nature of airway management and need to minimize aerosol generation has prompted the publication of guidance checklists for the safe airway management of COVID-19 suspected or positive patients.

These checklists focus on preparation and planning which includes thorough pre-anaesthesia assessment to anticipate any difficulties that may be made worse by the infective nature of the patient, effective communication and assignment of roles early with briefing, the usual pre-induction anaesthesia checks and equipment preparation with additional infection control measures (Fig. 5.16). Checklist used to ensure safety of healthcare personnel and minimize exposure/infection risk during airway management. Covers important steps to take during intubation and extubation [21].

5.10.1 Simulation Checklists

Simulation in medical training has long been valued as an effective tool to facilitate the practicing of clinical knowledge, skills and crisis management without the risk of patient harm in a similar real life scenario [22, 23]. Its roots have emerged from the aviation field, NASA space exploration and the military and advanced over the last few decades as technology has improved [24].

Simulation is a cost-effective approach to learning and also allows the assessment of competencies, communication, decision making and essential steps during patient care [22]. High fidelity mannequins are usually used to simulate clinical signs and assess interaction during various case scenarios.

Checklist used as a tool within the simulation setting is useful for standardizing care models during evaluation and treatment. Recently, a new electronic tool was developed called the CERTAIN (Checklist for Early Recognition and Treatment of Acute Illness) checklist. During a study into its effectiveness during simulated decompensated patients, it was shown that the use of a single team member to verbalize and prompt the algorithms improved not only performance but also satisfaction of the simulation experience during emergency simulated situations [25].

5.11 Conclusion

Checklists are an integral part of OR practice and their use is mandatory in some countries. They have been shown in numerous studies to reduce morbidity and mortality, particularly in the crisis and emergency setting. Simulation checklists as part of competency assessment and feedback during selected simulated clinical scenarios have also demonstrated a cost-effective means to improve communication, decision making and patient care. During the start of the COVID-19 pandemic, checklists for the safer conduct of airway and anaesthesia management in infected or suspected patients were created and still until now are being further developed to protect staff and improve patient safety outcomes.

Checklist use contributes to efficient and safer preparation for a surgical case and is often compared to the aviation industry. Human error can never be totally eliminated but checklist use can help reduce such errors and lapses greatly. Checklists in anaesthesia are more than just a list of inspections; it is a tool to be adapted to each local environment and used for every patient to help get things done right, all the time.

References

1. Saxena S, Krombach JW, Nahrwold DA, Pirracchio R. Anaesthesia-specific checklists: a systematic review of impact. Anaesth Crit Care Pain Med. 2020;39(1):65–73.
2. Nakarada-Kordic I, Weller JM, Webster CS, et al. Assessing the similarity of mental models of operating room team members and implications for patient safety; a prospective, replicated study. BMC Med Educ. 2016;16:229.
3. Snow J. On the fatal cases of inhalation of chloroform. Edinburgh Med Surg J. 1849;72(180):75–87.
4. Ludders JW, McMillan M, Appendix E. A brief history of checklists. Errors in veterinary anesthesia. 1st ed. New York: Wiley; 2017.
5. Food and Drug Administration. Anesthesia apparatus checkout recommendations. Anesthesia Patient Safety Foundation Newsletter 1986; 1.15.
6. Charlton JE. Checklists and patient safety. Anaesthesia. 1990;45:425–6.
7. American Society of Anesthesiologists: Standards and Guidelines 2008 ASA Recommendations for Pre Anesthesia Checkout. www.asahq.org/standards-and-guidelines. Accessed 25 July 2020.
8. Pugel AE, Simianu VV, Flum DR, Patchen DE. Use of the surgical safety checklist to improve communication and reduce complications. J Infect Public Health. 2015;8(3):219–25.
9. Cooper JB, Newbower RS, Kitz RJ. An analysis of major errors and equipment failures in anesthesia management: considerations for prevention and detection. Anesthesiology. 1984;60:34–42.
10. Hartle A, Anderson E, Bythell V, Gemmell I, Jones H, Mcivor D, Pattinson A, Sim P, Walker I. Checking anaesthetic equipment. The Association of Anaesthetists of Great Britain and Ireland; 2012.
11. Pronovost P, Needham D, Sinopoli D, et al. An intervention to decrease catheter related blood stream infections in the ICU. N Engl J Med. 2006;355:2725–32.
12. Burian BK, Clebone A, Dismukes K, Ruskin KJ. More than a tick box: medical checklist development, design, and use. Anesth Analg. 2018;126(1):223–32.
13. Jelacic S., Bowdle A., Nair BG., et al. Aviation-style computerized surgical safety checklist displayed on a large screen and operated by the anesthesia provider improves checklist performance. Anesth Analg 2020;130(2):382–390.
14. Gawande A. The checklist manifesto: how to get things right. 1st ed. India: Penguin Books India; 2010.
15. Ranasinghe, DN. 2000 Expiratory dates on anaesthetic gas cylinders Anaesthesia 2000; 55(12) 819–820.
16. The Association of Anaesthetists of Great Britain and Ireland (AAGBI) Safety Guideline Checklist for Anesthesia Equipment 2012.
17. Paulsen AW. Are there guidelines for adequate anesthesia suction? Newsletter. 2015;29(3):58–9.
18. American Society of Anesthesiologists: Standard and Guidelines- Standards for Basic Anesthetic Monitoring; 2015. https://www.asahq.org/standards-and-guidelines. Accessed 25 July 2020.

19. Saraogi A, Kumar A, Ravishankar M. Improvised device for negative-pressure leak test. Indian journal of. Anaesthesia. 2012;56(2):201–2.
20. World Health organization: WHO Surgical Safety checklist. https://www.who.int (2009) accessed on 27th July 2020. Accessed 25 July 2020.
21. World Federation of Societies of Anesthesiologists: COVID anaesthesia checklist. https://www.wfsahq.org (2020). Accessed 25 July 2020.
22. Cheng A, Duff J, Grant E, Kissoon N, Grant VJ. Simulation in paediatrics: an educational revolution. Paediatric Child Health. 2007;12(6):465–8.
23. Datta R, Upadhyay KK, Jaideep CN. Simulation and its role in medical education. Med J Armed Forces India. 2012;68(2):167–72.
24. Satish U, Streufert S. Value of a cognitive simulation in medicine: towards optimising decision making performance of healthcare personnel. BMJ Qual Saf. 2002;11(2)
25. Sevilla-Berrios R, O'Horo JC, Schmickl CN, et al. Prompting with electronic checklist improves clinician performance in medical emergencies: a high-fidelity simulation study. International. J Emerg Med. 2018;11(26)

Essential Anaesthesia Monitors and Equipment in the Operating Theatre

6

Nabil A. Shallik, Muhammad Firas Alhammad, Othman Al Hariri, Yusuf Kassim Al Refai, Mohamed Saad Elkhatib, Ayten Saracoglu, and Kemal Tolga Saracoglu

Contents

N. A. Shallik (✉) · M. F. Alhammad · O. Al Hariri
Y. K. Al Refai · M. S. Elkhatib
Anesthesia, ICU and Perioperative Medicine, Hamad Medical Corporation, Doha, Qatar
e-mail: nshallik@hamad.qa; MAlhammad@hamad.qa; oalhariri@hamad.qa; yalrefai@hamad.qa; melkhatib@hamad.qa

A. Saracoglu
Clinic of Anesthesiology and Intensive Care, Marmara University Pendik Training and Research Hospital, Istanbul, Turkey

K. T. Saracoglu
Clinic of Anesthesiology and Intensive Care, Health Sciences University Kartal Dr. Lutfi Kirdar Training and Research Hospital, Istanbul, Turkey

N. A. Shallik et al. (eds.), *Improving Anesthesia Technical Staff's Skills*,
https://doi.org/10.1007/978-3-030-88849-7_6

6.1 Introduction

Patients under anaesthesia need continuous monitoring, this includes monitoring the patient variables and the anaesthesia equipment, the importance of close and sufficient monitoring is due to the fact that patients under anaesthesia will have many changes in normal physiological function which emerge the need to early detection and timely manner intervention. In addition to the standard anaesthesia monitoring recommended by American Society of Anaesthesia (ASA), other necessary monitoring might be needed depending on the type of surgery and patients' comorbidities.

Keeping in mind the most important monitor in operating theatre is the presence of qualified anaesthesiologist. Many monitoring modalities have been developed recently, the up warding developing in anaesthesia monitoring have reduced the perioperative mortality and morbidity.

Anaesthesia monitors are numerous in number and various in types. Our chapter will concertante on the most common and critical monitors only but some other monitors and equipment are discussed in more details in other chapters within this book.

6.2 Autotransfusion Device and Cell Salvage

- Cell Salvage is a collection system used to recycle blood from patient's blood who is bleeding intraoperative.

6.2.1 Use of Autotransfusion Device and Cell Salvage Fig. 6.1

Indications

- Trauma patient especially in haemothorax injury intercostal catheter insertion in trauma patient is reasonable indication.
- Surgery:
  - If the expected blood loss is more than 1000 ml.
  - Severe anaemia in patient who refuse allogeneic blood transfusion like Jehovah's Witnesses.
  - Usually cell saver is used for major surgeries where significant bleeding is not avoidable such as cardiac surgery, orthopaedics, neurosurgery, vascular surgery, and urology.

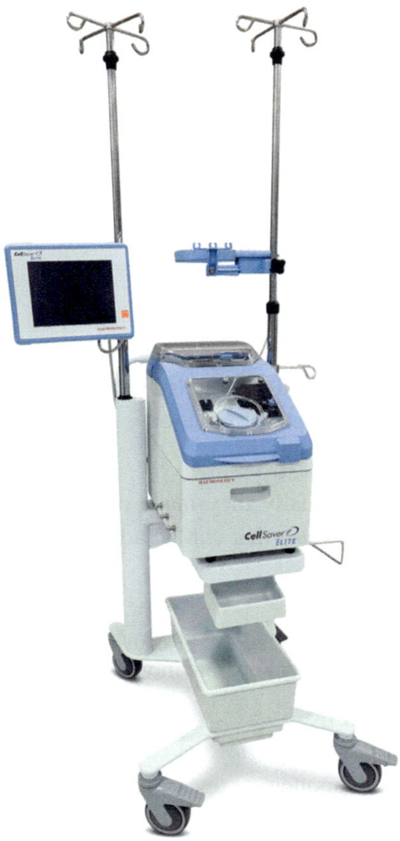

Fig. 6.1 Cell Saver (Image courtesy Dr. Nabil Shallik)

Contraindications
- If blood is suspected to be contaminated like penetrating chest injuries, with a stab or gunshot that might cause injury in stomach or colon.
- Also, in contaminated surgical field with infection or malignant tumour is being resected.
- If the patient refusing cell saver.

Description.

Intercostal catheter system component:
- Special collection system could be connected to the chest tube (autotransfusion canister).
- The shed blood will be collected to the canister.
- The collected blood will be filtered by a special filter.
- The filtered blood can be collected from a canister.

Cell salvage intraoperatively component
- a double-lumen suction device: the first one is a lumen that suctions blood from the surgical field while the other lumen adds a predetermined heparinized saline to the collected blood;
- blood filter;
- reservoir;
- cell saver which separates blood components using centrifuge principle;
- normal saline is used for washing process;
- collection bag for waste products this bag will be discarded;
- collection bag for washed RBCs (will be used for transfusion).

6.2.2 Method of Use

Intercostal catheter system
- The autotransfusion canister should be connected to the proximal end chest tube collection system close to the chest wall.
- Use an inline leukocyte depletion filter.
- At this step there is no need to add anticoagulation to the blood.
- Most systems can be used to re-infuse shed blood up to 6 hours after collection without heparin or other products.
- Follow-up the provider special instructions.

Cell salvage intraoperatively
- Double-lumen suction device suction blood from surgical field and mixes with heparinized saline.
- After mixing the blood passed through a special filter and collected in a reservoir.
- Centrifugation will separate the blood components.

- Washing process: after centrifugation the pure RBCs washed and filtered across a semi-permeable membrane in order to remove free haemoglobin, plasma, platelets, white blood cells, and heparin.
- Normal saline added to the salvaged RBCs (suspension) to reach relatively concentrated haemoglobin 50%–80%.
- The salvaged RBCs can be transfused to the patient within 6 hours.

Complications
- Blood loss when the connections are loose or there is a leak.
- Haemodilution (no significant rise in Hb).
- Thrombocytopenia and coagulopathy in large volumes transfusion.
- Contamination and infection.
- Contamination with medications and cleansing solutions.
- Inadequate washing or inadequate filtration may lead to contamination with activated leukocytes, cytokines, and other micro aggregates.
- RBCs mechanical destruction degradation over time due to suction non-immune haemolysis.
- Air embolus.

6.2.3 Other information

Composition of blood from intercostal catheter
- In chest tube the haemoglobin and haematocrit is lower than venous blood.
- In chest tube blood platelet count is very low.
- Potassium level is higher than blood (4.9 mmol/L).
- Factor V and fibrinogen are not detectable.

6.3 Bispectral Index (BIS) Monitoring

Overview
- BIS monitor was developed by Aspect Medical Systems Fig. 6.2.
- There are other methods to measure depth of anaesthesia like (Entropy).

Uses

- It is a method to monitor the depth of anaesthesia or depth of sedation.

Description
- Sensor: usually they made of disposable wet gel electrodes that can be attached directly to the patient.
- Cables.
- Monitoring module – integrated with anaesthesia machine or separate monitoring systems.

Method of use
- BIS is a monitor of the depth of the hypnotic arm component of anaesthesia.
- Multiple electrodes can be attached to patient frontoparietal area.
- After receiving the brain electrical activity signals the monitor generates a number.
- In general, high number associated with more activity and hence more awake level.
  - 100 = normal cortical activity (alert status)
  - 0 = cortical electrical silence.

BIS reading	40–60	60–80	Above 80
Clinical interpretation	Proper anaesthesia level	Sedation level	Awakes level

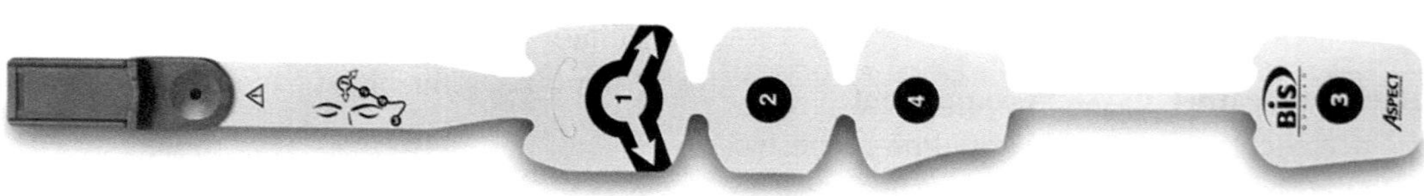

Fig. 6.2 Bispectral index single use lead (Image courtesy Dr. Nabil Shallik)

- Two signals are displayed EMG signal with represent the electrical activity of the frontal muscles, signal quality index which represents electro encephalographic.

The BIS algorithm

- EEG data had been recorded from healthy adults who received different anaesthetic regimens which change the level of consciousness and unconsciousness.
- Analysis identified features of EEG recordings that best correlated with clinical depth of sedation/anaesthesia the waves and complexity of the EEG reduces with deep anaesthesia.
- The results will be analysed by a model by multivariate logistic regression.
- The final algorithm will generate bispectral index readings.

Benefits

- BIS <60 results in very low chance of post-op recall.
- Using BIS might lower the consumption of anaesthetic medications.
- Slightly quicker awaking.
- BIS is considered safe to use with defibrillators and diathermy.

Problems

- Using opioids lead to changing in aesthesia depth which might not be detectable by BIS.
- Even though BIS monitor depth of anaesthesia however not able to predict movement in response to surgical stimulation.
- Variable readings.
- Using N2O or ketamine interfere with BIS reading.
- In small age group less than 5 years cannot be used.

Evidence in ICU

- Lower readings are associated with delirium.
- Currently no strong evidence to use in ICU.
- Useful in paralysed patient to monitor level of sedation.
- Possible out-of-hospital role like cardiac arrest cases.

6.4 Blood and Fluid Warmer

Overview

- Devices that warm blood or fluids before delivering to the patient.
- It can be used when rapid transfusion needed (e.g. >50 mL/kg/hr) to avoid hypothermia or in a special condition where cold fluid should be avoided like cold agglutinins.
- Massive transfusion protocol to avoid hypothermia.

Description.
Three main types/methods:

- Water-bath warmers.
- Dry heat plate warmers.
- Intravenous fluid tube warmers.

6.4.1 Water-Bath Warmers

- per-warmed water is used to warm the intravenous fluids without mixing, the maximum warming temperature is 38.0 °C,
- at high infusion rates is not efficient and other method should be used.

6.4.2 Dry Heat Plate Warmers

- Fluids can be warmed up to 41 °C.
- The Intravenous fluids are being warmed while passing a metal cassette between the heat plates.

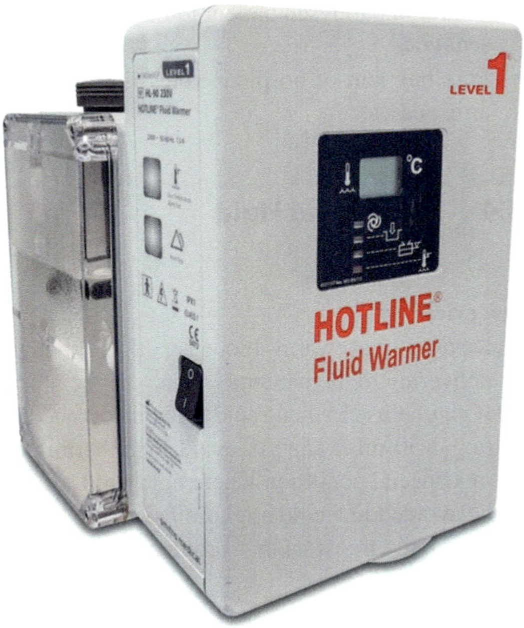

Fig. 6.3 Hotline Fluid Warmer (Image courtesy Dr. Nabil Shallik)

6.4.3 Intravenous Fluid Tube Warmers Fig. 6.3

- In this method warm water continuously circulate in an external layer around the intravenous tube line making a warm cover.
- Major disadvantage is that the tube is heavy and long also it is only efficient in low flow (20–30 mL/min).
- Special intravenous warmer coil is required.
- In general, the metals used methods are more effective conductors than the fluids used methods.

6.4.4 Method of Use

- unless blood warming is indicated, blood warming usually is not necessary,
- blood should not be heated above 41 °C special warming devices should be used not any other method,
- to avoid any complications regular service and maintenance for warming devices is a must.

Complications
- Overheating of the transfused blood or fluids heating blood to high degree have the risk of haemolysis.
- Air embolism is a possible complication when there is a leak in warming system.
- Hyperthermia can be happened especially if more than one technique is used for worming the patient.

6.5 Blood Gas Analyser

Uses
- Point-of-care measurement for arterial blood gases and electrolytes levels Fig. 6.4.

6.5.1 Description

Direct measurements
- pH, PCO2, and PO2.

Derived measurements
- HCO3–, BE (base excess), and O2 saturation.

6.5.2 Method of Insertion and/or Use

Direct measurements:

pH measurement
- Glass electrode.

Reference Electrode
- Capillary tube surrounded by buffer solution for the sample.
- The tube is pH sensitive glass that generate a potential difference, which is proportional to the pH.

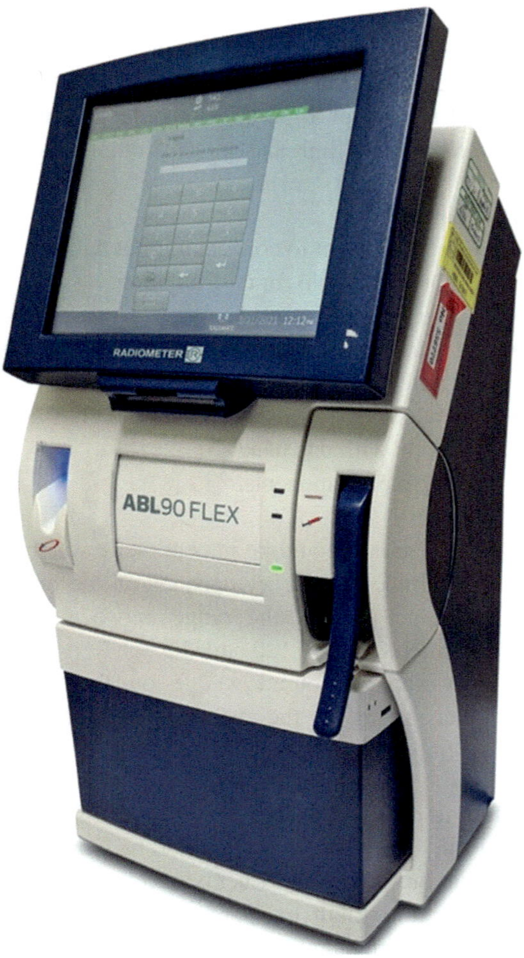

Fig. 6.4 Blood Gases Analyser (Image courtesy Dr. Nabil Shallik)

PCO2 measurement

- Modified glass electrode.
- CO2 permeable glass pH electrode.
- CO2 diffuses from the specimen into the HCO3 solution where it dissociates with a change in pH which is measured by the electrode.
- Potential difference is proportional to CO2 concentration.

PO_2 measurement

- Clark electrode or polarographic electrode.
- O2 molecules diffuse across a plastic membrane to small platinum or gold 2 nm diameter wire cathode in a glass rod immersed in a phosphate buffer with potassium chloride.
- O2 reduced by 2 hydroxyl ions by four electrons after application of 600–800 mV

$$O_2 + 2H_2O + 4e = 4\left(OH^-\right)$$

- This creates current flow between the cathode and silver/silver chloride anode.
- Increasing the voltage increases the current up to a plateau determined by the rate of supply of O2 molecules and proportional to the concentration of O2 in solution.

Direct measurements:

HCO3-

- Derived value which could be calculated by the machine from Henderson–Hasselbalch equation

$$[HCO3-] = [K\,[0.03] \times PaCO_2]/[H+]$$

where K is the combined CO_2 solubility constant and carbonic acid dissociation constant.which can vary with pH, temp, and ionic strength of solution.

- calculated actual HCO3- is assumed to by 24 mmol/L.

BE

- titratable acid in mmol/L required to titrate blood to a pH of 7.4 at a PCO2 of 40 mmHg,
- used to assess what changes in pH are due to PaCO2 changes,
- that is, at a pH of 7.4 the change in [HCO3-] from normal bicarb = the amount of HCl added.
- normal +2.5 to −2.5,
- large negative values = metabolic acidosis.

O2 saturation

- PaO2 ratio of oxyhaemoglobin to total haemoglobin.
- Normally 95–98%.

6.6 Cuff Pressure Gauge

Overview

- Cuff pressure gauge is known as ETT cuff manometre Fig. 6.5.

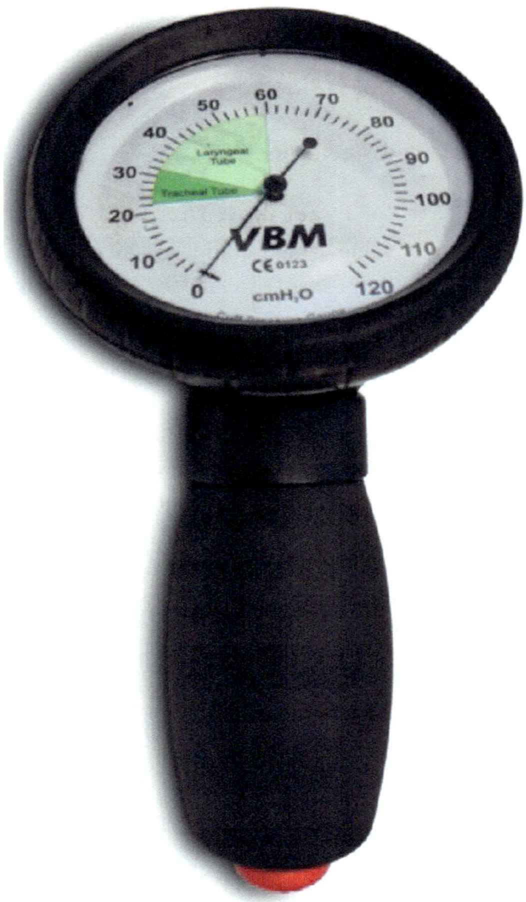

Fig. 6.5 Cuff Pressure Gauge (Image courtesy Dr. Nabil Shallik)

Uses

- Measuring the cuff pressure in Endotracheal Tube (ETT), Laryngeal Mask Airway (LMA), and Laryngeal Tube (LT) in order to ensure safe pressure limit and prevent complications.

Description

- Luer attachment to connect to pilot balloon.
- Rubber hand bulb for cuff inflation.
- Pressure display gauge.
- Pressure release valve on which allow releasing air.
- Ergonomic design to enable inflation and deflation with one hand.
- Latex free components.
- Gauges.
  - range unit could be in centimetre water or millimetre mercury depends on the brand model usually the range between 0–60 cmH2O and 0–120 cmH2O.
  - variable coloured wedge on the gauge according to the recommended pressure limits.

Method of insertion/use

- Firm attachment of the pilot balloon cuffs with pressure gauge Luer connector.
- To reduce high cuff pressure press release mechanism button.
- minimal leak technique: inflate ETT cuff, slowly deflate the air until bubbling sound could be heard on inspiration which indicate leak around ETT cuff, gradually re-insufflate cuff until leak disappears then check cuff pressure to ensure it is in the safe zone.

Complications

- It gives false reading if not attached properly.
- Loss of PEEP and micro-aspirate can be happened with over cuff deflation.

- Cuff size can variably fit in the trachea that is why the recommended safe zone should not always followed blindly and sometimes need to perform minimal leak technique in order to avoid serious complications like aspiration or inadequate ventilation.
- Exceeding proper pressure limit can lead to mucosal necrosis and subsequence tracheal complications like stenosis or stricture.

Other information

- In general, the pressure for balloon ETT between 20 and 30 cmH2O is safe.

  In shocked patients pressure limit for mucosal ischemia is lower than healthy patient as the mucosal perfusion is less.

6.7 Defibrillators

Uses

- Applying an electrical current across the heart can convert serious cardiac arrythmia (VF/VT) to sinus rhythm Fig. 6.6.

Description

- Essential modality in cardiac arrest case management.

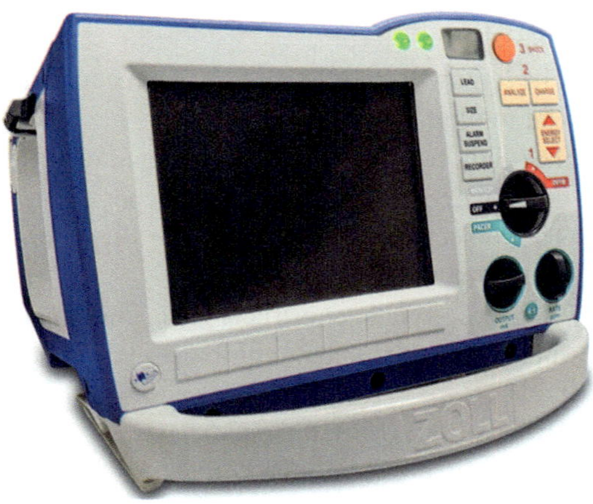

Fig. 6.6 Defibrillator (Image courtesy Dr. Nabil Shallik)

- Likelihood of abnormal rhythm to revert in to normal rhythm is inversely proportional to time which indicate as early as possible early defibrillation.
- Successful reversion decreases around 7–10% every minute min from onset of VF.
- The applied external electrical current causes synchronous contraction of cardiac muscle, which allows sinus rhythm to occur after refractory period.
- Inside the defibrillator, the capacitors make a potential difference between two plates and can reach up to 8000 V after discharging all currents.
  - estimated energy is 360 J for external defib patches while it is 50 J for internal defib which apply directly to the heart muscles.
- Thoracic impedance inversely proportional with number of shocks which means second shock will deliver greater energy and so on.
- The wave form during energy discharge release can be (monophasic or biphasic).

Monophasic

- Voltage rises rapidly and then returns to baseline (0, +ve, 0) consequently.

Biphasic

- Voltage rises, then reverses its direction below baseline before returning to baseline (0, +ve, 0, −ve, 0) consequently.
- The effective defibrillation of biphasic and monophasic are similar however the biphasic deliver lower energy.
- It is smaller than monophasic easy to carry and cheaper in price.

<u>Method of insertion and/or use</u>

- attach paddles to patients as recommended,
- charge,
- stand clear,
- discharge.

Other information

- pacemaker function,
- synchronized or non-synchronized shocks.

Complications

- DC more effective than AC also causes less damage.
- Repeated shocks can harm the myocardial muscle and cause damage.
- Safety for CPR team must be checked before any shock.
- Biphasic cause less myocardial injury than monophasic.
- Burning is possible, especially with high energy level.

6.8 Flexible Bronchoscope

Overview
- Flexible bronchoscope may be fibre optic (Fig. 6.7), video scope (Fig. 6.8) or hybrid systems.
  Uses

- Flexible bronchoscope has a great advantage in visualizing and direct examination of the tracheobronchial tree (Fig. 6.9).
- Provide excellent method for lesions biopsy in the broncho tracheal tree and bronchioalveolar lavage.

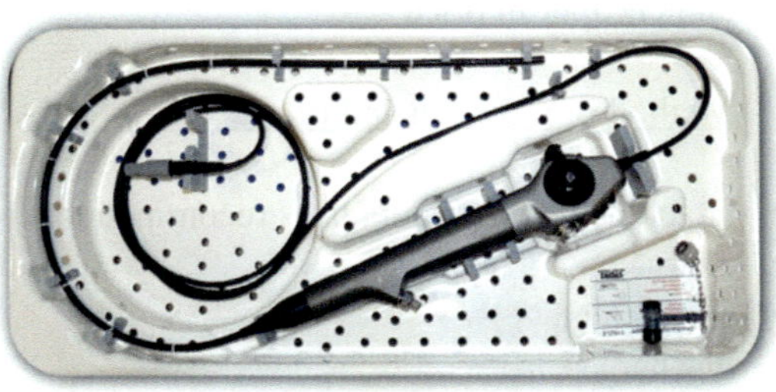

Fig. 6.7 Flexible bronchoscope in sterilization tray (Image courtesy Dr. Nabil Shallik)

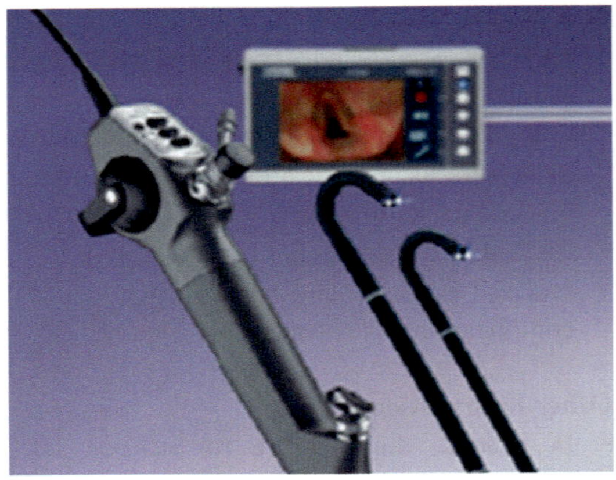

Fig. 6.8 Video scope system (FIVE and CEMOS technology) (Karle Storz, Germany)

- In anticipated difficult intubation can be utilized to perform awake or sleep fibreoptic intubation.
- Efficient suctioning secretions or blood in bronchoalveolar tree.
- Can be helpful in percutaneous tracheostomy placement, confirm double-lumen tube position and bronchial blockers position.
- Control bleeding if focal bleeding is active.

Physics:

- Flexible bundle contains (10.000 Glass fibre) (Fig. 6.10).
- Glass fibre 8–10 μm.
- The light will travel from light source to distal end to illuminate the object.
- The light from the object is reflected onto the objective lens at the tip of fiberscope.
- The objective lens focuses the light onto image transmission bundle.
- The eyepiece reconstructs the image and focused on the human retina.

Description: (Figs. 6.8 and 6.9)
- The flexible plastic tube containing the optic fibers which can be connected to a light source and.
- In order the view can obtain through an eyepiece or video cable which attached to the eyepiece.

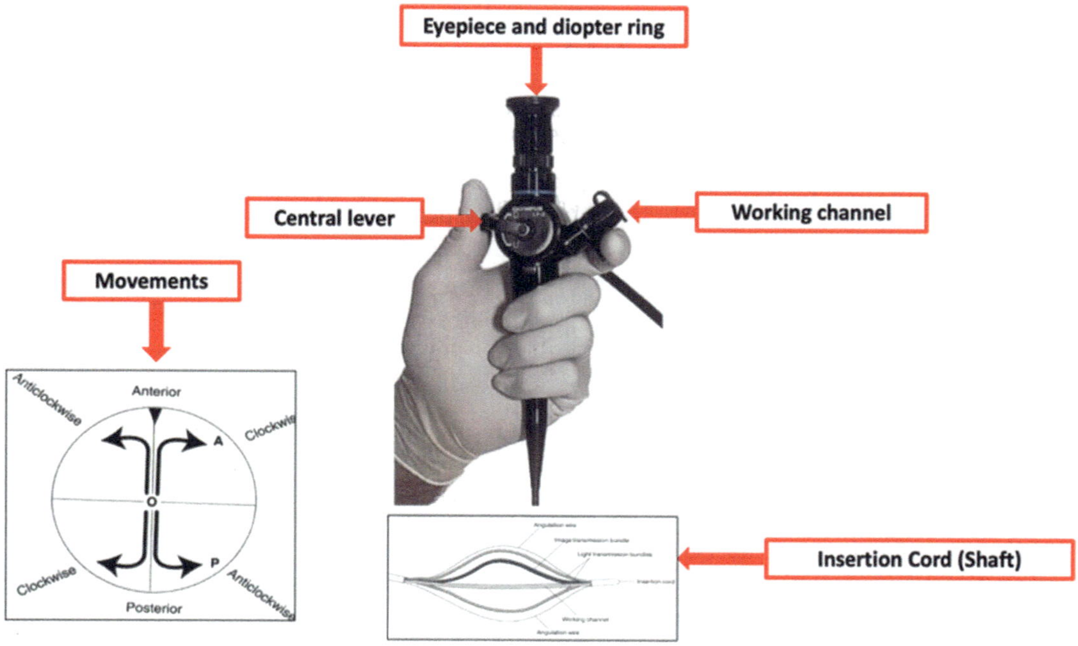

Fig. 6.9 Parts and movements of bronchoscope. (Image courtesy Dr. Nabil Shallik)

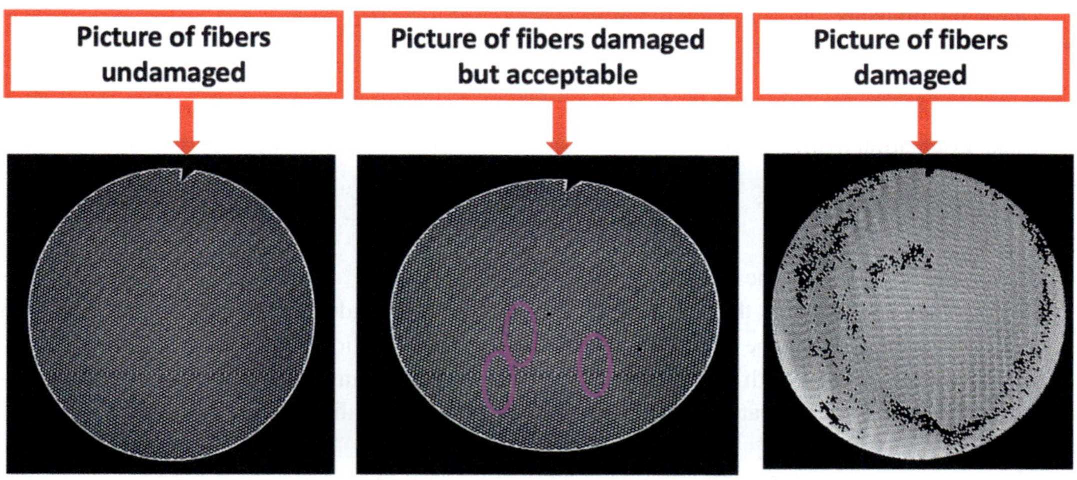

Fig. 6.10 The effect of fibres' damage on the images in old fibre optic system (Image courtesy Dr. Nabil Shallik)

- Flexible tip can be moved upward and downward through lever controlled by operator hand.
- Additional suction channel available to the tip and also can be controlled by the operator.
- Instrumentation port can be used to insert specific instruments like brush, biopsy forceps, or injecting medication and saline.
- 120° field of view with 180° up and 130° down angulation.
- Tip diameter can vary between 2.8 mm and 5.9 mm.
- Accessories can be either disposable or reusable.

Major Advantages of new fibroscope (Flexible Intubation Video Endoscope (FIVE) Fig. 6.8:

- Chip at the distal end (CMOS Chip).
- 5.5- and 4.0-mm outer diameter 2.3- and 1.5-mm diameter of the working channel.
- Smaller sizes started to appear in the market now.
- Documentation with pictures and movies.
- Integrated LED light source.
- Light weight (385 g).
- Excellent overview for intubation (4:3 image).
- Connected to the high-resolution monitor.
- Enables fast switch to the Video Laryngoscope.
- Less service – no image fibres!
- Suitable for intubation (ETT, DLT) and basic bronchoscopy procedure (bronchial lavage and lung exploration).

Checklist before using the fiberscope:

- Clean and disinfect every time to use.
- The movements of the tip before use.
- The suction port is working.
- Light source is working.
- Defog the tip using anti-fog, alcohol swap.
- Adjust sharpness of the pic. and white balance.
- Lubricate the shaft not the tip.
- Make orientation mark at 12.00 O'clock.

Method of insertion/use

- Make sure to assemble the flexible bronchoscope as recommended by the provider.
- Various techniques can be used to anesthetized patients' airway with local anaesthesia medications and deep sedation might also be used.
- Make sure the ventilator is ready to use and the variables adjusted according to the patient.
- Connect monitors as recommended by ASA.
- Suction should be ready to use.
- Insert a Y connector.
- Insert the distal tip.
- Manipulation can be done by flexion extension and rotation.

Complications

- airway trauma is possible complication especially in unexperienced providers,
- in case the inadequate anaesthesia the patient might cough or even bronchospasm might happen,
- oxygen desaturation might happen during the procedure especially in fragile patient and high flow nasal oxygen (HFNO) can be used to prevent oxygen desaturation,
- barotrauma,
- bronchoscope damage for example patient biting the scope,
- infection transmission could happen between the operator and the patient especially if inadequate respiratory precautions taken,
- accidental extubation while removing the scope.

6.9 Laryngoscope and Blades

Overview

- A device used during endotracheal intubation to visualize the vocal cords and facilitate intubation.

Use

- Facilitate endotracheal tube (ETT) insertion by visualization the vocal cords.
- Might help in gastric tube and transoesophageal echocardiography (TEE) probe insertion.

Description

- Blade base.
- Hook of blade.
- Curved (Macintosh) or straight blade (miller).
- Flange which containing web and light source.
- Handle tip contains batteries and electrical connection.

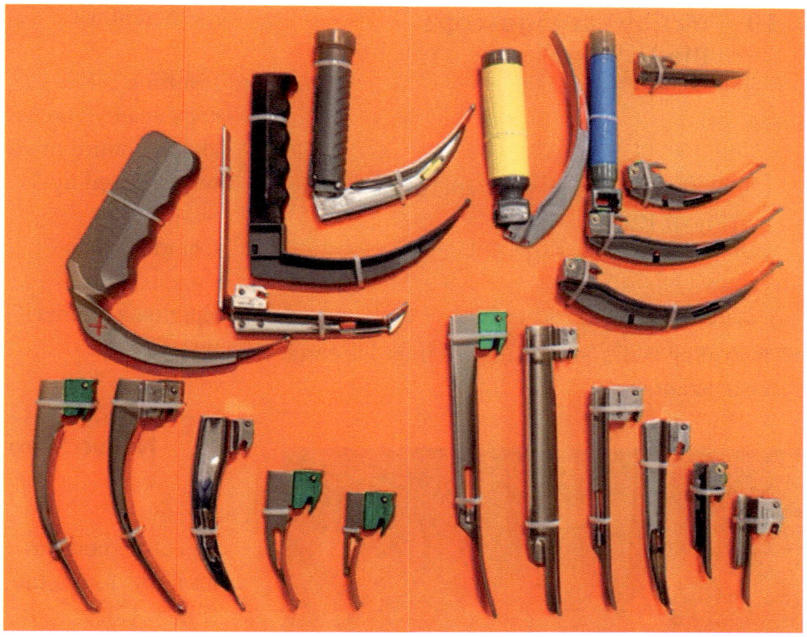

Fig. 6.11 Different types of laryngoscopes and blades available in the market (Image courtesy Dr. Nabil Shallik)

Method of insertion/use

- In curved blade the tip is placed in the vallecula behind the epiglottis.
- With a straight blade the tip is used to lift the epiglottis directly to reveal the cords, useful in paediatric age group because this group has large floppy epiglottis.

Complications

- Direct mechanical trauma including soft tissue, dental, cervical spine, and upper airway.
- Bleeding from tooth and mucosa.
- Laryngospasm in case inadequate anaesthesia level.
- Failure to perform procedure in case difficult intubation or inadequate experience.

Other information.
Handles

- Handle provided in Standard sizes (0.1.2.3.4).
- Short handle is useful for short necks, barrel chests, and large breasts such as obstetric or obese patients.

Blades

- Various types of blades.
  - Macintosh (commonest; blade attaches to handle at 90 degrees).
  - Kessel (like the Macintosh but the blade attaches at 110 degrees).
  - McCoy (Macintosh like blade with a moveable distal tip segment, flexed by a lever controlled by the thumb of the hand holding the handle to displace the larynx forwards).
  - Magill (straight blade with U-shaped cross section).
  - Miller and Wisconsin blades (straight blades with curved tips).
- Blads could be disposable metal, reusable metal or disposable plastic.
- Right-handed blades available for left-handed people (Fig. 6.11).

6.10 McCoy Laryngoscope Blade

Overview

- Laryngoscope blade with adjustable hinged tip (Fig. 6.12).

Uses

- Providing additional tip lift can improve cords visualization.

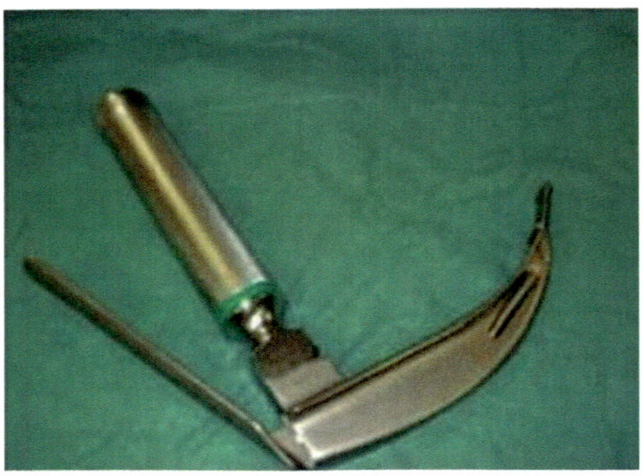

Fig. 6.12 McCoy Laryngoscope Blade (Image courtesy Dr. Nabil Shallik)

Method of use

- Insertion is like standard Macintosh laryngoscopy blade whoever lever adjacent to handle allows control of the flexible tip with extra lift when hinged tip.

Complications

- Epiglottis trauma if epiglottis stuck in hinge of movable tip.

6.11 Nerve Stimulator

Overview

- It is also known as train of four stimulator and train of four stimulator and nerve locator (Fig. 6.13).

Use

Provides an objective measure of neuromuscular blockade degree

- determine degree of neuromuscular blockade (e.g., during anaesthesia for a surgical procedure or for ICP control to titrate NMB dosing),

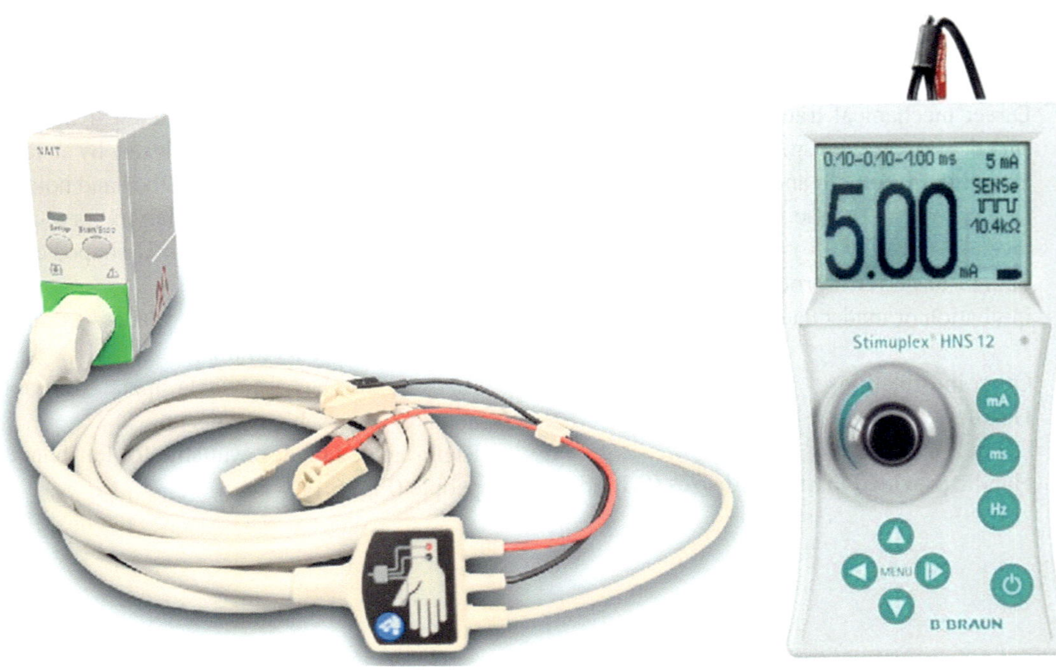

Fig. 6.13 Train of four stimulator and nerve locator (Image courtesy Dr. Nabil Shallik)

- exclude neuromuscular blockade prior to brain death assessment,
- may also be used for regional anaesthesia when performing nerve blocks (alternative or adjunct to ultrasound),
- nerve locator used to detect peripheral nerve for nerve block.

Description

- a peripheral nerve is stimulated by an electrical signal,
  - current = number of electrons supplied per stimulus,
  - twitch = muscle response to stimulus,
- usually, ulnar nerve can be stimulated and the accelerometer will measure number and speed of thumb movement; another used nerve is posterior tibial, facial and peroneal nerve,
- ECG dots (ensure good skin contact and current flow).
- Electrodes.
- Nerve stimulator module.

Method of use.
Ulnar nerve

- ECG dots placed.
  - first dot on the palmar aspect of the wrist 1–2 cm proximal to the wrist,
  - second dot in the same line 3 cm proximal to the wrist.
- Electrodes attached.
- black (negative) electrode is attached to distal dot close to the wrist,
- red (positive) attached to the proximal dot (must be in line to minimize nerve-muscle artefact and ensure maximal stimulation).
- stimulator is attached,
- voltage is slowly increased starting at 20 mA, voltage should not exceed 60 mA,
- red pulse light indicates voltage conduction,
- observe twitching of adductor pollicis (medial adduction of the thumb across the palm),
- "Train of four" (TOF) is commonly used (TOF)
- four electrical currents are delivered at intervals of 0.5 secs,
- 1–2 twitches indicate adequate neuromuscular blockade
- TOF is typically repeated hourly or as indicated.
- do not repeat within 10 seconds to allow recovery of the motor endplate.

Complications

- Painful in awake patient.
- Incorrect assessment may lead to serious complication.

Other information.
If no twitches seen check the following:

- Settings.
- Battery.
- Connections.
- Position and attachment of electrodes.
- Site (e.g., obese, thick skin, and oedema).

Pulse Oximeter.
Uses

- Device used to measure of arterial oxygen-haemoglobin saturation (SaO2) continuously denoted SpO2 when measured by pulse oximetry Fig. 6.14.

Description

1. Diodes.
   - produce light with special wavelengths (640–960 nm), usually in the red or infrared range as absorbance by body tissue is small compared to blood,
   - emitted light may alternate between wavelengths at several hundred Hz.

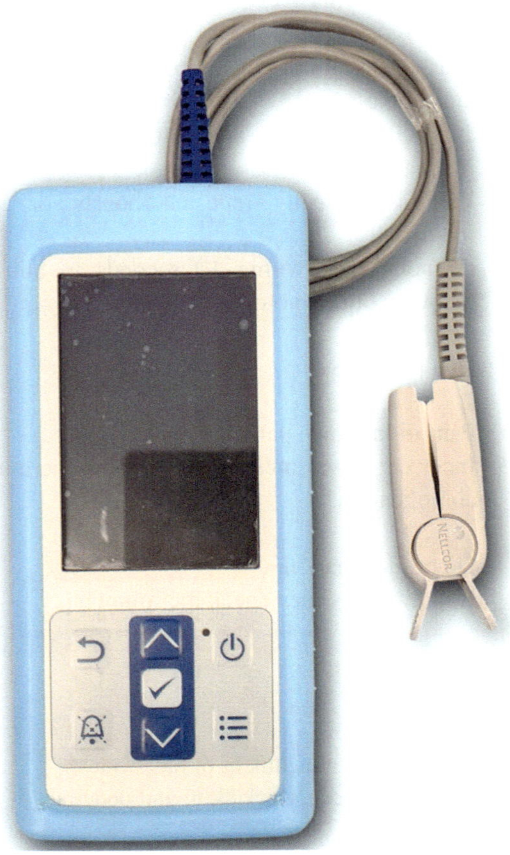

Fig. 6.14 Transportation Pulse Oximeter (Image courtesy Dr. Nabil Shallik)

2. Photodetector.
   - opposite to diodes is the photodetector which receive the transmitted light.
3. Signal converter.
   - Analysing the received light into two categories depending weather it is static or dynamic then convert this light signal to direct or alternative current.
   - DC component = tissue background, venous blood and the constant part of arterial blood flow.
   - AC component = pulsatile arterial blood flow.
   - In further analysis the DC component is omitted the AC component is amplified and averaged over a few seconds.
4. Display unit.
   - signal is displayed ideally as a continuous trace,
   - shows quality of signal as a waveform (plethysmography) and numbered value of SpO_2.

6.11.1 Method of Use

Pulse oximetry principle based on the fact that oxygenated haemoglobin and deoxygenated haemoglobin of pulsatile blood absorb infrared and red-light waveform.

Two light wavelengths are used: red (660 nm) and infrared (930 nm)

- signal is divided into two components,
  1. AC = pulsatile arterial blood.
  2. DC = tissue + capillary blood + venous blood + non-pulsatile arterial blood.

- > all pulse oximeters assume that only the pulsatile absorbance is arterial blood.

For each wavelength, the oximeter determines the AC/DC ratio

- the ratio (R) of these is calculated:

R = (ac absorbance/dc absorbance) red/ (ac absorbance/dc absorbance) IR

- R corresponds to SaO2.
- SaO2 100% = R 0.4.
- SaO2 85% = R 1.
- SaO2 0% = R 3.4.

6.11.2 Pules Oximetry Limitations

- SpO_2 and SaO_2 are not measures of blood or tissue oxygenation (if [Hb] and cardiac output known, then oxygen delivery (DO_2) can be calculated from SaO_2).
- insensitive to directional changes in PaO_2 above 80 mmHg,
- relatively insensitive to perfusion due to gain,
- reading failure,
- lag time as there is a delay for few seconds.

Source pulse oximeter misreading

- motion artifact, light artefact, anaemia, and pigmented skin intravenous dyes,
- nail polish, probe position, and ambient light,
- signal to noise ratio (shocked, hypothermia, and vasoconstrictors),
- dyshaemoglobinaemias (COHb indistinguishable from HbO2, Met Hb absorbance high - > R = 1.0),
- abnormal pulses (venous waves and ventilation) and non-pulsatile flow (bypass),
- low saturations (progressive inaccuracy below 80%),
- radiofrequency interference (MRI).

Complications

- measurement error may lead to inappropriate management,
- early intervention may be required before desaturation is detected due to oximetry lag time,
- pressure injuries from the probe even though it is not common.

False low reading causes

- Poor peripheral perfusion, ambient light, poor probe contact.
- Methylene blue as example of dyes.

False high reading causes

- COHb, MetHb or radiofrequency interference.

6.12 Rotameter (Flowmeter)

Overview.

Rotameters are devices that enable flow to be measured using a float that sits on a stream of gas within a glass tube and rise proportional to gas flow Fig. 6.15.

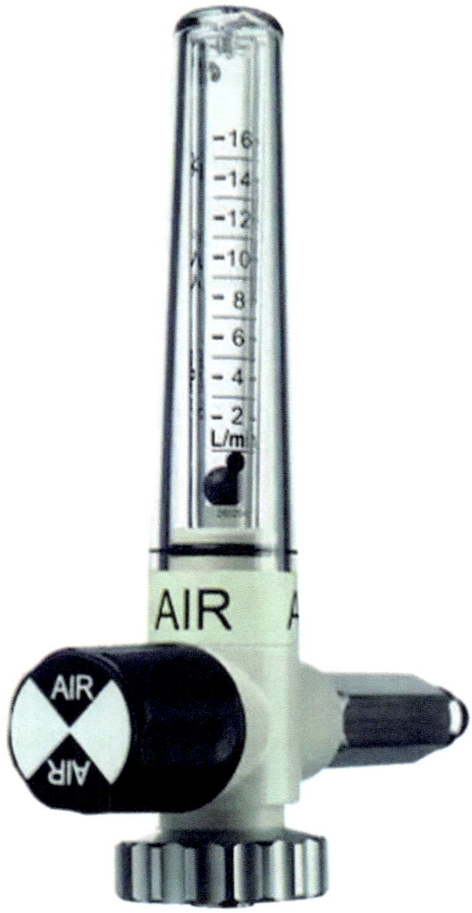

Fig. 6.15 Flowmeter (Image courtesy Dr. Nabil Shallik)

Use

- Controlled delivery of medical gases at appropriate flow rates.

Description

- glass tube containing a float which is elevated by a stream of moving gas,
- outlet for attachment of tubing,
- inlet from pressure regulator device attached to gas source,
- control knob,
- new digital Rotameter are used in the recent machines.

Method of use

- the float is raised in the tube as gas flow increases,
- cylinder markings allow determination of flow rate,
- reading is taken at the centre of the float,
- glass cylinder must be upright,
- float should spin (shows that it is not stuck).

Complications

- Incorrect function if not held vertically.
- float can stick if excess static electricity/debris and breakage of glass cylinder,
- malfunction of valve controlling flow.

Other information

- Different meters are required for different gases as flow rates depend on gas properties such as viscosity and density.
- Different flow meters are used for different purposes (e.g., paediatric 0–5 L/min and adult 0–15 L/min).

Thromboelastogram (TEG).

Overview.

Thromboelastography (TEG) is a viscoelastic haemostatic assay that measures the global viscoelastic properties of whole blood clot formation under low shear stress.

- Thromboelastography shows the interaction between platelets in blood and coagulation cascade like aggregation, clot strengthening, fibrin cross-linking, and fibrinolysis.
- Does not necessarily correlate with traditional blood tests that being used for to assess coagulation state such as INR, APTT, and platelet count knowing that these traditional tests are poor predictors.
- This part describes TEG® predominantly, ROTEM® is the alternative viscoelastic haemostatic assay that is widely available commercially.

6.13 Method

- TEG® measures the physical properties of the clot in whole blood via a pin suspended in a cup in a to 37 C temperature from a torsion wire connected with a mechanical-electrical transducer Fig. 6.16.
- The elasticity and strength of the developing clot changes the rotation of the pin, which is converted into electrical signals that a computer uses to create graphical and numerical output.
- Relatively it is quick that takes around 30 min.
- Can be repeated easily for comparing and follow up treatment plan.
- The TEG machine requires calibration almost three times daily.
- Trained staff has to perform the calibration.
- Sensitive to the technical variations.
- Activators used in TEG are: kaolin and more recently kaolin + tissue factor (TF) (Rapid TEG®).
- NATEM (TEG® using native whole blood) is slower.
- Other tests are available including functional fibrinogen, a measure of fibrin-based clot function, and multiplate which evaluates platelet function.
- This newer machine is using resonance instead of pin-in-cup technique.
- Where blood is exposed to a fixed vibration frequency range and the detector measures the

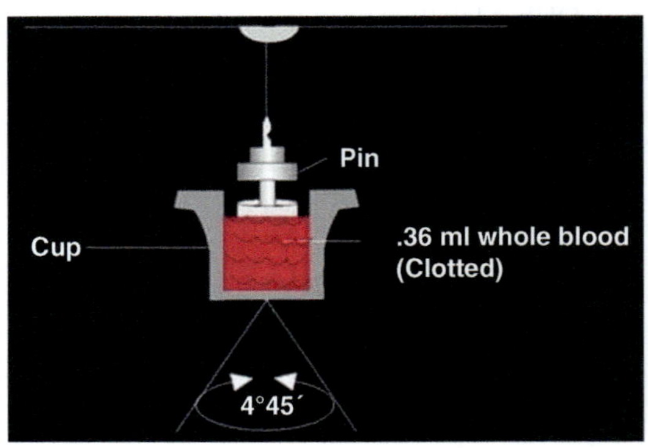

Fig. 6.16 TEG6s (Haemonetics)

vertical motion of blood meniscus under LED illumination and transforms that movement into tracing of clot dynamics.
- With pre-prepared cartridges, there is no longer any pipetting required!

Use
Indications

- Can predict the need of transfusion.
- Guide transfusion strategy.
- Studies show cost-effectiveness and reduction in blood products in:
- Open heart cardiac surgery, massive bleeding, massive trauma with major blood loss and liver transplantation.
- Maybe useful in:
- in trauma it reduces the need of blood product transfusion and seems like mortality reduced.
- obstetrics it might reduce the need of blood products transfusion which is controversial,
- it allows early detection of dilutional coagulopathy.

Hard to interpret in certain situations:

- Low molecular weight heparin (LMWH) and aspirin therapy.
- During and post cardiac cardiopulmonary bypass.
- Hypercoagulability or fibrinolysis.

6.14 Teg® Versus ROTEM®

Comparison

- Two commercial types of viscoelastic tests are available: thromboelastography = TEG® (developed in 1948, now produced in the USA) and rotational thromboelastogram = ROTEM® (from Germany).
- The main differences in diagnostic nomenclature for identical parameters between the two.
- TEG® operates by moving a cup in a limited arc (±4°45′ every 5 s) filled with sample that engages a pin/wire transduction system as clot formation occur.
- ROTEM® has an immobile cup wherein the pin/wire transduction system slowly oscillates (±4°45′every 6 s).
- Results are not directly comparable as different coagulation activators are used.
- ROTEM® is more resistant to mechanical shock, which may be an advantage in the clinical setting.

Equivalent variables for ROTEM® (Fig. 6.17)

- Clotting time (CT) = *R* value (reaction time).
- α angle and clot formation time (CFT) = *K* value and α angle.
- Maximum clot firmness (MCF) = Maximum amplitude (MA).
- Clot lysis (CL) = LY30.

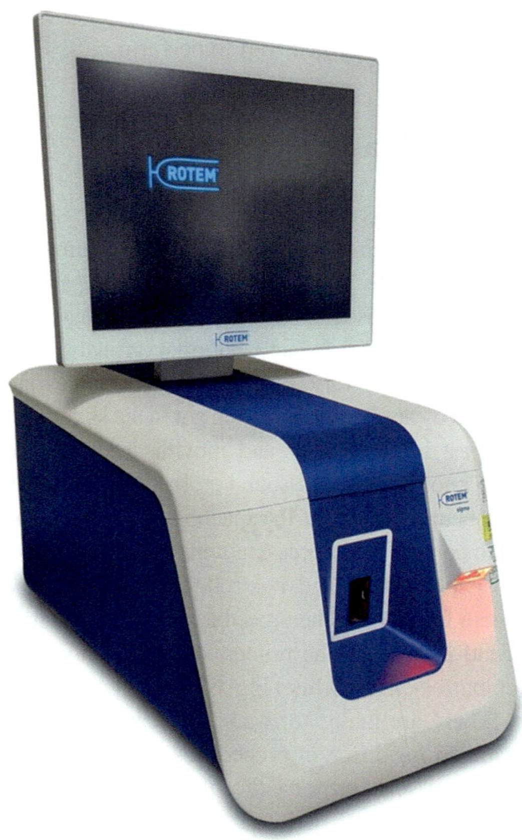

Fig. 6.17 ROTEM (Image courtesy Dr. Nabil Shallik)

Comparison with plasma clotting tests.
Pros of viscoelastic haemostatic assays

- assessment of global haemostatic potential provides more information than time to fibrin formation,
- can readily differentiate a coagulopathy due to low fibrinogen from one due to thrombocytopenia,
- point-of-care (POC) device with rapid turnaround times so that many results available within 5–10 min of starting the test.

Cons of viscoelastic haemostatic assays

- variable availability and user familiarity,
- marked inter-operator variability and poor precision,
- UK NEQAS data suggests coefficients of variance ranging from 7.1% to 39.9% for TEG® and 7.0% to 83.6% for ROTEM®.
- Might need trained staff to perform.

6.15 Ultrasound Machine

Ultrasound (US) is a procedure that utilize sound waves with high frequency (MHZ) above humanity hearing level to generate images of many parts of the body. Ultrasound (US) can check diseased or damaged tissues, locate abnormal growths, and identify a wide variety of conditions. Images are formed by applying lubricating gel to the skin to get the best image quality and moving a transducer, (also known as an ultrasound probe), over the body part being examined, the machine consists of the main control and processing unit, the control panel for patient entry and controlling the image, the screen for viewing the procedure process, the ultrasound probe, and the printer for images print out (colour/black and white) Fig. 6.18.

There are many software applications can be installed for different procedures such as nerves, blood vessels, orthopaedic, urology, paediatric, and small parts.

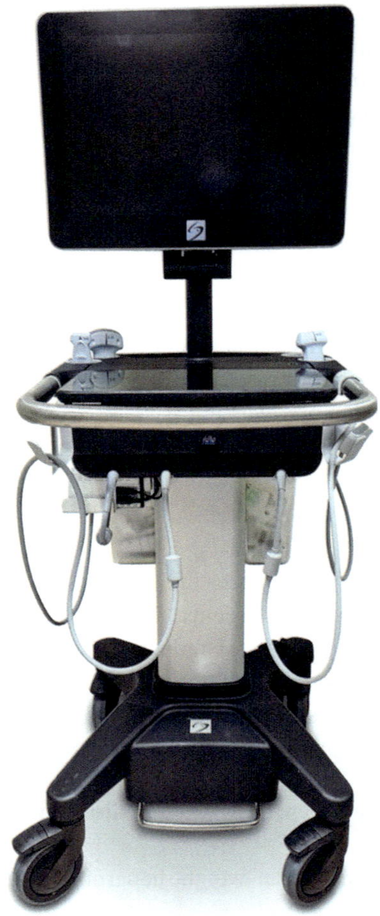

Fig. 6.18 Ultrasound machine (Image courtesy Dr. Nabil Shallik)

Doppler ultrasound uses high-frequency sound waves to obtain an image of blood flow through various vessels in the body. It is commonly used to diagnosis arteries and veins for the carotid artery in the neck or arteries and veins in legs and arms. It can detect diseased vessels and identify a wide variety of changing conditions.

A Doppler vascular ultrasound is performed the same way as US is performed. During portions of the exam, you will hear sounds similar to a heart sound or beat coming from the ultrasound machine while we are listening to the blood flow in your vessels.

US procedures can take up to 1 hour depends on the pathology or organ.

The ultrasound probe (US transducer) is the tool used by the ultrasound machine to get the image, it has a row of crystals emitting and receiving the ultrasonic wave, it comes with many shapes such as curved, linear, and vase array using for different procedures and different areas.

6.16 Vein Viewer

6.16.1 How Does it Work?

Vien viewer projects a near-infrared light which is absorbed by blood and reflected by surrounding tissue. The information is captured, processed, and projected digitally in real time directly onto the surface of the patient skin. It provides a real-time accurate image of the patient's blood pattern showing exactly where the vein is located for easy vascular access Fig. 6.19.

Vein viewer allows you to see blood patterns up to 15 mm deep and clinically relevant veins up to 10 mm. With vein viewer clinicians can see peripheral veins, bifurcations, and valves and assess in real time the refill and flushing of veins. With visualization pre-, during-, and post-procedure, clinicians can potentially avoid complications from accidental puncture and it improves the total vascular access process.

The reflected image size can be changed also the colour can be reversed.

Many vein viewers manufactures and they are varying in the colour, size, portability, and image control and image quality.

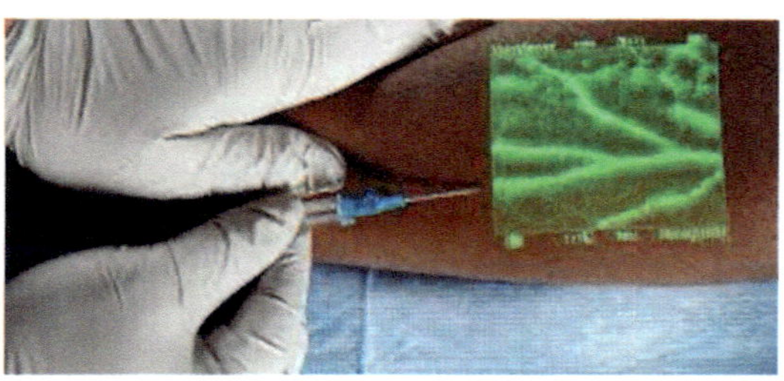

Fig. 6.19 Vein viewer (Image courtesy Dr. Nabil Shallik)

6.17 Body Warming Device

Overview

- Body Worming Device such as the Bair Hugger™ also known as patient warming system (Fig. 6.20).

Uses

- indicated when patient has low temperature < 35 °C or to prevent intra operative hypothermia.

Description

- the machine warms air then blows it over or under the patient using safe and effective heat distribution special blankets,
- Variable shapes and sizes of blankets can be used.

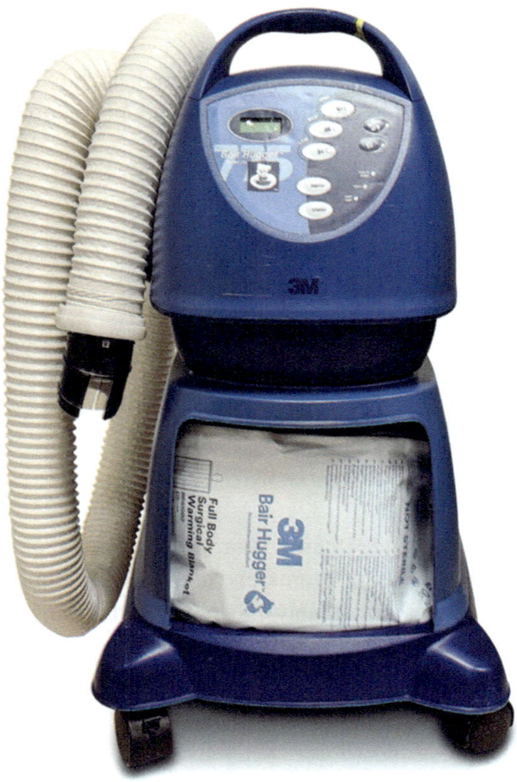

Fig. 6.20 Body Warming Device (Bair Hugger 3 M) (Image courtesy Dr. Nabil Shallik)

- typically consists of a silky polyester fabric with an inlay of nylon waterproof material to keep airflow circulating up towards the patient,
- Blankets can be used with all major brands of warm air convection units.
- All warming units regulate the air temperature at the end of the delivery hose and have audible and visual over temperature alarms.

Method of use

- Patient is covered with blanket and the hose inserted into the designated hole.
- Need to ensure that it is securely connected and no air is escaping.
- Hose is kept straight as excessive bends affect temperature performance.
- Blanket is inflated and checked for air leakage.
- Low/medium/high settings chosen according to the patient's temperature.
- Extra blankets should not be placed over the Bair Hugger™ as this can lead to uneven heat distribution.
- Head should always be covered in kids and neonates as this route may account for up to 50% of heat loss.

Complications

- Overwarming and complications of hyperthermia.
- Impaired detection of clinical signs (e.g., cyanosis and external bleeding).

Other information.
Concepts of heat transfer

- Heat is the thermal energy created by the movement of atoms and molecules within a substance that may be transferred from one system of atoms/molecules to another.
- Radiation (main mechanism) – energy transferred by electromagnetic (infrared) waves from a surface.
- Convection – energy transferred to air or liquid flowing past a surface.
- Evaporation – energy is lost as fluid on a surface is converted to gas.
- Respiration – energy is lost in exhaled humidified gas from the lungs.
- Conduction (least important mechanism) – energy is directly transferred between two surfaces in direct contact.

6.18 Conclusion

Many monitoring modalities have been developed recently, the upwarding developing in anaesthesia monitoring have reduced the perioperative mortality and morbidity.

One of the responsibilities of the ATs is to assist in preparation of the anaesthesia or induction room. This includes making sure of the availability of preparing and maintaining functioning equipment including patient monitoring devices.

Anaesthesia monitors are huge in number and various in types. Our chapter will concentrate on the most common and critical monitors only but some other monitors and equipment are discussed in more details in other chapters within this book.

Suggested Readings

1. Cook TM, Tuckey JP. A comparison between the Macintosh and the McCoy laryngoscope blades. Anaesthesia. 1996;51(10):977–80. [PMID 8984878].
2. Anesthesia Equipment. 3rd Edition. Principles and Applications. Authors: Jan Ehrenwerth James Eisenkraft James Berry. eBook ISBN: 9780323775496 July 2020.
3. Daniel Aston, Angus Rivers, Asela Dharmadasa. Equipment in Anaesthesia and Critical Care: A complete guide for the FRCA 1; 1999. (ISBN: 9781907904059).
4. Andrew Davey Ali Diba. Ward's Anaesthetic Equipment 6th Edition. December 2011.

Infection Control and Prevention in Operation Theatre

7

Nabil A. Shallik, ElSayed ElKarta, Shakshanam Mirishova, Ilhem Othmani, Ghazi Miladi, and Hamad Mohammad Suleiman

Contents

N. A. Shallik (✉) · E. ElKarta · S. Mirishova
H. M. Suleiman
Anesthesia, ICU and Perioperative Medicine, Hamad Medical Corporation, Doha, Qatar
e-mail: nshallik@hamad.qa; eelkarta@hamad.qa; HSuleiman@hamad.qa

I. Othmani · G. Miladi
Anesthesia, Hamad Medical Corporation, Doha, Qatar
e-mail: iothmani1@hamad.qa; Gmiladi@hamad.hamad.qa

N. A. Shallik et al. (eds.), *Improving Anesthesia Technical Staff's Skills*,
https://doi.org/10.1007/978-3-030-88849-7_7

7.1 Introduction

From the ancient time and Middle Ages, representatives of different cultures suspected the importance of cleaning and decontamination. As early as in Hippocrates time, cleaning techniques with boiled water or wine were used. Following Pasteur's discoveries, Joseph Lister became true Father of Modern Antisepsis in 1860.

Ralph Milton Waters (1883–1979) was an American anaesthesiologist who reported the need for infection prevention techniques in operation theatre in 1930s.

Hospital-acquired infection (HAI) is a huge global public health concern which causes high mortality and rehospitalization rates, impacting important preventable costs [1, 2].

Research of Maslyk has found significant anaesthesia work area bioburden with both commensal and pathogenic bacteria, including coagulase-negative Staphylococci, Bacillus spp., Streptococci, Staphylococcus aureus, Acinetobacter spp., and other gram-negative bacilli [3].

Research data demonstrated that bacterial transmission in the OR anaesthesia work area was associated with 30-days postoperative infections, affecting as many as 16% of patients undergoing surgery. Unfortunately, microorganism including multidrug-resistant ones may be spread in the Operating Room (OR) via anaesthesia providers. Indeed, up to 30% of bacterial transfer occurred between cases and was linked to an anaesthesia work area that was not completely decontaminated with routine cleaning [4].

The highest risk of the anaesthesia work area contamination occurs during induction and anaesthesia emergencies [4, 5].

Hence, the clear comprehension and the strict compliance, as well as the applications of infection control recommendations in the OR by anaesthesia providers; will decrease efficiently those risks.

7.2 Cleaning and Reprocessing Basis

7.2.1 Cleaning

It is defined as the physical removal of organic material and/or soil, generally by using water with detergents. This process is designed to remove organisms rather than killing them. Cleaning must precede high-level disinfection and sterilization.

Disinfection: It is a process capable of destroying most microorganisms, not bacterial spores (Fig. 7.1)

- High-level disinfection: Heat automated.
  - Pasteurization.
  - Liquid (chemical sterilant).
    - 2% glutaraldehyde
    - 1.12% glutaraldehyde and 1.93% phenol
    - 1% hydrogen peroxide and 0.08% peracetic
    - Hydrogen peroxide.
    - Ortho-phthalaldehyde.
    - Formaldehyde.
- Intermediate level disinfection.
- The destruction of viruses, mycobacteria, fungi, and vegetative bacteria (but not bacterial spores).
- Intermediate Level Disinfection Techniques.

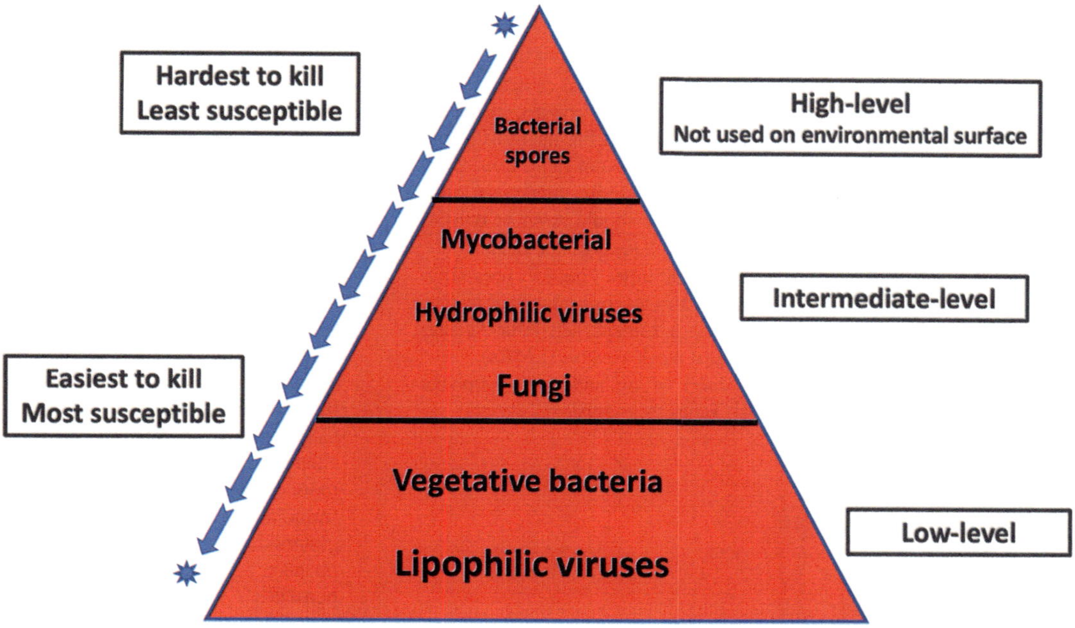

Fig. 7.1 Microorganism disinfection levels in anaesthesia workspace

- Chlorine and phenol products for a minimum of 1 min.
- Alcohols.
- Low level disinfection.
- The destruction of vegetative bacteria (but not M. tuberculosis), some fungi and virus but not spores.
- Low Level Disinfection Techniques.
- Includes chlorine-based products, phenolics, quaternary ammonium compounds, and 70–90% alcohol.
- Quaternary Ammonium Compounds.

7.2.2 Sterilization

A process that renders an object completely free of all viable infectious agents by eliminating all forms of microbial life.

Critical devices must be sterile at the time of use.

Sterilization Techniques:

- Steam.
- Dry Heat.
- Ethylene Oxide.
- Peracetic Acid.
- Plasma Gas (vaporized hydrogen peroxide).
- 2.4% Glutaraldehyde.

7.3 Spaulding's Classification

In 1939, Dr. Earle Spaulding proposed a simple and rational strategy through the microbiology department at Philadelphia Temple University to classify and treat properly medical instruments and equipment based upon how a device was used (Table 7.1):

- Critical items were destined for the use in sterile body tissue, cavities, or the vascular system.
- Semi-critical items are coming in contact with mucous membranes or non-intact skin.
- Non-critical items come in contact with intact skin (not mucous membranes).

On 1968, his approach was approved by the worldwide medical community and still in use today known by Spaulding's Classification System. This classification was updated on 1991

Table 7.1 The updated Spaulding's Classification of Anaesthesia equipment and Workspace surfaces

Category	Description	Anaesthesia workspace surfaces and items	Required processing
Critical	Sterile body tissue, cavities, or the vascular system	Intravenous and arterial catheters, tubing, stopcocks, needles, syringes, medication vials, and ampules. For the most part (with the exception of multi-dose vials), these items are sterile, single use, and disposable and should never be reused	Sterilization (all anaesthesia critical items are single use and should never be reused)[a]
Semi critical	Contact mucous membranes or non-intact skin.	Endoscopes, laryngoscope blades, endotracheal tubes[b], masks[b], breathing circuits[b], airway connectors[b], fibre-optic endoscopes, forceps, self-inflating bags, laryngeal mask airways (LMAs), transducer tubing, and trans-oesophageal (exp: Temperature probes), stylets	Sterilization: – through the use of steam sterilization or other low-temperature process such as ethylene oxide, hydrogen gas plasma, – liquid chemical sterilant. Germicides categorized as chemical sterilant include 2.4% or more of glutaraldehyde-based formulations, 0.95% glutaraldehyde with 1.64% phenol/phenate, 7.5% stabilized hydrogen peroxide, 7.35% hydrogen peroxide with 0.23% peracetic acid, 0.2% peracetic acid, and 0.08% peracetic acid with 1.0% hydrogen peroxide – high-level disinfection (at minimum) through the appropriate use of glutaraldehyde, hydrogen peroxide, ortho-phthalaldehyde, and peracetic acid with hydrogen peroxide
Non-critical	Direct contact with intact skin	Cables that are in physical contact with patients: Pulse oximeter, ECG leads, NMT, BIS, blood pressure cuffs, ultrasound probes, laryngoscope handles	Disinfection: – intermediate-level disinfection (eliminates tuberculosis bacilli, non-enveloped viruses and fungi) – low-level disinfection (eliminates most vegetative bacteria and enveloped viruses)
	Anaesthesia Environmental surfaces	The anaesthesia machine work surface, gas flow controls, vaporizer dials, adjustable pressure limiting valve (APL), control knobs, monitors, supplies cart's drawers, cupboards handle, medication dispensers, cables, IV stands, fluid and body warmers, computer keyboard and mouse, ultrasound machines, video laryngoscopes screen	

[a]The reuse of single-use devices (SUDs) can affect their safety, performance, and effectiveness, exposing patients and staff to unnecessary risks. This table displays the legal implications based on conspiracy to commit adulteration and Medicare fraud, leading to imprisonment for up to 10 years and/or a maximum fine of 50,000 $ with administrative action up to suspension of practice license. (Senate Bill 528/Public Act 25 and 26 of 2010) [6, 7]

[b]According to the Food and Drug Administration (FDA) guidance, the risk categories of some types of SUDs that may re-sterilized by the user and reused following the manufacturer's instructions for use, following Medicines & Healthcare Products Regularity Agency regulations. The items mentioned are supposed to be disposable but in some regulated circumstances they may be reprocessed and reused. Consequently, third-party reprocessing is allowed by the FDA as the device manufacturer reprocessed is considered as defined under the Code of Federal Regulations Title 21 Part 82 [6–8]

by the US Centres for Disease Control and Prevention. After that, they added a new category designated as environmental surfaces which is subdivided to housekeeping surfaces and medical equipment surfaces. Well, it is a fact that anaesthesia providers are a potential vector of cross contamination between medical equipment surfaces and patients.

7.4 Recommendations

Association of Anaesthetists of Great Britain and Ireland (AAGBI) have put up the following recommendations in their latest guidelines [9].

1. There should be a named Lead Consultant in each Department of Anaesthesia who is responsible for liaising with their Trust Infection Prevention and Control Team and Occupational Health Department to ensure relevant specialist standards are established and monitored in all areas of anaesthetic practice.
2. Precautions to prevent the transmission of infection between patient and anaesthetist or between patients should be routine practice. All anaesthetists should comply with local infection control policies, including the safe use and disposal of sharps.
3. When performing invasive procedures, the correct skin cleaning solution should be used. For neuraxial procedures, 0.5% chlorhexidine gluconate in 70% alcohol is recommended. For invasive vascular procedures, 2% chlorhexidine in 70% alcohol is recommended.
4. Protocols should be followed to minimize infection risk associated with indwelling invasive devices. These include correct dressing application, cleaning before access, flushing, changing of administration sets, regular review of device condition, and assessment of continuing need.
5. Single-use equipment should be used wherever transmission of infective agents is a risk. Techniques exist for the reprocessing of some single-use equipment, in which case nationally recommended policies for their decontamination and/or sterilization, and based on the manufacturers' advice, should be followed and audited.
6. Appropriate infection control precautions should be established for procedures such as spinal and epidural insertions, epidural blood patches, blood cultures, and urinary catheters.
7. Anaesthetists should administer antimicrobials according to local protocols in order to preserve their future effectiveness.

7.4.1 Standard Precautions

Most anaesthesia societies recommend adhering to standard precautions, which is in most cases are simple Personal Protective Equipment (PPE) (gloves, masks, eye protection shields, and gown). These are recommended for every patient when contact with bodily fluids including blood, mucus membranes are anticipated. Special precautions should be taken when there is possibility of splatter of body fluids [9, 10].

7.4.2 Hand Hygiene (HH)

Hand hygiene is a cornerstone in reducing the risk of hospital-acquired infection (HAI). According to the WHO it should be performed ideally in five crucial moments at a hospital environment Fig. 7.2:

1. before touching a patient (e.g., attaching the monitor cables);
2. before clean/aseptic procedures (e.g., inserting CVC, inserting arterial catheters, drawing medications, and spiking IV bags);
3. after body fluid exposure/risk (e.g., intubation, inserting LMA, induction, oral and tracheal suction);
4. after touching a patient (e.g.: removing the body warmer);
5. after touching patient surroundings (after entering/exiting the OR and even removing gloves).

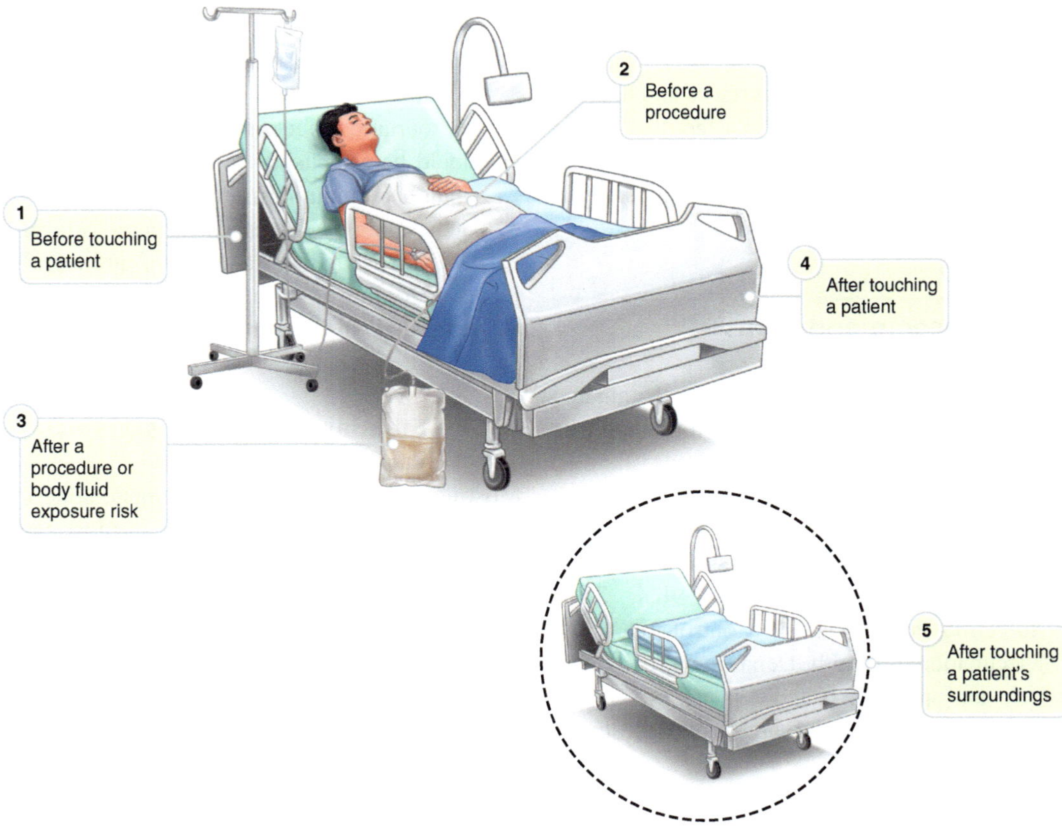

Fig. 7.2 The WHO recommendations for hand hygiene (HH) during patient care

7.4.3 Technique

The following are the steps of proper hand-washing (Fig. 7.3):

1. **Step 1:** Wet the hands with lukewarm water (35–45 °C) and apply soap, create lather.
2. **Step 2:** Rub your palms in clockwise and anticlockwise.
3. **Step 3:** Link the fingers and rub the back of your hand with palms of second hand, then alternate.
4. **Step 4:** Put both palms facing together and link fingers, clasp hands, then rub them.
5. **Step 5:** Cup the fingers keeping one hand over another, interlock fingers and rub the backs against palms, alternate hands.
6. **Step 6:** Encircle one hand around the thumb of another, keep rubbing in rotating motion, then alternate.
7. **Step 7:** Open the palm of one hand and rub the fingers of another hand in circular motion, then repeat with swapping to another hand.

Joint Commission International (JCI) is recommending 40–60 s for hand washing with plain soap duration, and 20–30 s for hand rub with alcohol-based hand rub (ABHR) and better to follow the manufacturer guidelines. [11].

Applying Alcohol Based Hand Rub (ABHR) on gloves being worn during a case, instead of removing them and performing hand hygiene between doffing and donning is not advised. Because, there is no sufficient researches ensuring glove's integrity after application of foam/gel. Actually, gloved hands are usually assumed to be contaminated, however, bare hands are assumed to be clean following appropriate HH. Indeed, the.

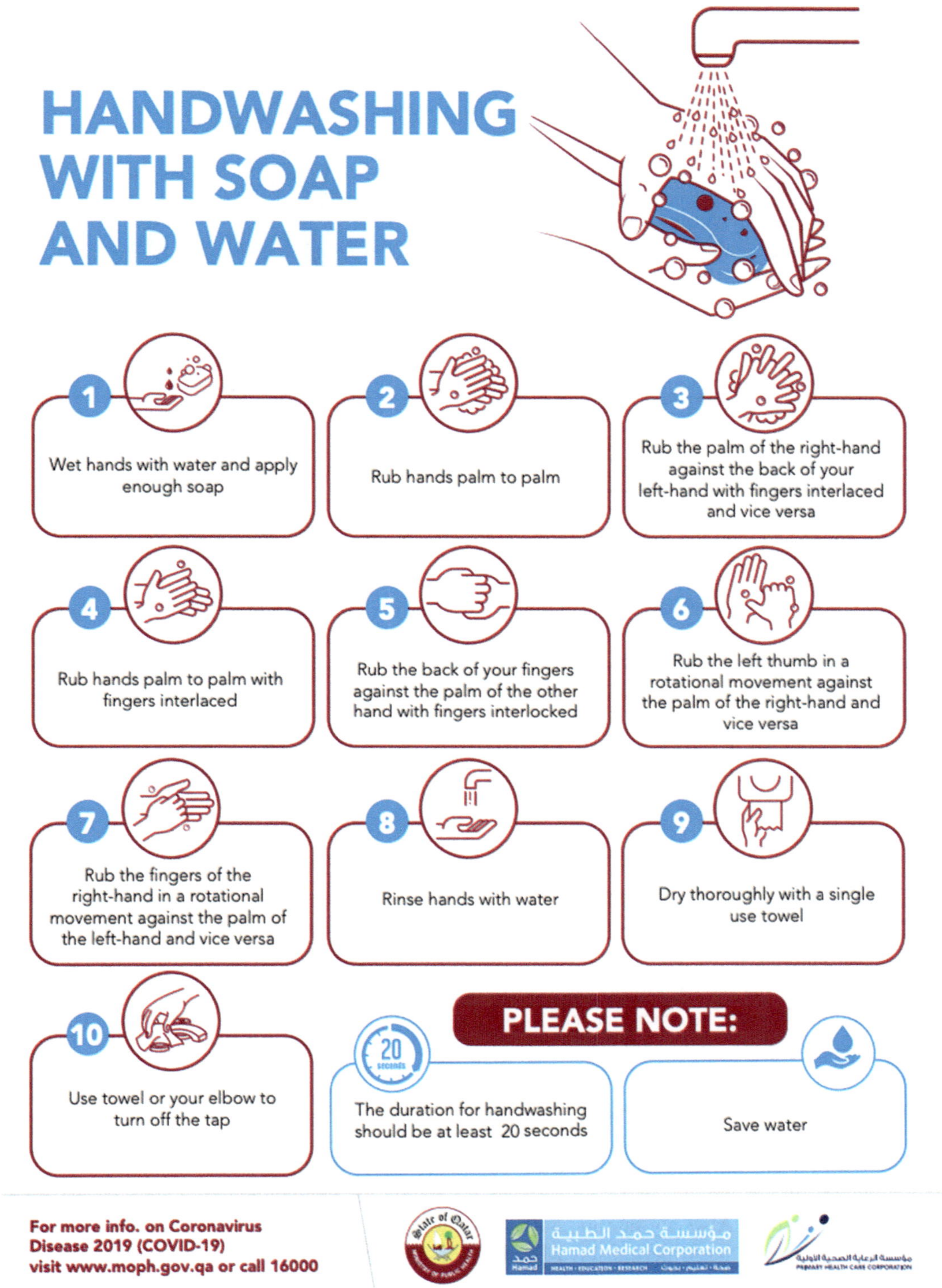
HANDWASHING WITH SOAP AND WATER
1
Wet hands with water and apply enough soap
2
Rub hands palm to palm
3
Rub the palm of the right-hand against the back of your left-hand with fingers interlaced and vice versa
4
Rub hands palm to palm with fingers interlaced
5
Rub the back of your fingers against the palm of the other hand with fingers interlocked
6
Rub the left thumb in a rotational movement against the palm of the right-hand and vice versa
7
Rub the fingers of the right-hand in a rotational movement against the palm of the left-hand and vice versa
8
Rinse hands with water
9
Dry thoroughly with a single use towel
10
Use towel or your elbow to turn off the tap
PLEASE NOTE:
20 seconds
The duration for handwashing should be at least 20 seconds
Save water
For more info. on Coronavirus Disease 2019 (COVID-19) visit www.moph.gov.qa or call 16000
State of Qatar
Hamad Medical Corporation

Fig. 7.3 Steps of proper handwashing

Centres for Disease Control (CDC) and WHO guidelines recommend removing gloves before performing HH as standard practice.

The wearing of the full maximal sterile barrier (full PPE that includes: face mask, cap, sterile gown, sterile gloves) and a large sterile drape, should be used by the anesthesia provider during operation theatre technique before inserting Central Intravenous Catheters (Fig. 7.4). Also, it is a must to use of a cap, mask, sterile gloves, and a small sterile fenestrated drape; in case of placing peripheral arterial lines. Meanwhile, those measures should be followed whenever a catheter is exchanged over a guidewire.

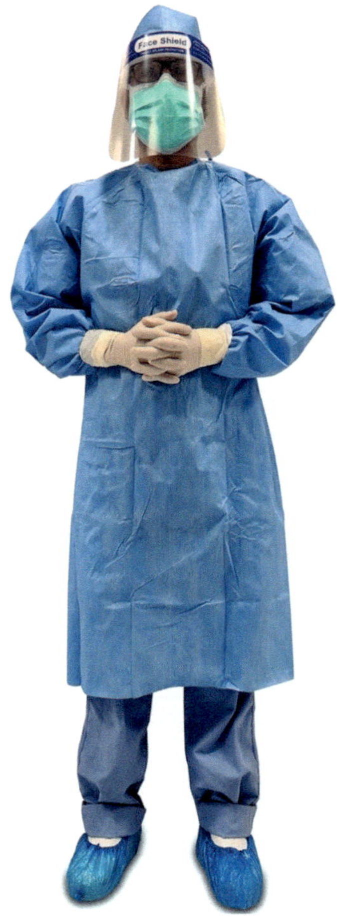

Fig. 7.4 Full Personal Protection Equipment (PPE)

7.5 Cleaning of the Operating Theatre

After each patient, the operation theatre should be thoroughly cleaned, applying local protocols for bodily fluids cleaning on the area, including the floor, which should be disinfected in between the cases. Cleaning should also take into account type of identified pathogens, for example, MRSA, VRE, and Clostridia. Regular cleaning schedule should be in place and take into account recommendations from infection control team.

7.5.1 Anaesthesia Workspace

Parts of current anaesthetic equipment cannot be made single use; this increased the risk of cross contamination. Appropriate cleaning and avoiding reusing single-use items should be strictly implemented.

Anaesthesia workspace surfaces should be wiped between each case including the anaesthesia supply cart (Fig. 7.5). That is why, it is preferable to avoid storage supplies on its top surface, as much as possible. Also, its interior must be cleaned on a tailored basic period fixed by the facility. Regarding its drawers and bins, anaesthesia providers should perform HH before opening them and handling their contents.

This general rule of cleaning anaesthesia workspace surfaces with hospital approved disinfectant between cases is applied as well on computer keyboard, mouse, and touchscreen, anaesthesia workstation (including monitors, APL valve, knobs, vaporizers, and monitor cables.) Moreover, disinfection is indicated whenever there is obvious soiling or contamination.

Indeed, several studies have demonstrated the potential for contamination of anaesthesia equipment and workspaces and possible transmission of a variety of microorganisms within the anaesthesia environment.

Thereby, especially after COVID-19 pandemic, facilities are encouraged to consider dis-

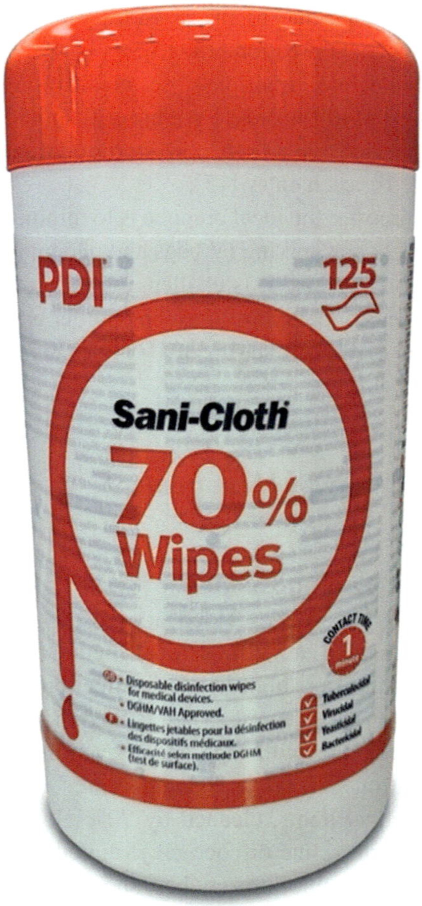

Fig. 7.5 Cleaning wipe

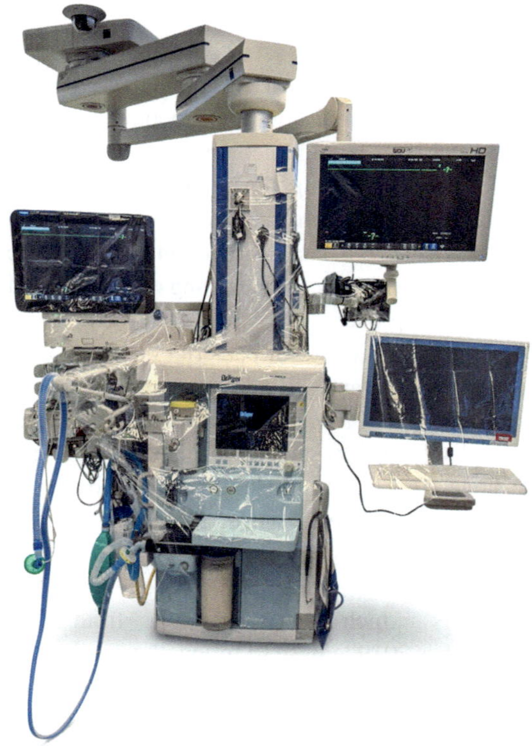

Fig. 7.6 Disposable plastic coverage of anaesthesia machine

posable coverage anaesthesia machines, as it has a rational impact on reducing contamination also facilitate cleaning and disinfection (Fig. 7.6).

On the other hand, internal components of anaesthesia ventilators including Airway Breathing System (ABS), reusable soda lime canister and valves, must be cleaned and disinfected per manufacturer's instructions and the hospital infection control policies. Filter is usually used to protect anaesthesia machine and circuit, which may prevent cross contamination. Modern filters allow humidification and heat exchanged and basically two kinds of designs are used. Type one includes mechanical filters, they stop particles larger than its pores. Second type is electrostatic filters which attract and hold charged particles. To retain heat and moisture, inert, sponge form material is added.

Actually, Mycobacterium Tuberculosis (TB) can survive for 3 h in soda-lime and 40% of bacteria can pass through it. Therefore, the High-Efficiency Particulate Air (HEPA bacterial) filters must be used in the respiratory circuit or at least on the expiratory limb because their efficiency is not affected during wet conditions. The anaesthesia provider may add another filter on the inspiratory limb if it is not increasing respiratory pressures [12] **(for more details, please refer to the end of this chapter under filter subtitle).**

Indeed, vials' rubber stoppers and necks of anaesthesia drugs ampules are not sterile. Hence, it should be a standard practice of disinfection by scrubbing them with 70% alcohol prior to each use.

Aiming to reduce the contamination of peripheral intravenous tubing stopcocks (triple ways) and injection ports that are used for medication administration during intraoperative use, with potential pathogenic bacteria due to lower compliance rates of provider HH and higher numbers of intravenous medication. It is recommended, to wipe those ports with alcohol ports for 10–15 s followed by a drying time immediately before each injection. However, during induction and emergencies, passive disinfection using sterile alcohol-containing caps is turning out as the most practical approach.

To reduce the risk of bacterial contamination of the syringe and syringe contents; needleless syringes should be capped with a sterile cap that completely covers the Luer connector on the syringe. This technique should be used to administer multiple doses of a drug to the same patient after each administered dose (Fig. 7.7) [13].

The United States Pharmacopeia (USP) Chapters which were effective from first December 2019, advise to follow the beyond use dating of OR intravenous drugs and solutions list classified upon the contamination level risk and the product stability [9, 10].

Mainly, they recommend to discard prepared intravenous medication and solution in the OR, after each case even not used, especially those which have not been prepared in air environment less than ISO class 5 (e.g., Pharmacy IV drug room). So, they discourage anaesthesia providers to return back to stock unused commercial prefilled syringes even with have intact security locking caps due to the possibility of external surface contamination [14, 15].

Meanwhile, multiple-dose medication vials must be used for only 1 patient and should only be accessed with both new sterile syringe and needle for each entry [15].

Moreover, the ideal practice is to minimize the time between spiking IV bags and patient administration and also it is challenging in urgent circumstances including lifesaving surgeries which require advanced set-up of IV fluids like Level one.

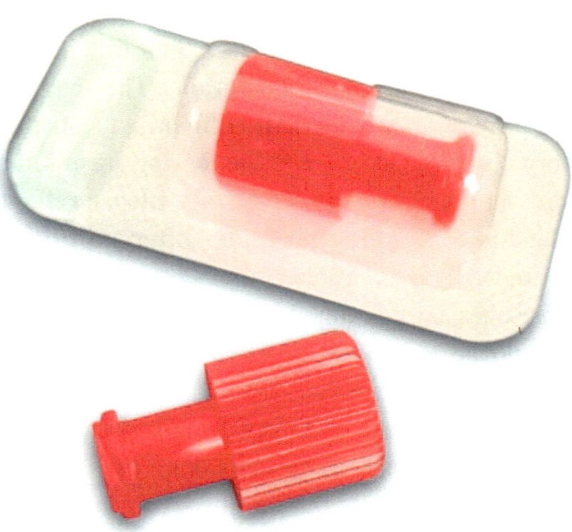

Fig. 7.7 Sterile cap for Luer lock

7.5.2 Airway Management Equipment

7.5.2.1 Laryngoscopes

Metal laryngoscopes /video laryngoscopes blades are classified as semi-critical items requiring sterilization or high-level disinfection (at the minimum) prior to use. Then, stored in appropriate packaging with tags and preventing recontamination. Though handles are classified non-critical items, cleaned by 70% alcohol and 2% chlorhexidine or coco alkyl dimethyl benzyl ammonium chloride, studies show shown that 40–50% of laryngoscope handles become contaminated with blood during airway management [16] (Fig. 7.8).

Therefore, reusable laryngoscope handles should be disassembled and autoclavable in a monthly basis, plus in case of resistant microor-

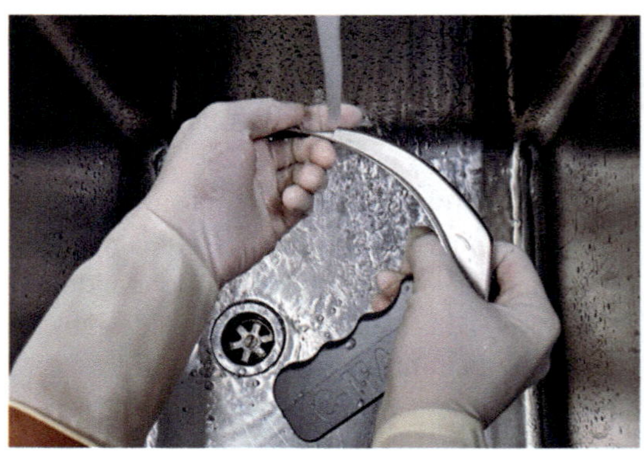

Fig. 7.8 Washing the laryngoscope handles before sterilization

ganism risk. The sterilization process makes their reprocessing potentially costly. That is why, it is recommended to consider using single-use laryngoscopes due to their performance, costing less than high-level decontamination for reusable laryngoscopes also, with possibility of recycling [11].

Currently, many options of single-use video laryngoscopes are available, for example, the Cobalt GlideScope® video laryngoscope (cGVL). It is composed of reusable video baton and a disposable clear plastic blade that is placed over it. The disposable blade can be discarded after each use and a new one placed on the video baton for subsequent intubations, eliminating the need for disinfection of the cGVL blade and reducing the potential risk of cross-contamination of infectious material between patients. The cGVL video baton must, however, undergo low-level disinfection after each patient use, and if it becomes visibly contaminated with gross material, high-level disinfection of the baton must be performed. Other brands of single-use video laryngoscopes are available in the market and each brand has its advantages and disadvantages (Fig. 7.9).

7.5.2.2 Fiber-Optic Endoscopes

After using the fiberoptic endoscopes, precleaning through removing the patient's secretions is a compulsory step. In fact, it should be performed at the point of use in the operating room, before

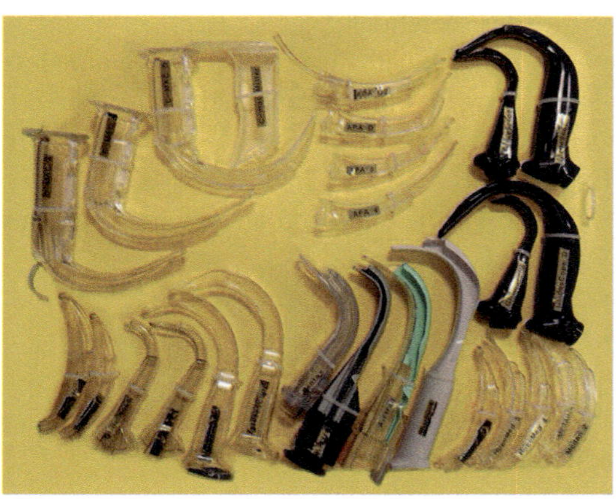

Fig. 7.9 Example of disposable video-laryngoscopic blades

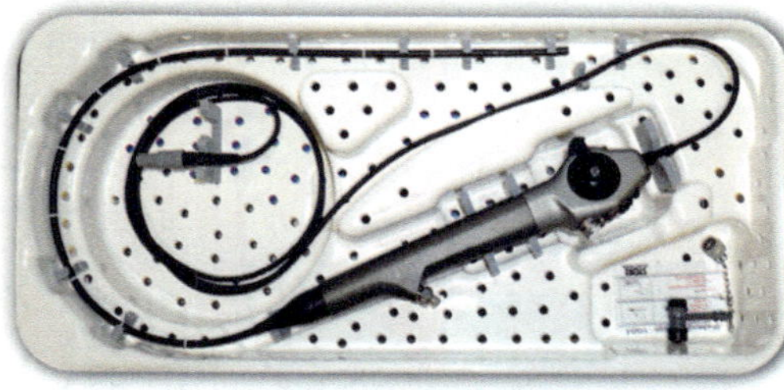

Fig. 7.10 Fibre-optic endoscope ready for sterilization

bioburden has an opportunity to dry. The second step is wiping the exterior of the endoscope with the appropriate fiber optic endoscopes detergent solution (never use alcohol wipes it will destroy its membrane). Glutaraldehyde 2% solution is the recommended agent for chemical disinfection of fiber-optic bronchoscope and it should be placed in the solution for 10–30 min.

For using gas sterilization, five hours' exposure to Ethylene Oxide (EO) is recommended for sterilization of instruments (Fig. 7.10).

7.6 Anaesthesia Breathing Circuit Filters, Types Fig. (7.11)

1. Electrostatic.

In electrostatic filters, the use of polarized material in the electromagnetic field, which attracts and captures the charged microbes and viruses, and it holds them within a loosely woven. It has bigger pores comparing to the second type but ensures better air quality with less airway resistance.

2. Mechanical (HEPA).

As its name indicates High-Efficiency Particles Air (HEPA), which physically, stops and prevents pathogens from passing through its miniscule pores. It consists on pleated hydrophobic glass fibres.

In fact, HEPA filters tended to outperform electrostatic filters since the latter can lose their effectiveness with humidity during the use of a

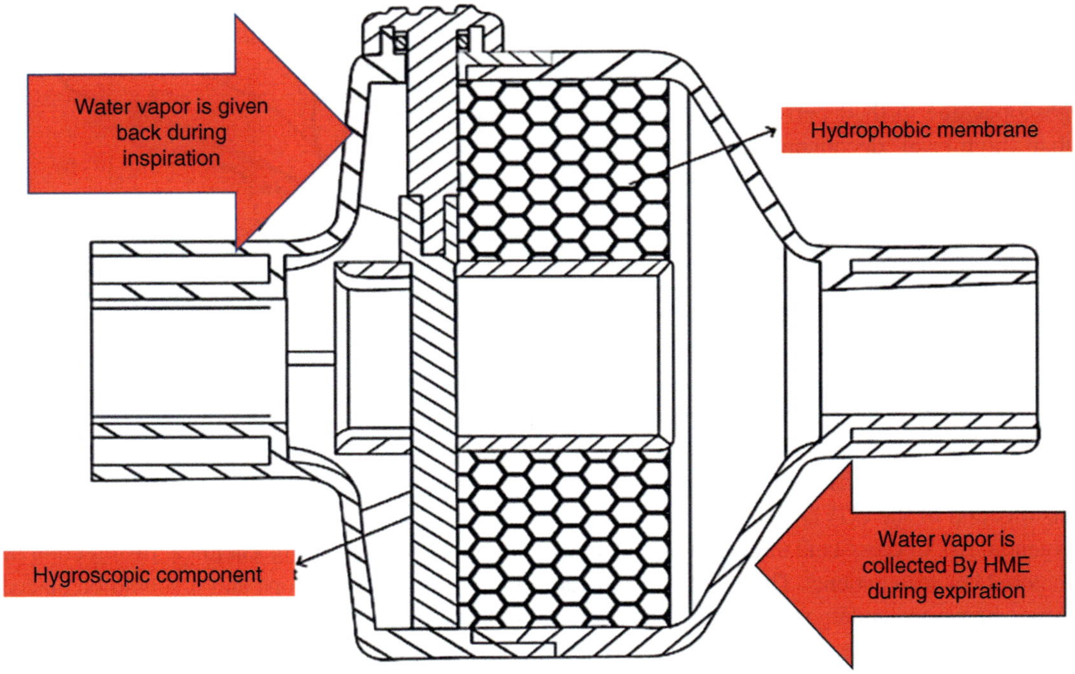

Fig. 7.11 Cross section in filter

circle system with active humidification. Actually, HEPA filters capture efficiency = 0.01 micron; meanwhile; the size of SARS COV-2 = 0.125 micron.

All filters efficient filters have to be subject of ISO 23328-1 and ISO 9360-1 standards; by means of standardized test performing a minimal Viral Filtration Efficiency (VFE) of 0.3-micron particle challenge.

3. Heat Moisture Exchanger Filter (HMEF).

These filters (either electrostatic or HEPA) may be modified by inserting sponge material sometimes chemically coated to perform additional functions like conservation of heat and moisture content of inhaled respiratory and anaesthetic gases and thus function as Heat, Moister Exchanger Filters (HMEF)

(a) Indications.
  - The upper airway provides 75% of the heat and moisture supplied to the alveoli during invasive mechanical ventilation, humidification is mandatory to supply this missing heat and moisture.
  - HMEF filters capture heat and moisture by around 50% of the patient exhaled moisture passively to prevent hypothermia, disruption of the airway epithelium, bronchospasm, and atelectasis.

(b) Contraindication.
  - Patients with frank bloody or thick, copious secretions.
  - Patients with an expired tidal volume less than 70% of the delivered tidal volume.

Example:
- Those with large bronchopleurocutaneous fistulas.
- Tracheal tube cuff malfunction.
- Presence of uncuffed endotracheal tube.

(c) HMEF Positioning Fig. 7.12:
- Connection to the expiratory hose:
  - It is prohibited to place a filter with HME characteristics between the circuit and

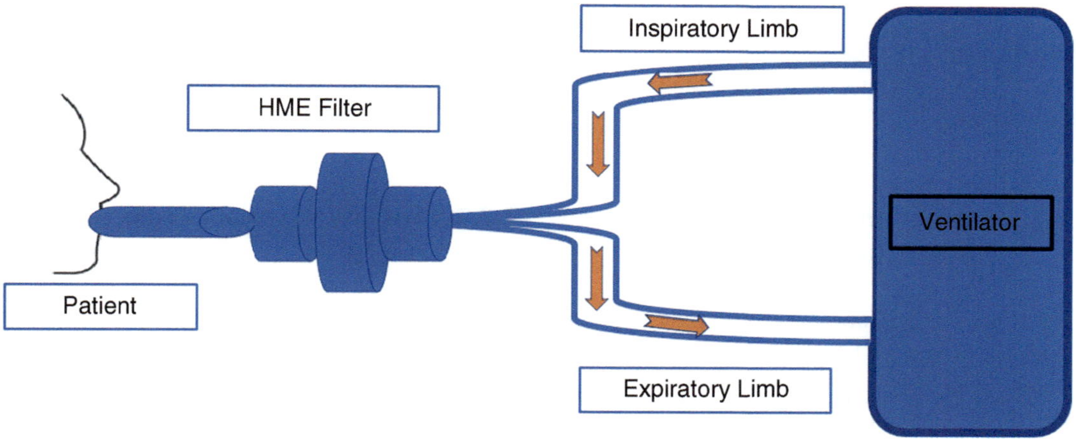

Fig. 7.12 HME Position in Ventilator circuit

the soda lime absorber (on the expiratory hose) due to the risk of biohazards by creating a microenvironment in circle absorber systems that predisposes an accumulation of carbon monoxide and other toxic metabolites such as Compound A.

  - This compound is one of the several products formed when sevoflurane is in the presence of strong bases in soda lime and barium hydroxide lime, especially at higher temperatures. Compound A is the most common sevoflurane degradation product in anaesthesia machines. Unfortunately, these compounds have been demonstrated to be nephrotoxic in mice.

- Connection to the Inspiratory hose or Endotracheal Tube port (ETT):
  - HME/filters are designed to retain exhaled moisture on the patient side of the HMEF. They can only contribute to an effective patient humidification if they are placed directly in contact with ETT port.
  - This assembly is indicated as well, in order to avoid contamination of the gas measurement unit and consequently the entire anaesthesia device.
  - If placed in distal position (on the inspiratory hose), it will decrease the absolute humidity and temperature of the ingoing gas with faster condensation of the water trap.
- Breathing circuit filters (without humidifier) Positioning.
  - All antiviral and antibacterial filters (either HEPA or electrostatic) have to be placed between breathing circuit and the expiratory hose, as a second barrier, to protect the anaesthesia machine from any potential pathogenic risk during disconnection and/or replacement of the filter at the patient side.
  - It is strongly recommended to use HEPA filters, because their VFE is not affected by wet conditions like electrostatic ones. However, they may exceed breathing resistance.

7.7 Ultraviolet Germicidal Irradiation (UVGI)

UV irradiation produces ultraclean air in operation theatres (OT) and highly effective way to reduce microbial contamination in the OT. It is much more cost-effective than the laminar air system and its efficiency is not less. The most commonly used technologies are: low pressure mercury lamps or pulsed xenon lamps. The efficacy of disinfection depends on the distance of the light source and surface, because intensity of light decreases exponentially with increasing distance from the light source. Currently, portable UV devices are available which are safe, easy to use.

7.7.1 Infection Control during Anaesthetic Procedures

Performing procedures in operation theatre alone does not guarantee lowering the risk of infection unless appropriate guidelines are followed and strictly implemented.

For Ultrasound guided procedures:

1. Use sterile protective cover for each patient.
2. If the probe comes into contact with blood, it should be sent for proper sterilization following manufactures recommendations.

Following are the steps of probe cleaning:

1. Disassemble.
2. Remove the probe cover.
3. Clean probe immediately by using a low lint cloth and pre-cleaning solution listed in the ultrasound manufacturers' IFU.
4. Rinse with tap water.
5. Dry with cloth/towel or air dry.
   - The drying step is imperative. As with debris and gel, residual water can mitigate the disinfection process. Whereas the former can act as barriers, water can dilute the disinfectant. Always perform MRC (Minimum Required Concentration) testing of HLD solution before reprocessing to ensure efficacy.
6. Visually inspect entire transducer to make sure that it is clean, no visible residual biofilm or bioburden remains, and there are no defects in the transducer housing or cables, which could potentially cause harm to the patient [17].
7. New ultrasound probes cleaning machines are offering fast and easy, also cost-effective way of high-level disinfection. These systems are automated and programmed, providing consistency. Other advantages of such systems are free of toxic fumes, they are able to kill resistant organisms such as Human Papillomavirus (e.g., Trophon EPR) [18].

7.7.2 For any Vascular Access

1. Use a sterile pack.
2. Use "no touch" technique.
3. Wear non-sterile gloves after hand washing for peripheral venous access, sterile gloves for arterial line placement, and full PPE for central line insertion.
4. Clean skin entry site with 2% chlorhexidine gluconate in 70% alcohol and wait to dry before proceeding. For patients sensitive to chlorhexidine, povidone iodine may be used.
5. Use whenever possible upper extremity for catheters.
6. Secure the catheter with sterile dressing.
7. The lines should be assessed frequently and removed as soon as possible.

7.7.3 Peripheral Nerve Blocks

1. Complications are rare but disastrous.
2. Use aseptic technique and 0.5% chlorhexidine gluconate in 70% alcohol (should be avoided to reach subarachnoid space).
3. Follow regional anaesthesia practice guidelines for neuraxial procedures (e.g., tunnel epidural catheters if prolonged need is there).

7.7.4 Considerations for High-Risk Patients

The particular group of patients will require extra efforts of infection prevention due to concurrent existing conditions such as immune suppression or they might possess high risk for other people, e.g., tuberculosis patients. For immunocompromised patients most procedures should be with high level of aseptic techniques. In case of infected patients, staff should protect themselves and avoid cross contamination between patients.

7.7.5 Considerations for Patients with Known Prion Diseases

Prions are infectious proteins and extremely resistant to most sterilization techniques. Patients suspected or known of prion disease require additional effort and adherence to national guidelines. Following are the list of precautions to be taken [15]:

1. Clear operation theatre of any unnecessary equipment.
2. Schedule the case last on list.
3. Ensure all staff wears full PPE.
4. Try to use single-use equipment.
5. Destroy instruments exposed to high-risk tissues (brain, spinal cord, and posterior eye).
6. Try not to use ventilators, and if they are used in definitive cases—quarantine the anaesthetic machine.
7. Recover the patient in operation theatre.

7.7.6 Considerations for Patients Known, or Suspected, to Be Infected with New Pathogens

Most recently new infectious agents have emerged, e.g., COVID-19, necessitating rapid change of current practice and prompt development of local policies and procedures to protect operation theatre team.

All surgical team members involved in COVID-19 cases should take contact and droplet precautions, such as N95, FFP2 or similar masks, goggles or face shields, gowns, gloves, and shoe covers. During transportation patients also must wear face masks and all contact and droplet precautions should be undertaken.

Dedicated operation theatres for COVID-19 patients should be chosen in such way with less flow of staff and ideally with negative pressure ventilation, high ventilation rate and its doors should be closed till the end of the case. Minimal number of staff should attend such cases. After finishing the case of a patient with COVID-19, operation theatre sit should be performed if there was aerosol generating procedures (APG) such as intubation, keeping doors closed for 30 min. After sit time passed the room and instruments may undergo standard cleaning and sterilization process. Further information should be obtained in local practice guidelines for each individual health organization.

7.7.7 Perioperative Antibiotic Prophylaxis

One of the most effective means to decrease postoperative infection is to administer antibiotics preoperatively. Antibiotics should be administered routinely in surgeries involving implants, bone grafts, or when surgical trauma expected to be large. The optimal timing for antibiotic administration is 30–60 min before surgery, achieving the goal of maximum concentration in the tissues [19]. Some antibiotics (e.g., Vancomycin, levofloxacin) require slow administration, usually within 120 min and must be started earlier, ideally before entering operation theatre. Even if patient already receiving antibiotic for another reason, an extra dose should be administered within 1 h of surgery. Redosing requires attention to half-life of the particular antibiotic used, and factors altering the half-life (renal dysfunction, burns, long surgery, and extensive blood loss).

Attention should be given if tourniquet is being applied, then antibiotics should be given before inflating it. The selection of type antibiotics depends on what body part is undergoing operation, making sure to cover the most common organisms in that location with narrowest spectrum. We should keep into consideration the cost, safety, antibiotic resistance in the particular hospital as well.

Antibiotics should be stopped after 24 h, except source of infection persists.

7.7.8 Audit and Quality Improvement Guide

Each health institution should prioritize the practice of routine audits raising staff awareness and adherence to impeccable hand hygiene, safe disposal of sharps, correct aseptic precautions for invasive procedures, managing contaminated equipment (e.g., airway equipment, breathing circuits, and bacterial/viral filters), compliance with antibiotic prophylaxis protocols [14].

7.7.8.1 Tips and Tricks

- To reduce the risk of contamination in the OR, anaesthesia providers should wear double gloves during airway management then should discard the outer gloves immediately after airway manipulation. As soon as possible, they should remove the inner gloves and perform HH.
- The optimum practice in order to promote frequent HH and decrease the incidence of Hospital-acquired infection (HAI) is to locate alcohol-based hand rub (ABHR) dispensers at the entrances to ORs and near anaesthesia providers inside the OR.
- Performing rinsing of processed items before using or storing them, with sterile water rather than from tap water to prevent contamination,s is a crucial step.

Because, high-level disinfectants can cause allergic reactions and tissue burns when they come in contact with human tissue.

- Placing one layer of cotton bandage roll between the patient arm and the blood pressure cuff is not only a barrier minimizing direct contact surface with the skin but also reduce the skin irritation due to the continuous pressure.
- The management of turnaround time between cases in the OR (which is varying between 10 and 20 min depending on the surgeries nature plus facility's policies) turns out very challenging for anaesthesia providers and assistants. Consequently, it is wise to start cleaning and disinfection of items being in direct contact with patient like monitor cables presenting high-risk vector for cross infections.

Summary and Take-Home Message To reduce hospital-acquired infection (HAI) prevalence rate in the anaesthesia workspace: Hospital's stakeholders should implement updated infection control policies tailored to their needs and their capacities. Then, communicate clearly and promote those standards among anaesthesia team.

In addition, we encourage the quality improvement projects related to infection control in the OR by identifying SMART goals, collecting data, facilitating the use of process measures to identify variations adjusting them, then sustaining the whole process.

Thus, rather than spreading a culture of blame, the anaesthesia frontlines should cooperate with infection control department to implement a real compliance to its requirements ensuring a positive change in both behaviour and the daily practice.

Finally, we encourage observations, feedback programs, and audits including blinded ones (to avoid the Hawthorne effect, in which the awareness of being observed changes one's behavior) to improve the infection control policies and guidelines in all health care facilities.

Finally, to optimize adherence to recommended disinfection practices, providers may enrol educational activities with combined theories, simulated workshops, and evaluation tests.

References

1. https://academic.oup.com/cid/article/65/4/644/3788023
2. https://www.cambridge.org/core/journals/infection-control-and-hospital-epidemiology/article/estimating-the-proportion-of-healthcareassociated-infections-that-are-reasonably-preventable-and-the-related-mortality-and costs/85B4290844BF00DF4530EBB2E5BEDC2D
3. Maslyk PA, Nafziger DA, Burns SM, Bowers PR. Microbial growth on the anesthesia machine. AANA J. 2002;70:53–6.
4. Loftus RW, Koff MD, Birnbach DJ. The dynamics and implications of bacterial transmission events

arising from the anesthesia work area. Anesth Analg. 2015;120:853–60.
5. Rowlands J, Yeager MP, Beach M, Patel HM, Huysman BC, Loftus RW. Video observation to map hand contact and bacterial transmission in operating rooms. Am J Infect Control. 2014;42:698–701.
6. f Medicines & Healthcare Products Regularity Agency: Single-use_medical_devices_v2.3_Oct-19 p3-4-5-6.
7. https://www.legislature.mi.gov/documents/2009-2010/billanalysis/Senate/htm/2009-SFA-0528-N.htm
8. Reprocessing-and-Reuse-of-Single-Use-Devices-Guidance-for-Industry-and-FDA-Reviewers.pdf_p27.
9. Radhakrishna S, Bailey c. Guidelines infection prevention and control 2020. Anaesthesia. 2020;
10. https://www.usp.org/compounding/general-chapter-797?fbclid=IwAR1ZsoFU3ivrVhsOeWQBWvDDHkyQ5Y5vwCUQ8hjLwCiQZkkSjVE-AZy7orU
11. https://www.usp.org/compounding/general-chapter-hazardous-drugs-handling-healthcare?fbclid=IwAR30rAlJ_POsCMQYD8oTaNedb8k7SznUO7gXeqllrbR6DFGC0erJNpCyulM
12. SHEA Expert Guidance Infection prevention in the operating room anesthesia work area Infection Control & Hospital Epidemiology (2019), 40, 1.
13. Association of perioperative Registered Nurses. Recommended practices for cleaning, handling and processing anesthesia equipment, 2010 perioperative standards and recommended practices. Denver, CO: Author; 2010. p. 379–88.
14. Spaulding E. The role of chemical disinfection in the prevention of nosocomial infections. In: Proceedings of the international conference on nosocomial infections, 1970. Chicago, IL: American Hospital Association; 1971. p. 247–54.
15. Farling P, Smith G. Anaesthesia for patients with Creutzfeldt-Jakob disease. A practical guide Anaesthesia. 2003;58:627–9.
16. Call T, Auerbach F, Riddell S, et al. Nosocomial contamination of laryngoscope handles: challenging current guidelines. Anesth Analg. 2009;109:479–83.
17. AIUM Guidelines for Cleaning and Preparing External- and Internal-Use Ultrasound Transducers Between Patients & Safe Handling and Use of Ultrasound Coupling Gel, https://www.aium.org/officialStatements/57
18. Ryndock E Robison R Meyers C, "Susceptibility of HPV16 and 18 to high level disinfectants indicated for semi-critical ultrasound probes." J Med Virol, Vol. 88, Issue 6, pages 1076–1080, June 2016.
19. Tarchini G, Liau KH, Solomkin JS. Antimicrobial Stewardship in Surgery: Challenges and Opportunities. Clin Infect Dis. 2017 May 15;64(suppl_2): S112-S114.

Anesthesia Machines and Anesthetic Breathing System

8

Kemal Tolga Saracoglu, Berk Cimenoglu, Recep Demirhan, Ayten Saracoglu, and Gamze Tanirgan

Contents

K. T. Saracoglu (✉)
Department of Anesthesiology and Reanimation, Health Sciences University Kartal Dr. Lutfi Kirdar Training and Research Hospital, Istanbul, Turkey

B. Cimenoglu · R. Demirhan
Department of Thoracic Surgery, Health Sciences University Kartal Dr. Lutfi Kirdar Training and Research Hospital, Istanbul, Turkey

A. Saracoglu
Department of Anesthesiology and Reanimation, Marmara University Pendik Training and Research Hospital, Istanbul, Turkey

G. Tanirgan
Department of Anesthesiology and Intensive Care, Marmara University Medical School, Istanbul, Turkey

N. A. Shallik et al. (eds.), *Improving Anesthesia Technical Staff's Skills*,
https://doi.org/10.1007/978-3-030-88849-7_8

8.1 Introduction

Anesthesia machine provides the control of patient's gas exchange. In addition, anesthesia maintenance is carried out by applying inhalation anesthetics. Morton identified ether in 1846. In 1912, Gwathwey described continue flow anesthetic machine. Then, Boyle modification was reported in 1917. Anesthesia machine reduces the pressure of desired gases to a safe level. Volatile anesthetics are vaporized into the final gas mixture. It controls the flow of oxygen and nitrous oxide. Positive pressure ventilation is provided by anesthesia machine. The risk of delivering hypoxic gas mixture to a patient is avoided.

8.2 Basic Components of Anesthesia Machine (Figs. 8.1 and 8.2)

- Gas supply.
- Flowmeter.
- Vaporizers.
- Breathing circuits.
- Ventilator.
- Scavenging System.
- Monitors.

The anesthesia machine can be divided into three parts as high, intermediate, and low pressure systems. The high pressure system includes cylinders and pressure regulators. Oxygen pressure is kept between 2200 and 45 psig. Nitrous oxide (N_2O) pressure ranges from 750 to 45 psig. The high pressure system provides more constant and proper gas transport to the flowmeter.

The intermediate pressure system starts from pressure regulators and continues to the flow control valves. The pressure of gas supplied from cylinder to the anesthesia machine is 45 psig, while the approximate pipeline pressure is about 50–55 psig. The anesthesia machine receives medical gases from piping network and cylinders. The cylinders are generally used as a back-up supply in case of pipeline failure.

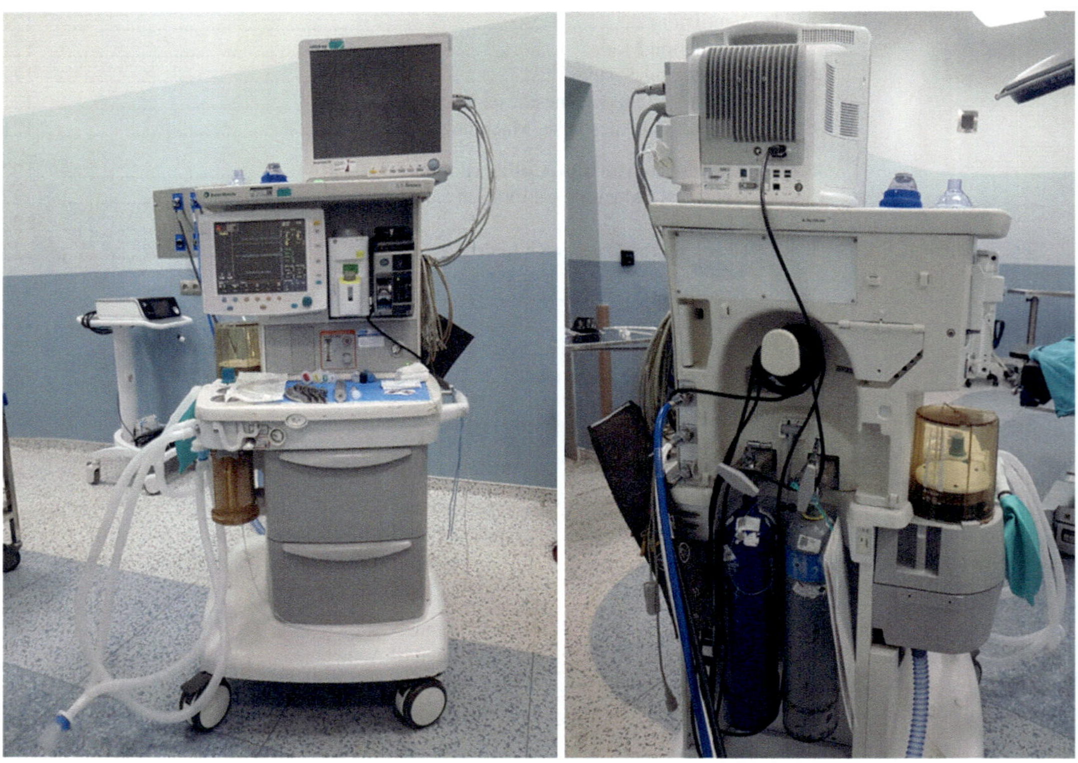

Fig. 8.1 Basic features of anesthesia machine

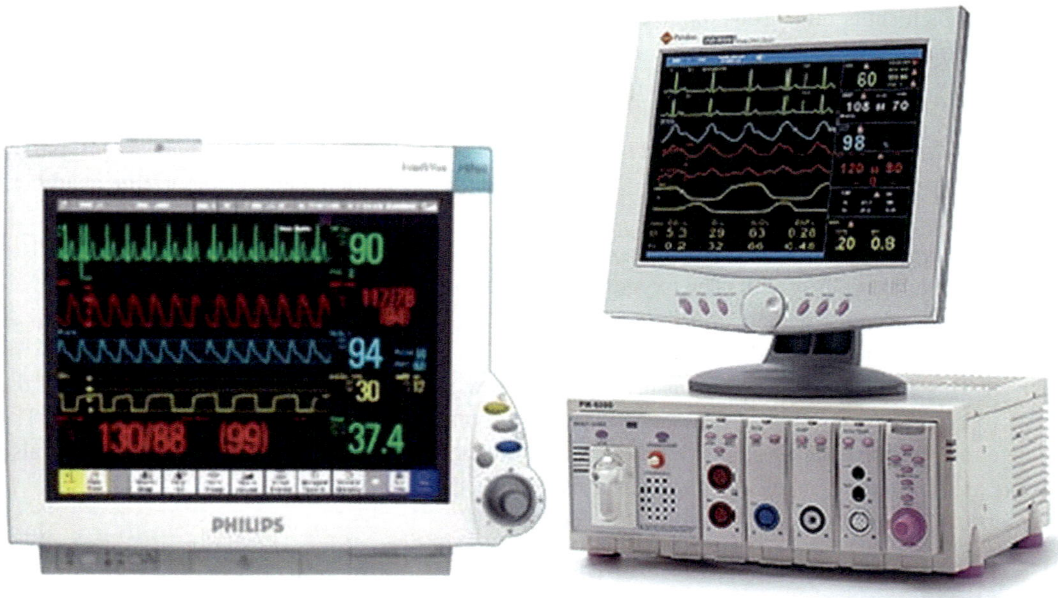

Fig. 8.2 The monitors of anesthesia machine

8.2.1 Oxygen Flush Valve

It is located in the intermediate pressure system with 45–60 psig pressure. It allows the delivery of 35–75 L/min of 100% oxygen flow to breathing circuit. Malfunction of oxygen flush valve may result in barotrauma or awareness during anesthesia. It dilutes the anesthetic agent concentrations.

The hose attachment to the anesthesia machine is specific for each supplied gas. Connectors have safety features such as non-interchangeable screw thread (NIST). Moreover, there are different universal colored flexible hoses for each gas to prevent incorrect connection.

The low pressure system contains the flowmeter tubes, vaporizers, unidirectional valves, and components up to the common gas outlet. The low pressure section is the section distal to the flow control valves. Flowmeter and flow control valves separate intermediate and low pressure systems. Flowmeter regulates the amount of gas that will pass into the low pressure system.

The unidirectional valves prevent gas flow back to the vaporizer during positive pressure ventilation. The tubes have an antistatic coating on both surfaces, preventing the effect of static electricity. There could be electronic flowmeters in the low pressure system as well. There are electronic flowmeters in modern anesthesia machines. In these machines, the data are displayed graphically or numerically on the screen.

8.2.2 Fail-Safe Systems

Fail-safe systems prevent the delivery of a hypoxic mixture of gas to the patient. These systems include pneumatic and electronic alarm devices. When the oxygen pressure drops below a limit set by the manufacturer, it gives an alarm within 5 seconds. This is called 2000 ASTM F1850–00 standard. In addition, the oxygen concentration in the common gas outlet should not be below 19%. Modern anesthesia machines have many safety equipment. The aim is to minimize the risk of hypoxic gas mixture. Fail-safe system is present in all gas lines except oxygen. When oxygen pressure drops, other gases are either completely shut down or their ratio is reduced in proportion to oxygen. Datex-Ohmeda machines feature pressure sensor shut off valve. It works on the off-or-on principle. North American Drager machines have oxygen failure protection device

(OFPD), which shuts off nitrous oxide or allows its proportional flow.

8.2.3 Safety Systems to Prevent Hypoxic Gas Mixture

There is oxygen/nitrous oxide ratio controller in Datex-Ohmeda Link 25 system. The oxygen gear is connected to nitrous oxide gear. When oxygen flow decreases, nitrous oxide flow is directly reduced. This arrangement helps to ensure a minimum oxygen concentration of 25%. The disadvantage of proportional systems is that their sensors are not oxygen specific. This poses a risk of incorrect gas connections. Therefore; it is necessary to use an oxygen analyzer.

8.2.4 Causes of Flowmeter Malfunction

- They could provide wrong measurements because of debris in the flow tube, static electricity or sticking inside the tube.
- Scales may be mixed.

8.2.5 Vaporizers

Vaporizers are the devices which convert liquid anesthetics into vapor and deliver volatile anesthetics to the breathing circuit. Vapor pressure is not affected by atmospheric pressure; it only depends on the characteristics of the volatile agent and the temperature. A liquid's boiling point is the temperature at which its vapor pressure is equal to the atmospheric pressure. Boiling points at 760 mmHg are 22.5 for desflurane, 48.5 for isoflurane, 50.2 for halothane, 56.5 for enflurane, and 58.5 for sevoflurane. All modern vaporizers are agent specific. They are capable of delivering a constant concentration of the agent regardless of temperature changes or flow through the vaporizer.

Electrically heated special vaporizers must be utilized for desflurane because it boils at room temperature. According to the working principle of agent-specific variable by-pass vaporizers, anesthetic gas mixture passes through the vaporizing chamber. The gas flow directed to the vaporizing chamber is saturated with liquid anesthetic agent. These vaporizers are agent specific. In flow over vaporizers, the carrier gas passes over the inhalation agent in vaporizing chamber.

8.2.6 Factors Affecting the Vaporizer Output

Flow rate, temperature and characteristics of the volatile agent affect on vaporizer output. The characteristics of the carrier gas are also effective.

8.2.7 Points to Pay Attention in Vaporizers

- Filling vaporizers with the incorrect anesthetics.
- Contamination.
- Excessive tilting of vaporizers.
- Overfilling.
- Insufficient filling.
- Filling with multiple agents.
- Leaks.

8.3 Carbon Dioxide (CO_2) Elimination

The exhaled CO_2 is chemically bound with granules consisting of alkaline metal and earth metal hydroxides. Sodalyme and barolyme are the most commonly used absorbents. 100 g sodalyme absorbs 26 L CO_2. On the other hand, 100 g barolyme absorbs 18 L of CO_2. When the color change reaches 60–70%, the absorbent is replaced (Table 8.1).

When sodalyme and sevoflurane are combined, Compound A and formaldehyde are formed. Carbon monoxide formation increases with desflurane. New absorbents significantly reduce Compound A formation with Sevoflurane use. Spherasorb does not contain KOH and Amsorb does not contain NaOH and KOH.

Table 8.1 Active substances in the structure of CO2 absorbents which play a role in color change

Active substance in absorbent	Color change
Ethyl violet	White to purple
Cresyl violet	Red to yellow
Ethyl orange	Orange to yellow
Mimosa Z	Red to white
Phenolphthalein	White to pink

8.3.1 Ventilators

Ventilators are classified as single-circuit and double-circuit systems according to the movement mechanism. Modern ventilators are timed and electronically controlled. In a double-circuit ventilator, the driving gas activates the pneumatic system that pushes the bellows. Oxygen or a mixture of oxygen and air are used as pressurized gas. Single-circuit ventilators have special electrically driven motors. They can work more precisely and computer-controlled. This type of ventilator requires no driving gas. An ascending bellows is safer. When the fresh gas flow is cut off, the ascending bellow will collapse; it prevents breathing of hypoxic gas mixture.

8.3.2 Ventilation Modes

In order to provide optimum mechanical ventilation, the pressure, volume, and flow parameters on the ventilator should be adjusted in accordance with the patient's respiratory system. Modes of mechanical ventilation can be classified according to the control of tidal volume. In this regard, volume controlled and pressure controlled modes are available. Volume controlled modes include Continuous mandatory ventilation (VC-CMV), Synchronized intermittent mandatory ventilation (VC-SIMV), and Autoflow. On the other side pressure controlled modes are Continuous mandatory ventilation (PC-CMV), Synchronized intermittent mandatory ventilation (PC-SIMV), Pressure control with volume guarantee (PC-CMV-VG), Pressure support ventilation (PC-PSV), Biphasic positive airway pressure (PC-BIPAP), and Airway Pressure Release Ventilation (PC-APRV). In VC-CMV, there is a constant flow. Peak inspiratory pressure varies according to lung mechanics. In both VC-SIMV and PC-SIMV, the mandatory breaths are synchronized with the patients' breathing effort.

8.3.3 Scavenging System

It consists of two parts: active and passive. In the passive system, gases are discharged with their own pressure. The positive pressure valve is sufficient. In the active system, there is a connection to the hospital's vacuum system. The negative pressure reducing valve protects against the negative pressure of the vacuum system. The positive pressure reducing valve protects against the positive pressure caused by clogged replaceable hoses.

The scavenging system extends the anesthesia circuit. Obstruction in the circuit may occur. In case of obstruction, excessive positive pressure is applied to the respiratory tract, which may cause barotrauma.

8.3.4 Alarm Systems in Anesthesia Machine

There are several safety features in anesthesia machines. These are connected with alarm systems. Oxygen pressure failure system works as a standard to activate an audible alarm when oxygen pressure falls below a safe threshold. The oxygen failure safety system detects failure on pressure and provides an alarm to warn the low level of oxygen. Integral monitor alarms are other types for patient safety.

8.3.5 Monitors of Anesthesia Machine

The monitors provide valuable information about ventilation, oxygenation, hemodynamic parameters, and temperature. Ventilation monitoring includes pulse oximeter, end tidal carbon dioxide measurement, and respiratory rate analysis. Electrocardiogram (ECG), non-invasive and invasive blood pressure monitoring give information about circulation.

8.4 Anesthesia Machine Calibration and Checklist

8.4.1 Anesthesia Machine Calibration

Today, modern anesthesia machines are different than simple pneumatic devices. Anesthesia workstation is consist of vital electrical, electronic, and mechanical components such as computer equipped microprocessors. Therefore, their complex structure makes the calibration, maintenance, and cleaning more complicated. The calibration includes the physical and electrical components of workstation, oxygen supply and the monitor, flowmeters, ventilators vaporizers, and panel connectors. The calibration of oxygen sensor should be performed with both 21% and 100% oxygen. The control of anesthesia device and related equipment should include routine maintenance and calibrations by authorized services. Weekly maintenance and daily checks should be performed by nurse anesthetists or anesthesiologists. It is mostly applied as checklists and should be checked at appropriate time intervals.

8.4.2 Checklist

The American Society of Anesthesiologists (ASA) issued a pre-anesthetic checkout procedure in 2008 as a guide. The items are presented in Table 8.2.

Table 8.2 The list of items to be completed daily

Item to be completed
Item #1: Verify auxiliary oxygen cylinder and self-inflating manual ventilation device are Available & Functioning
Item #2: Verify patient suction is adequate to clear the airway
Item #3: Turn on anesthesia delivery system and confirm that ac power is available.
Item #4: Verify availability of required monitors, including alarms.
Item #5: Verify that pressure is adequate on the spare oxygen cylinder mounted on the anesthesia machine
Item #6: Verify that the piped gas pressures are $\geq$ 50 psig
Item #7: Verify that vaporizers are adequately filled and, if applicable, that the filler ports are tightly closed.
Item #8: Verify that there are no leaks in the gas supply lines between the flowmeters and the common gas outlet
Item #9: Test scavenging system function.
Item #10: Calibrate, or verify calibration of, the oxygen monitor and check the low oxygen alarm.
Item #11: Verify carbon dioxide absorbent is not exhausted
Item #12: Breathing system pressure and leak testing.
Item #13: Verify that gas flows properly through the breathing circuit during both inspiration and exhalation.
Item #14: Document completion of checkout procedures.
Item #15: Confirm ventilator settings and evaluate readiness to deliver ANESTHESIA care. (ANESTHESIA TIME OUT)

8.4.3 Checking the Oxygen Cylinder

Oxygen can be dangerous if not used correctly. Therefore, the check of the cylinder has a vital importance for both patients and health care workers. As oxygen may cause explotion and burns, the safety guidelines should be followed. First, the pressure gauge is checked to prevent the lack of oxygen. Then, the gauge should be checked when the valve is turned on. Afterwards the flowmeter is adjusted. Connections to oxygen delivery devices and oxygen cylinders should be checked for leakage at least once monthly.

8.5 Breathing Systems

8.5.1 Classification

- Open systems.
- Semi-open systems.
- Semi-closed systems.
- Closed systems.

There is no anesthetic gas reservoir balloon in open systems. There is no rebreathing of exhaled gases. These systems are simple and cheap. No breathing resistance occurs. It is used with insufflation by open drop or mask method.

Semi-open systems are flow-controlled, valve-free, and non-rebreathing systems. There are types as Mapleson A, B, C, D, E, and F. The Mapleson circuits are simple, lightweight, and easy to clean. There is low breathing resistance. The disadvantages are that they require high flow rate, there is high heat and moisture loss and there is excessive anesthetic agent mixing into the operating room air.

Mapleson A is named as Magill circuit. It requires very high fresh gas flow to prevent rebreathing in controlled ventilation. Mapleson C is named as Waters' "to and fro" circuit. Mapleson D is Bain circuit. Mapleson E is called as Ayre's T-piece. Mapleson F is Jackson modification. The disadvantage is that it requires high fresh gas flow and waste gas excretion is not sufficient. Advantages are minimal dead space, minimal resistance to breathing, and economy during controlled ventilation.

Bain circuit has coaxial modification. There is fresh gas inlet tubing inside breathing tube. Exhalation occurs via outer tube. During spontaneous ventilation, a fresh gas flow of 200–300 mL/kg/min is required for normocarbia. On the other side, during controlled ventilation, a fresh gas flow of 70 mL/kg/min is needed to prevent rebreathing. The advantages of Bain circuit are that it retains heat and humidity. The disadvantages are unnoticed disconnection, the possibility of kinking of inlet tubing, high flow requirement, and increase in physiological dead space.

Sorting by advantages in spontaneous ventilation is like A > D > C > B; in controlled ventilation it is like D > B > C > A.

8.5.2 Semi-Closed Breathing Systems

It is the most commonly used breathing system in adults and older children. There is CO_2 absorbent. Their disadvantage is that they are large, less potable, and more complex. Resistance is higher in spontaneous ventilation due to valves. Humidity is minimized when the fresh gas flow >5 L/min. Bacteria filter is required. Its advantages are low cost, protection of humidity and heat, reduction in environmental pollution, increased rebreathing with the decrease of fresh gas flow, and very low levels of fresh gas flow.

8.5.3 Closed Breathing Systems

If the fresh gas volume delivered into the system is exactly equal to the amount received by the patient in a certain period of time, this system is called a closed system. The entire volume of expiratory gas returns to the patient after CO_2 is absorbed. Maintaining sufficient gas volume in the system is ensured by the fact that excess gas discharge valve is closed and no leak from the system is present. Closed breathing systems have some hazards such as giving 02 in unknown and insufficient concentrations and administration of potent anesthetic inhalation agent at unknown and excessively high concentrations.

8.6 Conclusion

As a result, anesthesia administration started with open systems using ether. Today, modern devices with increased safety are being used and they address different patient types. Mastering the components of these devices, which play a critical role in anesthesia practice, is crucial for physicians working in this field.

Airway Management and Equipment

9

Massimiliano Sorbello

Error is in the artist, not in the art.

Isaac Newton.

Contents

9.1 Introduction

Airway management is a core skill and a mandatory competence for any physician involved in operatory room, intensive care unit, any invasive or non-invasive procedure requiring sedation (Monitored Anaesthesia Care – MAC, and Non-Operating Room Anaesthesia – NORA), emergency department, and out-of-hospital emergency. Many of the anaesthesia-related accidents are still associated with failed or poor airway management [1, 6] and such an evidence calls for adoption of dedicated guidelines and their implementation, for the need of training and development of dedicated teams, skills, and safety programmes.

M. Sorbello (✉)
Anaesthesia and Intensive Care, AOU Policlinico San Marco, Catania, Italy

N. A. Shallik et al. (eds.), *Improving Anesthesia Technical Staff's Skills*,
https://doi.org/10.1007/978-3-030-88849-7_9

Nevertheless, the statement form Sir Isaac Newton opening this chapter underlines that having guidelines and all necessary devices may not be enough to grant a successful airway management and to provide our ultimate goal, which is patients' safety.

Evidence suggests that many accidents, if not the majority, are not due to a missing device, but rather to a missed planning or preparation of a suitable strategy for a specific patient. Out of any doubt, devices are the key for success, providing they are located in the frame of a safe and effective planning, including rescue options, and that the artist knows exactly how to use the tools.

Finally, we should never forget that the ultimate goal of any airway management strategy should be granting adequate oxygenation to our patients, independently on the device we use, switching the paradigm of airway management from device to a sole target: oxygenation [7].

9.2 Which Equipment and for Which Purpose

The process of managing the airway could be structured into three different phases: ventilation, intubation, and oxygenation. Each of these phases could be considered as elective procedure or emergency (rescue) procedure.

As a result, a possible classification of airway management devices might be designed as indicated in Table 9.1.

Starting from the classification provided in Table I, we will analyse the single devices for airway management, including their role and position in the decisional process of elective procedures and rescue manoeuvres.

9.2.1 Facemask

This device is a simple interface to be interposed between the patient's face and the oxygen/respiratory gas delivery circuit. Different kinds of masks are available, provided in different materials (rubber, PVC, silicon, etc.) and with different designs (anatomical, inflatable, etc.). Many of them could be used for either spontaneous breathing, for anaesthetic induction, emergency ventilation, anaesthetic delivery or non-invasive ventilation. Some specifically designed facemasks include dedicated ports for gas sampling, for sensors placement and sealed ports to allow passage of endoscopic instruments. This is the cases of dedicated endoscopy masks which might

Table 9.1 classification of airway management devices and role in elective/emergency procedure

	Ventilation	Intubation	Oxygenation
Facemask	√□		√□
Oral airway	√□		√□
Nasal airway	□		√
High flow nasal oxygen	(√)		√□
Supraglottic airway	√□		√□
Intubating second generation SAD	√□	√	√□
Laryngoscope		√	
Videolaryngoscope		√	
Tracheal introducer (bougie)		√	(√)
Airway exchange catheters		√	(√)
Flexible bronchoscope		√	
Optical/video stylets		√	
Cricothyrotomy <4 mm ID			√□
Cricothyrotomy >4 mm ID	√□		√□

√ elective procedure.
(√) possible.
□ emergency procedure.

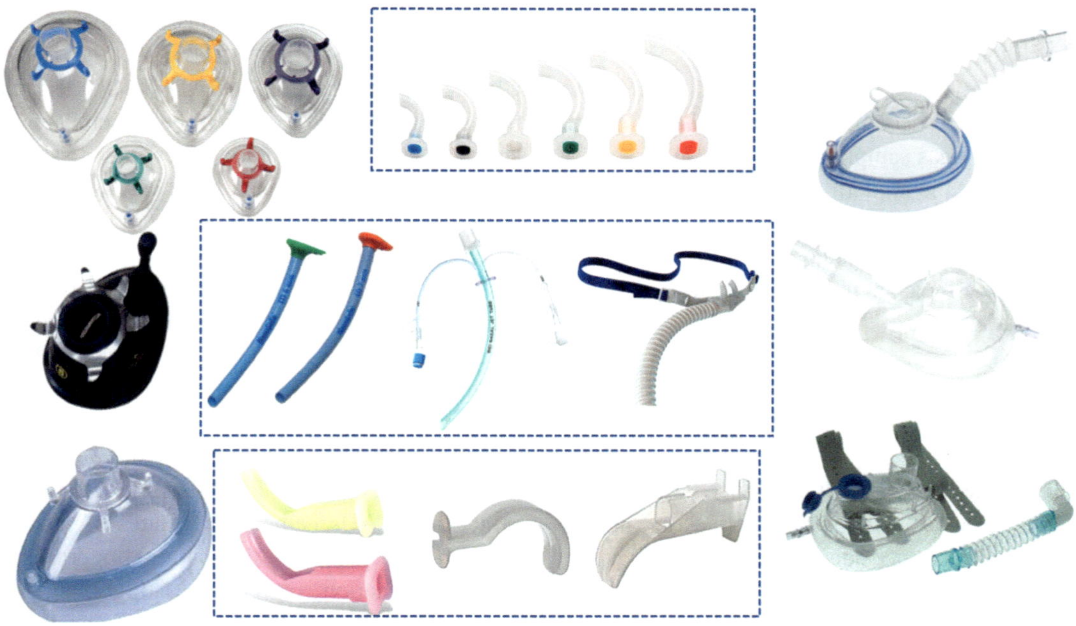

Fig. 9.1 Different models of facemasks (left). Different models of oral airways (middle, top), nasopharyngeal airways (middle, centre), and modified oral airways for bronchoscopic intubation (middle, bottom). Modified facemasks for endoscopic procedures (right)

be used for airway and gastrointestinal endoscopy or to provide extra oxygen administration during bronchoscopies, including flexible bronchoscope intubation [8] (Fig. 9.1).

General anaesthesia might also be delivered via a facemask, which could be an option in a failed intubation scenario with ongoing surgical emergency (in example emergency caesarean delivery), taking account of the increased risk of pulmonary aspiration, given that no facemask may provide adequate airway protection or isolation [9].

In some patients, anatomical and physiological factors may impede adequate facemask ventilation [10, 11], which could be aided adding an oral or nasal airway, and which might end up in a cannot – intubate/cannot – oxygenate (CI-CO) scenario in case of consensual failed intubation.

Facemask ventilation is an important skill, which should be learnt and regularly practiced, as it may represent an easy rescue manoeuvre in case of failed laryngoscopy and intubation [12], during cardiac arrest or for emergency surgery.

Most of the modern facemasks are disposable devices, so they do not get commonly disinfected or sterilized. Care needs to be paid to integrity of packaging, expiring date, and disposal after use.

9.2.2 Oral and Nasal Airways

The purpose of these airway devices is to grant and maintain airway patency during ventilation, might it be spontaneous, assisted, or controlled. Different devices are available modified for different purposes: some of them include gas sampling ports for $EtCO_2$ detection, some of them include drug delivery ports and some others include shafts and guides to facilitate intubation, as for example Berman airway for flexible bronchoscopic intubation. A male 15 mm connector may be included in the oral or nasal airway for direct connection with breathing circuit, and these devices are usually coupled with a facemask for optimized ventilation.

These devices may be used also as an aid for endoscopic procedures, especially if they are provided with gas sampling ports (Fig. 9.1).

Most of the modern oral and nasal airways are disposable devices, so they do not get commonly disinfected or sterilized. Care needs to be paid to integrity of packaging, expiring date, and disposal after use.

9.2.3 High Flow Nasal Oxygen

HFNO has been recently introduced as a valuable airway device for many purposes; initially designed to provide delivery of humidified warmed oxygen, HFNO is nowadays used for preoxygenation, procedural apnoeic oxygenation (the so-called *trans-nasal humidified rapid insufflation ventilatory exchange*, THRIVE), ventilation of the obstructed airway, support for airway instrumentation including flexible bronchoscope intubation and postoperative oxygen delivery, thanks to the ability of HFNO to generate a minimal positive airway pressure [13, 14]. Many uses have still to be validated by robust data, but some evidence addresses to extended applications of this technique. The device consists of soft nasal cannulas, provided in recent version with carbon dioxide sampling line, of a dedicated circuit including an electronic machine providing humidification and warming of inhalatory mixture, with possibility to provide a 5–70 litres per minute flow.

9.2.4 Supraglottic Airway Devices

The laryngeal mask, introduced by Dr. Archie Brain in the last decade of the past century, has probably represented one of the few revolutions airway management, acting as something in between a facemask and endotracheal intubation. The LMA was the first of a new species, with so many different devices from many manufacturers available today, each of them with specific and more or less valuable characteristics. In such a large availability of supraglottic airway devices (SADs) [15], a tentative classification might include first generation SADs (like the LMA Classic), second generation SADs (characterized by a gastric access for gastric tube placement and stomach emptying and a higher sealing pressure), and specific second generation SADs (which some authors address as third generation SADs) with particular features, including dedicated devices for specific procedures (such as gastrointestinal dedicated SADs as LMA-Gastro – Teleflex Medical, or Gastro-laryngeal Tube – VBM Medizintechnik) and advanced intubating features [16].

Particularly, if compared with the very first intubating SAD, the LMA-Fastrach, modern intubatable SADs gather the features of second generation SADs with intubation opportunity. This combination represents a high-valuable option when facing a difficult or failed intubation, with or without concurrent ventilation difficulty. In such a case, a second generation intubatable SAD might be placed, granting ventilation, airway control, and airway protection and allowing a subsequent flexible bronchoscope aided intubation through the SAD, with option to maintain ventilation and oxygenation thorough the procedure [17] (Fig. 9.2).

Noticeably, the most important difference between first and second generation SADs, as supported by literature data, and particularly the National Audit Project 4 from UK [1], is the ability of these latter to provide a higher degree of airway protection, including reduction of potential for aspiration. These feature poses second generation SADs as the first-line rescue device in case of failed intubation with maintained or compromised facemask ventilation, allowing rescue of patient's oxygenation and providing a controlled airway suitable for continuing emergency cases; this might be the classical scenario of failed intubation in emergency obstetric case, where a second-generation SAD could be used to continue surgery. If a second generation intubatable SAD is positioned, at any time an endotracheal intubation with bronchoscopic aid may be performed [18].

More recent supraglottic devices are disposable devices, so they do not get commonly disin-

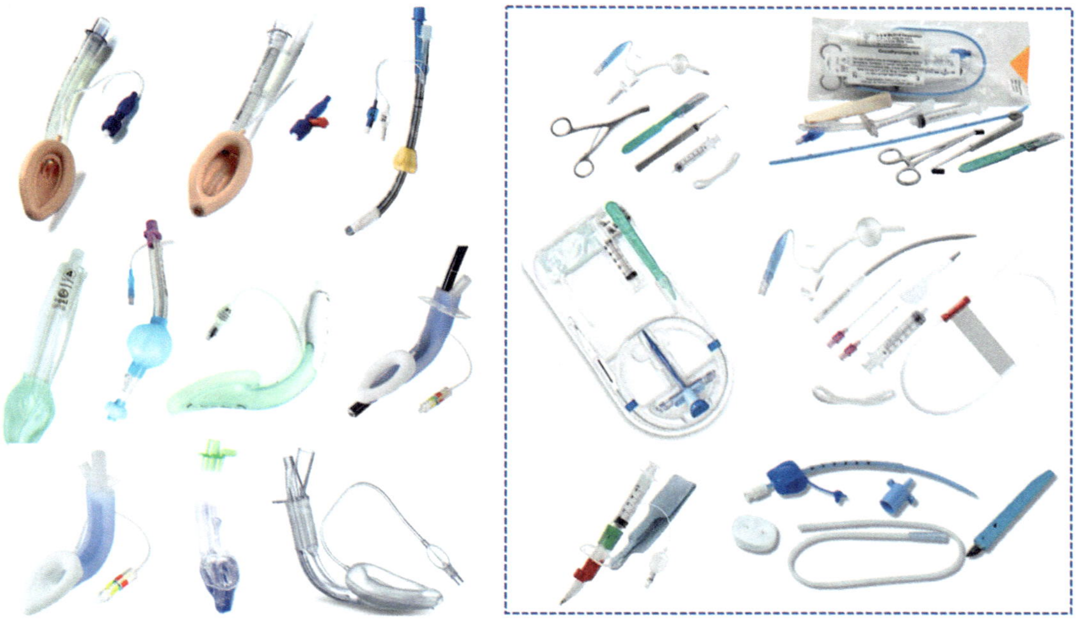

Fig. 9.2 Different models of supraglottic airway devices: first and second generation; intubatable; modified for endoscopy (left). Different models for cricothyrotomy (eFONA) with different techniques (right)

fected or sterilized. Care needs to be paid to integrity of packaging, expiring date, and disposal after use.

Some devices remain reusable, with a limited number of sterilizations allowed; the procedure needs to be carefully performed and monitored, using dedicated checklists to track the number of sterilisations and the efficiency of the process.

9.2.5 Laryngoscopy and Videolaryngoscopy

Laryngoscopy, introduced by Sir Macintosh, has been considered one of the most important contributions towards safety in general anaesthesia.

Direct laryngoscopy is based on achievement of the *line of sight* [19], which is aligning the operator's eye with the laryngeal inlet. Due to anatomical factors [20] and to operator's experience [21] such an achievement might not always be possible, thus resulting in a certain failure range of laryngoscopy and intubation. In the last years, new devices for laryngoscopy have been introduced in clinical practice: videolaryngoscopes (Fig. 9.3). They are provided with normal or the so-called hyper-angulated blades and a video system allowing to move the operator's eye inside the patients' airways, with result of a global improvement in laryngoscopy, and a sort of difficulty shift, also named "visual paradox," towards intubation difficulty rather than laryngoscopy difficulty.

In a certain, though small, number of cases, in front of an optimal or suboptimal laryngoscopy, difficulties in addressing the tube in trachea might be encountered.

There is great enthusiasm and evidence favouring use of videolaryngoscopes, with special emphasis to rescue a failed conventional (direct) laryngoscopy, if not as first choice for any intubation [22].

Further studies will address precise answers, including an exhaustive classification of these devices (Macintosh blade vs. hyper-angulated blade; channeled vs. unchanneled devices), a clear definition of difficult videolaryngoscopy predictive indexes, and univocal recommendations and guidelines for their use. Noticeably, no videolaryngo-

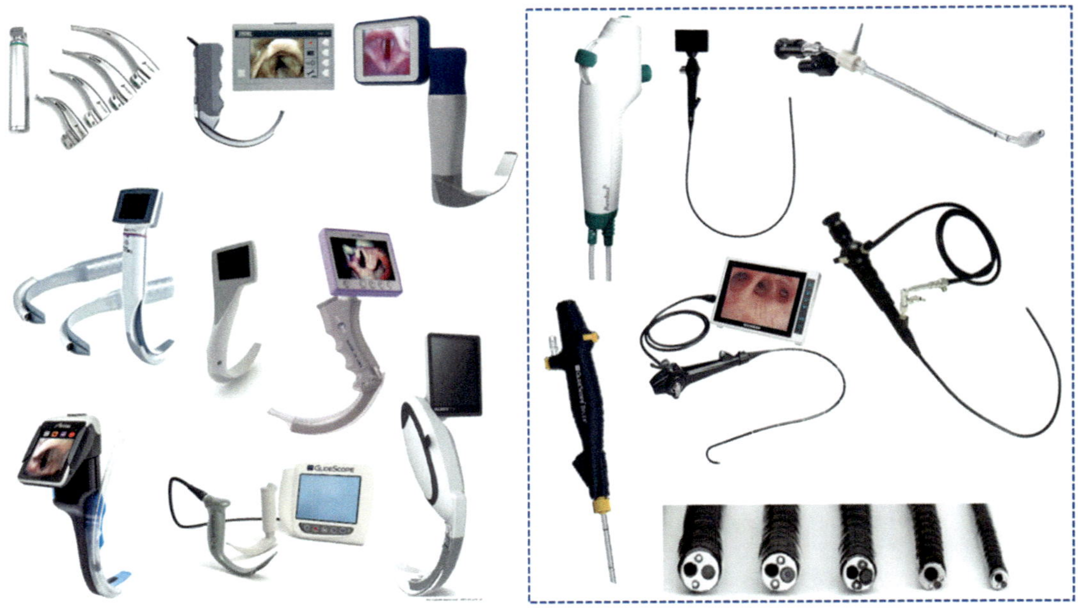

Fig. 9.3 Different models of videolaryngoscopes (channeled, unchanneled, portable) and on top left a classic Macintosh laryngoscope (left). Different models of flexible bronchoscopes (optical, video-endoscopes) and optical stylets (right)

scope can provide patients' oxygenation, so they cannot be considered as a rescue tool for difficult ventilation or severely desaturating patients [23].

Interestingly, recent studies indicate the possibility to use videolaryngoscopes for awake intubation, after adequate topicalization of the airway and eventual sedation of the patient: available information show that performance, appraisal, and success are similar to flexible bronchoscope awake intubation but with higher operator's satisfaction and confidence [24].

As a further remark, videolaryngoscopes are a promising tool, with improved success rate for laryngoscopy, a different learning curve, opportunity for targeted help, team-based decision making, education (given the opportunity of a shared video output) and, probably, implications for a better patients' outcome [25].

Both laryngoscopes and videolaryngoscope may come as reusable or disposable devices. Depending on the characteristics, a different care is needed either for adequate check of package integrity, expiring date and disposal after use or monitoring and tracking of sterilization processes.

9.2.6 Tracheal Introducers (Bougie) and Airway Exchange Catheters

The first prototype of a bougie was made out of a urinary catheter and it was designed to aid intubation with a straight laryngoscopic blade in mid '900 s. Since then, the bougie (tracheal introducer) was largely used as intubation aid. It consists of a guide, longer than a stylet, usually malleable and with an angled or coudè tip designed to aid intubation with limited laryngeal exposure (glottis partly visible).

The original Eschmann guide was a reusable bougie, later joined by many devices from different manufacturers, but made out of plastic materials (PVC, PET, Teflon, etc..) with different features (hollow, different colours, etc..) but all based on the same principle of the Eschmann guide.

Between these devices, designed as disposable and single-patient, the Frova introducer seems to outperform other devices.

Given their stiffness, particular care should be adopted in their use, oxygen administration through hollow introducers should be avoided, also in low flows, and their use requires at least a partial view of the larynx (Cormack-Lehane grades I, II, IIe, III).

Tracheal introducers are now experiencing a second youth, in light of recent studies suggesting the possibility to couple them with videolaryngoscopes, with evidence of improving success rate of these devices [26, 27].

Other airway catheters, known as airway exchange catheters are also available: they are longer than an introducer, and often hollow to permit (prudent) oxygen administration (no more than one litre per minute). They were designed to allow tube exchange manoeuvres with aim to maintain airway control, and the same precautions recommended for tracheal introducers should be adopted.

Use of a laryngoscope (or better a videolaryngoscope) is recommended thorough the tube exchange manoeuver, and particular care should be adopted for depth of insertion. Some catheters, including introducers, are packed with dedicated connectors for oxygen administration [28].

Airway exchange catheters, including modified versions, have been designed also to allow a "protected" or "staged" extubation: inserted in the tracheal tube before removal, they are left in place for a certain time period in the awake recovered patient, acting as a guide for re-intubation should it be needed [29]. Same precautions and prudence should be adopted also in this use [30], maintaining a recuse plan in case of re-intubation failure [31].

All modern airway catheters are disposable devices, so they do not get commonly disinfected or sterilized. Care needs to be paid to integrity of packaging, expiring date, and disposal after use.

9.2.7 Flexible Bronchoscope and Optical Stylets

The idea of bringing the doctor's eye inside the human body took shape when medical research became familiar with optical fibres and cold light systems. The original design of flexible optical systems included an optical fibres bunch (coherent and incoherent) embedded in a protective sheet and connected to an ocular and a light source, with dedicated leverage system to manoeuvre the instrument's tip (Fig. 9.3).

This principle has been maintained for many years and updated and modernized, with different calibre instruments allowing precise leveraging and orientation, dedicated working and suction channels, opportunity to be connected to external screens, and electronic data storage systems.

Recently, the optical fibres have been substituted with video sensors and electronics, so that the instrument do maintain their familiar design and functions, while being much more resistant and less keen to rupture or damage, with no need of external light sources, immediate digital data storage, and easy transportability. The new devices are nowadays named *flexible video-endoscopes* and their use is significant in airway management.

This evolution has also allowed production of reasonable cost single use devices, which can be used minimizing cross-infection risks and reducing the costs of procedures of disinfection, sterilization and re-packaging [32]. They are available from different manufacturers, in different sizes and with specific features.

Flexible bronchoscopes are used in ICU for percutaneous tracheostomy, bronchial suctioning, and bacteriological sampling, for visual inspection of the airway; they are used in airway surgery and lung separation procedures, and they can be used also for preoperative evaluation, still representing the gold standard for awake tracheal intubation in severe difficult airways with risk of difficult/impossible ventilation [33].

For the last application, a careful evaluation and preparation of the patient are of utmost importance; airway topicalization must be adequately granted (use of swabs, dedicated atomizers and distillers, dedicated oral/nasal airways, and nerve blocks), and titrated and monitored sedation might be applied [34]. Supplemental oxygen may be delivered during the procedure, including HFNO, and intubation may also be performed trough dedicated airways or, mostly in asleep patients, through intubatable SADs [35].

Based on a similar principle, but combining the familiar use of a stylet with direct vision, optical and video stylets represent other alternative resource in airway management. In these devices, the device's body is typically rigid, and like a stylet it can be malleable or steerable, with embedded video system. The tube is preloaded on the stylet and it is subsequently addressed through the larynx into the airway. More evidence is needed to support their routine use, which remains strictly operators' experience dependent [36], but they are getting diffusion and they are available from different manufacturers with specific functions, portability, steerable options and embedded monitor system.

Both reusable flexible scopes and optical/video stylets need to be cleaned and sterilized between uses: precise and device-specific procedures need to be undertaken, with a special emphasis for electronic parts and operative channels and protective sheets, not to compromise devices' integrity and to grant patients' safety.

When using fibre-optical devices, special care is needed in handling, cleaning, sterilizing, and storage procedures, given the risk of glass-fibres breakage (resulting in poor vision quality) and external sheath tear or rupture (resulting in the loss of integrity, risk of contamination, and malfunction). Any device has mechanical parts (levering and tip control) which may also be damaged in case of improper handling, sterilisation and storage procedures.

9.2.8 Cricothyrotomy

In exceptional circumstances, a contemporary difficult if not impossible ventilation and intubation may occur, resulting in the so called cannot intubate – cannot oxygenate (CI-CO) scenario. In such a situation, emergency oxygenation needs to be urgently delivered to the patient, before hypoxic brain damage occurs.

The fastest and most effective way to achieve this goal is performing an emergency front of neck access (eFONA). Different techniques have been described, but they can be separated in surgical and percutaneous. The first may require a set of surgical instruments, or, as from recent indications, a simple scalpel, a bougie/stylet, and a small bore tracheal tube (so-called scalpel-bougie-technique).

The second is usually performed with dedicated cricothyrotomy sets which might be distinguished in Seldinger-based or non-Seldinger-based techniques (Fig. 9.2).

Seldinger devices come with a needle and a Seldinger guide on which a dilator and a cricothyrotomy cannula are subsequently railroaded once the guide is positioned in the tracheal lumen through the cricothyroideal membrane. A potential advantage of this approach is the separation of airway identification and cannula insertion.

The non-Seldinger techniques are based upon Trocar-like devices, with needle or sharp introducer assembled with the cannula, which enters the trachea directly without a guide intermediate passage. A potential advantage is the less time needed to perform the technique.

There is no evidence, nor probably may ever be, that one technique is superior to the other [37]: what we know today is that most of eFONA are performed too late, and many of them derive from human error and non-technical issues [38]. It is, thus, of paramount importance to prepare an adequate airway plan and strategy so to avoid any CI-CO scenario; should it occur, early FONA is a life-saving procedure, and all the airway team is called to know the devices adopted and to be familiar with the procedure, acting in a collective approach aimed to avoid FONA or to perform it quickly and timely if needed [39].

Cricothyrotomy kits are usually disposable, so special care needs to be adopted during disposal procedures, with special emphasis on needles and sharp devices which may result in healthcare providers injuries.

9.2.9 Other Airway Management Devices

Many other devices are available as airway management tools; some of them need to be adequately tested, and many more will come, starting from new SADs models to new videolaryngoscopes or stylets or revolutionary tools.

Some other devices are not primarily airway management devices, but their function is strictly related to safety of airway management procedures or to extended applications:

- Dedicated patients' positioners or supports (such as ramped position pillows for obese patients [40], jaw-trust performing devices for difficult ventilation or assistance of spontaneous breathing [41], etcetera) (Fig. 9.4).
- Capnography: delayed or unrecognized oesophageal intubation remains one of the leading causes of airway management related accidents [1–6, 42]. Tube position confirmation may be obtained with direct visualization (shared and double-checked if a videolaryngoscope is used) of tube between vocal cords or with endoscopic examination of the airway with consensual view of endotracheal tube and trachea (which is not routine practice). The gold standard remains detection of normal morphology, repeated capnographic waves; this finding, though with different morphology, is obtained also during cardiopulmonary resuscitation[1], and its absence should be assumed as failed or oesophageal intubation.
- Ultrasounds: point of care ultrasound is a largely available, easy to perform and non-invasive tool gaining room also in airway management practice. It has been extensively described either as adjunct for preoperative airway evaluation [43] and as a tool to confirm directly or indirectly a correct endotracheal intubation [44]. Aside from ultrasounds, we list also the virtual endoscopy techniques as supporting tools to assist preoperative airway evaluation [45].
- Robotic intubation: in a parallel with surgical robots, in recent years some prototypes have been developed to assist intubation [46]. No systems are actually validated, but they may be proposed in the forthcoming years as intubation support.

Extra-Corporeal Membrane Oxygenation (ECMO): this advanced and invasive extracorporeal support technique, originally designed for cardiac surgery, has recently been used for treatment of severe respiratory failure in already intu-

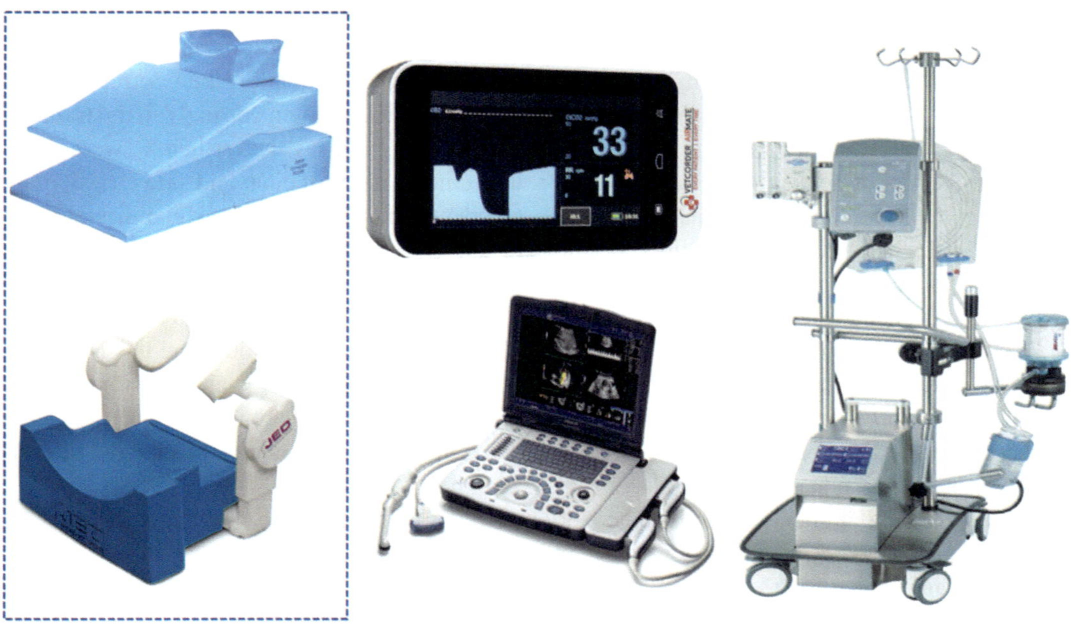

Fig. 9.4 Other devices used in airway management: patients' positioning systems (left). Capnography monitor, ultrasound machine, and ECMO machine

bated patients in Intensive Care Unit, and it has also been recently proposed as adjunct or surrogate for tracheal intubation in patients with "impossible airways" such as severe and/or extended tracheal stenosis, inaccessible airways, critical patients or conflictual surgical field [47]. The technique is invasive, it requires dedicated personnel and skills and its use is a niche which needs anyway to be listed between airway management devices (Fig. 9.4).

9.3 Roles and Tasks of Anaesthesia Technicians, Technologists or Anaesthesia Nurses

Anaesthesia technicians, technologists, and nurses play an important role in airway management. They need to know the equipment, so to provide adequate preparation, storage, disinfection or sterilization, and to provide meaningful, oriented, and targeted help to physicians in charge of airway management.

Maintaining a dedicated (difficult) airway trolley is of utmost importance, as this is a key point to manage adequately any airway management scenario and emergency. A standardized and uniform storage of all airway devices is functional to their easy finding and retrieval during any procedure, with the motto *everything in its place, a place for everything*. Storage may respect a local policy or a sequential scheme, which should be team-discussed and shared. Use of checklists is highly recommended either to double check availability and restoring of any device and to optimize handover procedures.

Disinfection and sterilization of reusable devices is a critical process, conditioning safety of healthcare providers and patients. Strict respect of standardized procedures is mandatory, and local sterilization/handling procedures may be developed. Similar attention needs to be paid also for disposable devices, checking integrity of packaging and expiry date. These tasks are becoming more important, given the diffusion of disposable devices (such as laryngoscopes, videolaryngoscopes, and video-endoscopes) and in case of pandemic events such as the recent COVID-19 surge.

In such a setting, an airway cart may be equipped also with Personal Protective Equipment (PPE) storage and with portable monitors to allow tube position control or other procedures.

Education and knowledge of devices and techniques are extremely important, because the best way to prepare the crisis is getting trained with regular and daily practice. In this perspective, new tools such as high-fidelity simulation and non-technical skills development are extremely important and they should become part of any training and educational process in airway management, so to develop a perfectly working team structure and activity, a clear communication, and all conditions to manage adequately either elective and emergency airway management scenarios [7].

9.4 Conclusions

Many devices and techniques are available for airway management, with either basic and advanced techniques for both elective/planned and emergency/rescue airway control.

Knowledge of devices is mandatory and of utmost importance to allow their correct use and above all to locate them correctly in the frame of a decisional pathway. Nevertheless, we need to underline that a proficient and safe airway management is not based upon availability and use of any device, for advanced and performing it may be [48].

We need to focus on the main target, which is always patients' oxygenation, and this is the first and only goal we need to achieve with maximal priority. Once oxygenation is granted, any technique may be used providing availability of tools and knowledge and skill.

Teamwork, effective communication, planning, definition of a strategy, multidisciplinary collaboration are the keys of a successful airway management, accidents, and critical events being most frequently associated with non-technical issues.

Despite any device, only good sense, prudence, and adequate planning seem to be the most effective techniques, the only irreplaceable airway management tool remaining our brain.

References

1. Cook TM, Woodall N, Harper J, Benger J. Fourth National Audit Project. Major complications of airway management in the UK: results of the fourth National Audit Project of the Royal College of Anaesthetists and the difficult airway society. Part 2: intensive care and emergency departments. Br J Anaesth. 2011;106:632–42.
2. Joffe AM, Aziz MF, Posner KL, Duggan LV, Mincer SL, Domino KB. Management of Difficult Tracheal Intubation: a closed claims analysis. Anesthesiology. 2019;131:818–29.
3. Rosenstock CV, Nørskov AK, Wetterslev J, Lundstrøm LH. Danish Anaesthesia database. Emergency surgical airway management in Denmark: a cohort study of 452 461 patients registered in the Danish Anaesthesia database. Br J Anaesth. 2016;117(Suppl 1):i75–82.
4. Fornebo I, Simonsen KA, Bukholm IRK, Kongsgaard UE. Claims for compensation after injuries related to airway management: a nationwide study covering 15 years. Acta Anaesthesiol Scand. 2017;61:781–9.
5. Woodward ZG, Urman RD, Domino KB. Safety of non-operating room Anaesthesia: a closed claims update. Anesthesiol Clin. 2017;35:569–81.
6. Robbertze R, Posner KL, Domino KB. Closed claims review of anaesthesia for procedures outside the operating room. Curr Opin Anaesthesiol. 2006;19:436–42.
7. Sorbello M, Afshari A, De Hert S. Device or target? A paradigm shift in airway management: implications for guidelines, clinical practice and teaching. Eur J Anaesthesiol. 2018;35:811–4.
8. Aoyama K, Yasunaga E, Takenaka I, Kadoya T, Sata T, Shigematsu A. Positive pressure ventilation during fibreoptic intubation: comparison of the laryngeal mask airway, intubating laryngeal mask and endoscopy mask techniques. Br J Anaesth. 2002;88:246–54.
9. Bacci A, Lewis G, Baltag V, Betrán AP. The introduction of confidential enquiries into maternal deaths and near-miss case reviews in the WHO European region. Reprod Health Matters. 2007;15:145–52.
10. Sato S, Hasegawa M, Okuyama M, Okazaki J, Kitamura Y, Sato Y, et al. Mask ventilation during induction of general Anaesthesia: influences of obstructive sleep apnea. Anesthesiology. 2017;126:28–38.
11. Kheterpal S, Healy D, Aziz MF, Shanks AM, Freundlich RE, Linton F, et al. Multicenter perioperative outcomes group (MPOG) perioperative clinical research committee. Incidence, predictors, and outcome of difficult mask ventilation combined with difficult laryngoscopy: a report from the multicenter perioperative outcomes group. Anesthesiology. 2013;119:1360–9.
12. Petrini F, Accorsi A, Adrario E, Agrò F, Amicucci G, Antonelli M, et al. Gruppo di studio SIAARTI "vie Aeree Difficili"; IRC e SARNePI; task force. Recommendations for airway control and difficult airway management. Minerva Anestesiol. 2005;71:617–57.
13. Mir F, Patel A, Iqbal R, Cecconi M, Nouraei SA. A randomised controlled trial comparing transnasal humidified rapid insufflation ventilatory exchange (THRIVE) pre-oxygenation with facemask pre-oxygenation in patients undergoing rapid sequence induction of anaesthesia. Anaesthesia. 2017;72:439–43.
14. Sorbello M, Mir F, McNarry AF. THRIVE? The answer, my friend, is blowing in the (high flow) wind! Trends Anaesth Crit Care. 2018;22:63.
15. Sorbello M. Evolution of supraglottic airway devices: the Darwinian perspective. Minerva Anestesiol. 2018;84:297–300.
16. Sorbello M, Pulvirenti GS, Pluchino D, Skinner M. State of the art in airway management during GI endoscopy: the missing pieces. Dig Dis Sci. 2017;62:1385–7.
17. Sorbello M, Cortese G, Gaçonnet C, Skinner M. A modified Bailey's manoeuvre for supraglottic airway continuum using LMA protector™. Indian J Anaesth. 2019;63:78–80.
18. Frova G, Sorbello M. Algorithms for difficult airway management: a review. Minerva Anestesiol. 2009;75:201–9.
19. Cooper RM. Laryngoscopy — its past and future. Can J Anesth. 2004;51(Suppl 1):R21.
20. Levitan RM, Heitz JW, Sweeney M, Cooper RM. The complexities of tracheal intubation with direct laryngoscopy and alternative intubation devices. Ann Emerg Med. 2011;57:240–7.
21. Mulcaster JT, Mills J, Hung OR, MacQuarrie K, Law JA, Pytka S, Imrie D, Field C. Laryngoscopic intubation: learning and performance. Anesthesiology. 2003;98:23–7.
22. Piepho T, Cavus E, Noppens R, Byhahn C, Dörges V, Zwissler B, Timmermann A, German Society of Anesthesiology and Intensive Care Medicine. S1 guidelines on airway management. Anaesthesist. 2015;64:859–73.
23. Sgalambro F, Sorbello M. Videolaryngoscopy and the search for the holy grail. Br J Anaesth. 2017;118:471–2.
24. Alhomary M, Ramadan E, Curran E, Walsh SR. Videolaryngoscopy vs. fibreoptic bronchoscopy for awake tracheal intubation: a systematic review and meta-analysis. Anaesthesia. 2018;73:1151–61.
25. Lewis SR, Butler AR, Parker J, Cook TM, Schofield-Robinson OJ, Smith AF. Videolaryngoscopy versus direct laryngoscopy for adult patients requiring tracheal intubation: a Cochrane systematic review. Br J Anaesth. 2017;119:369–83.

26. Aziz MF, Brambrink AM, Healy DW, Willett AW, Shanks A, Tremper T, Jameson L, Ragheb J, Biggs DA, Paganelli WC, Rao J, Epps JL, Colquhoun DA, Bakke P, Kheterpal S. Success of intubation rescue techniques after failed direct laryngoscopy in adults: a retrospective comparative analysis from the multicenter perioperative outcomes group. Anesthesiology. 2016;125:656–66.
27. Driver BE, Prekker ME, Klein LR, et al. Effect of use of a Bougie vs endotracheal tube and stylet on first-attempt intubation success among patients with difficult airways undergoing emergency intubation: a randomized clinical trial. JAMA. 2018;319:2179–89.
28. Axe R, Middleditch A, Kelly FE, Batchelor TJ, Cook TM. Macroscopic barotrauma caused by stiff and soft-tipped airway exchange catheters: an in vitro case series. Anesth Analg. 2015;120:355–61.
29. Loudermilk EP, Hartmannsgruber M, Stoltzfus DP, Langevin PB. A prospective study of the safety of tracheal extubation using a pediatric airway exchange catheter for patients with a known difficult airway. Chest. 1997;111:1660–5.
30. Sorbello M, Frova G. When the end is really the end? The extubation in the difficult airway patient. Minerva Anestesiol. 2013;79:194–9.
31. Corso RM, Sorbello M, Mecugni D, et al. Safety and efficacy of a staged-Extubation-set in patients with difficult airway: a prospective multicenter study [published online ahead of print, 2020 mar 6]. Minerva Anestesiol. 2020; https://doi.org/10.23736/S0375-9393.20.14105-1.
32. Mouritsen JM, Ehlers L, Kovaleva J, Ahmad I, El-Boghdadly K. A systematic review and cost effectiveness analysis of reusable vs. single-use flexible bronchoscopes. Anaesthesia. 2020;7:529–40.
33. Heidegger T, Schnider TW. "awake" or "sedated": safe flexible Bronchoscopic intubation of the difficult airway. Anesth Analg. 2017;124:996–7.
34. Cabrini L, Baiardo Redaelli M, Ball L, et al. Awake Fiberoptic intubation protocols in the operating room for anticipated difficult airway: a systematic review and meta-analysis of randomized controlled trials. Anesth Analg. 2019;128:971–80.
35. Zou T, Huang Z, Hu X, Cai G, He M, Wang S, Huang P, Yu B. Clinical application of a novel endoscopic mask: a randomized controlled, multi-center trial in patients undergoing awake fiberoptic bronchoscopic intubation. BMC Anesthesiol. 2017;17(1):79.
36. Gravenstein D, Liem EB, Bjoraker DG. Alternative management techniques for the difficult airway: optical stylets. Curr Opin Anaesthesiol. 2004;17:495–8.
37. Onrubia X, Frova G, Sorbello M. Cricothyrotomy: a narrative review. Trends Anaesth Crit Care 2018. https://doi.org/10.1016/j.tacc.2018.06.001.
38. Timmermann A, Chrimes N, Hagberg CA. Need to consider human factors when determining first-line technique for emergency front-of-neck access. Br J Anaesth. 2016;117:5–7.
39. Chrimes N, Cook TM. Critical airways, critical language. Br J Anaesth. 2017;118:649–54.
40. Petrini F, Di Giacinto I, Cataldo R, Esposito C, Pavoni V, Donato P, et al. Perioperative and periprocedural airway management and respiratory safety for the obese patient: 2016 SIAARTI Consensus. Minerva Anestesiol. 2016;82:1314–35.
41. Altschul DJ, Vats T, Unda SR, Osborn I, McHenry J, Zampolin R. Jaw elevation device: tool for neck immobilization to facilitate recovery in endovascular Thrombectomy via Transcervical access. World Neurosurg. 2020;140:109–13.
42. Honardar MR, Posner KL, Domino KB. Delayed detection of esophageal intubation in Anaesthesia malpractice claims: brief report of a case series. Anesth Analg. 2017;125:1948–51.
43. Falcetta S, Cavallo S, Gabbanelli V, Pelaia P, Sorbello M, Zdravkovic I, et al. Evaluation of two neck ultrasound measurements as predictors of difficult direct laryngoscopy: a prospective observational study. Eur J Anaesthesiol. 2018;35:605–12.
44. Rahmani F, Parsian Z, Shahsavarinia K, Pouraghaei M, Negargar S, Mehdizadeh Esfanjani R, Soleimanpour H. Diagnostic value of sonography for confirmation of endotracheal intubation in the emergency department. Anesth Pain Med. 2017;7(6):e58350.
45. Ahmad I, Millhoff B, John M, Andi K, Oakley R. Virtual endoscopy--a new assessment tool in difficult airway management. J Clin Anesth 2015; 27: 508–513.
46. Biro P, Hofmann P, Gage D, et al. Automated tracheal intubation in an airway manikin using a robotic endoscope: a proof of concept study. Anaesthesia. 2020;75(7):881–6.
47. Malpas G, Hung O, Gilchrist A, Wong C, Kent B, Hirsch GM, Hart RD. The use of extracorporeal membrane oxygenation in the anticipated difficult airway: a case report and systematic review. Can J Anaesth. 2018;65:685–97.
48. Sorbello M, Petrini F. Airway spider or airway spiders? Anaesthesia. 2018;73:953–4.

Scavenging, Medical Gas Pipelines, and Vacuum Systems

10

Nabil A. Shallik, Wael Abdulmajeed Eldegowa,
Mohammed Omar Zekri,
and Muhammad Firas Alhammad

Contents

N. A. Shallik · W. A. Eldegowa (✉) · M. O. Zekri
M. F. Alhammad
Department of Anesthesia, ICU and Perioperative Medicine, Hamad Medical Corporation, Doha, Qatar
e-mail: nshallik@hamad.qa; WEldegowa@hamad.qa; MZekri@hamad.qa; MAlhammad@hamad.qa

N. A. Shallik et al. (eds.), *Improving Anesthesia Technical Staff's Skills*,
https://doi.org/10.1007/978-3-030-88849-7_10

10.1 Introduction

Scavenging system is necessary to prevent contamination and pollution of the operating theater via collecting excess anesthetic gases and vapors from the breathing system and disposing them outside the working environment.

10.2 Definitions

Scavenging system is defined as a system for collecting and removing of vented anesthetic gases from the Operating Room (OR). In fact, these anesthetic gases and volatile anesthetics are exceeding the amount needed for the patient.

10.3 A Complete System Consists of Four Parts: (Fig. 10.1)

1. *Collecting tubes:* It is usually connected to APL valve and relief valve to collect any extra anesthetic gases and volatile anesthetics.
2. *Transferring tubes* (Fig. 10.2).
3. *Scavenging interface:* It is acts as a safety part and it protects the breathing circuit from any positive or negative pressure change.
4. *Disposal tubing:* It carries gas from interface to disposal assembly. *Gas disposal assembly*: which has two types, active or passive (old one), nowadays days active is the most common and it utilizes the hospital suction system.

10.4 Types of Scavenging Systems

10.4.1 Active Anesthesia Gas Scavenging Systems (AGSS)

There are several versions of the active Anesthesia Gas Scavenging System (AGSS) available depending on the hospital's type of waste gas disposal system. Each version has a 1-L reservoir to capture peak exhaust flows that briefly exceed the extract flow.

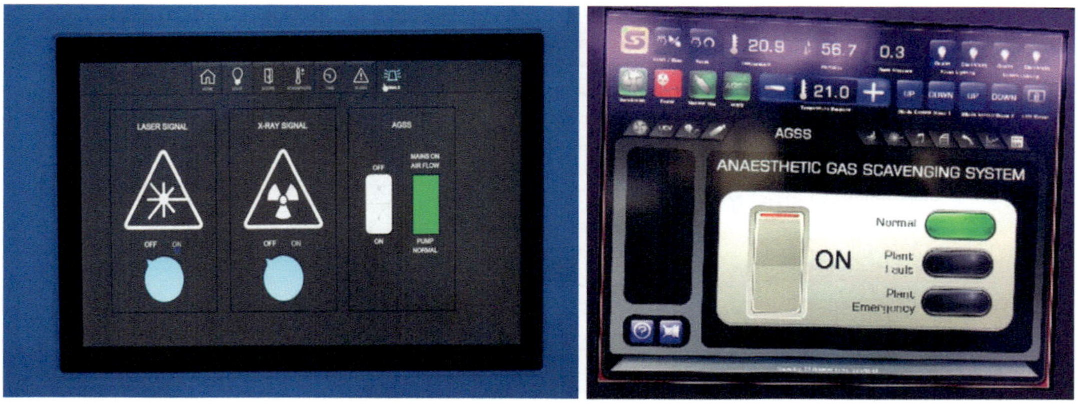

Fig. 10.1 Anesthesia gas scavenging system control panel

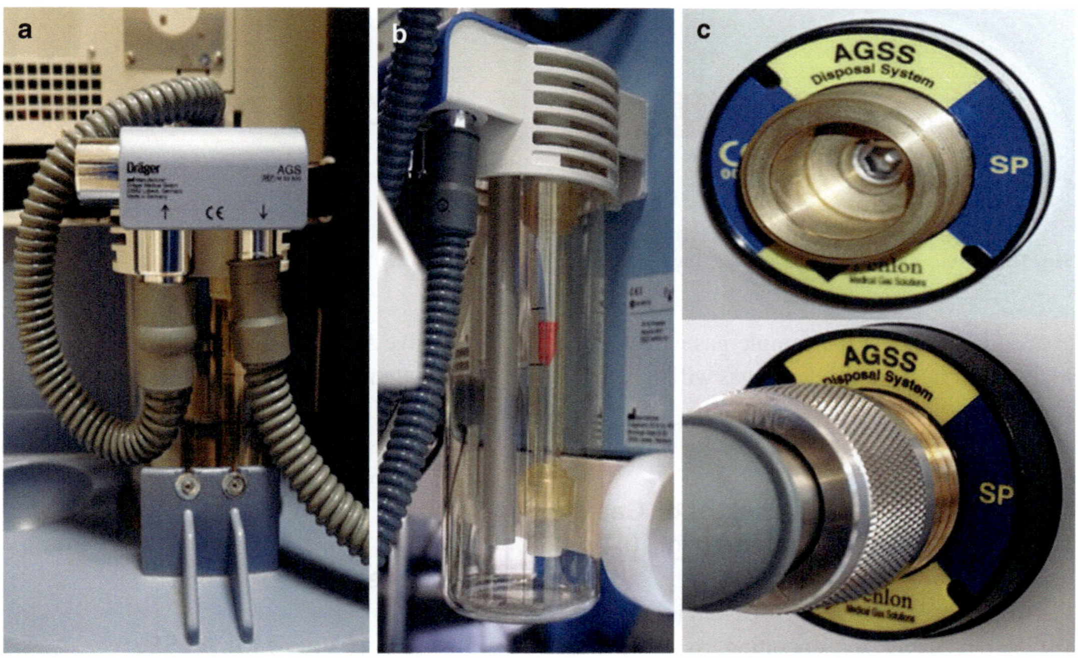

Fig. 10.2 (**a**, **b**) Scavenging system outlet at the back of anesthesia machine. (**c**) Scavenging system outlet

10.4.2 Active Adjustable Flow

It provides the capability to adjust the flow with a needle valve and a visual indicator bag which should be properly inflated. To ensure adequate scavenging, you have to adjust the needle valve. so, the visual indicator bag puffs out slightly with each breath. The bag should not be completely collapsed (close the needle valve slightly) nor completely inflated (open the needle valve slightly) (Fig. 10.3).

Active Adjustable Flow gas scavenging can cause a high PEEP alarm. Make sure the scavenge hose is connected to suction. Make sure that the needle valve is open enough that the scavenger bag moves with inspiration and expiration.

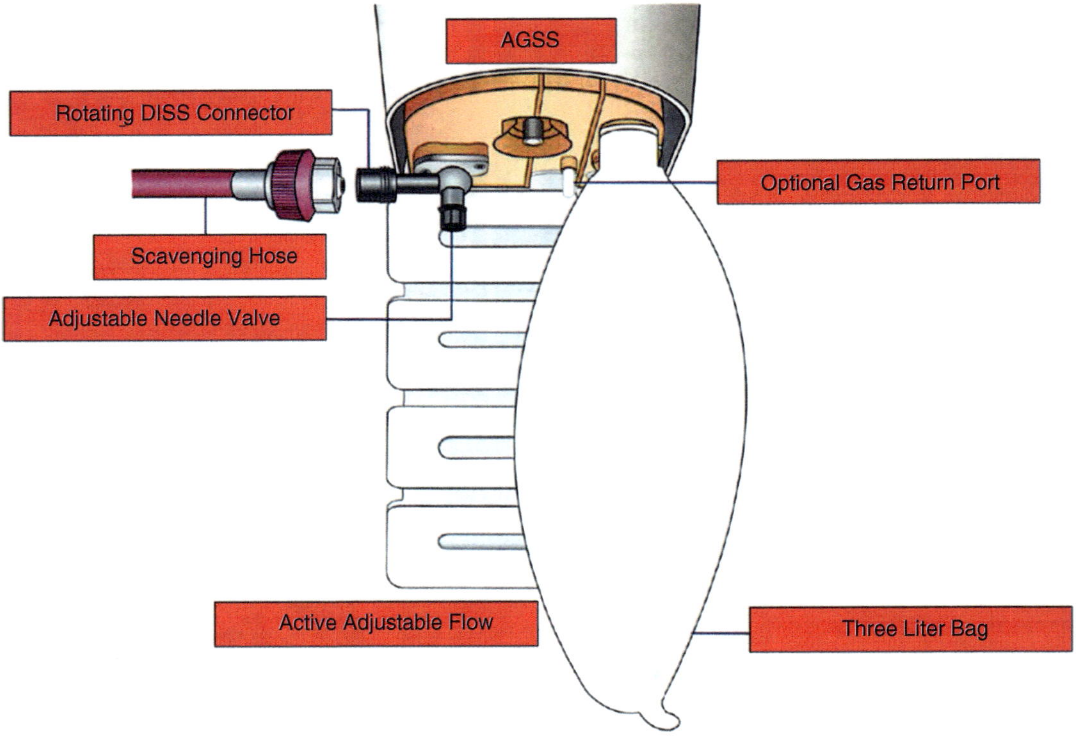

Fig. 10.3 Active anesthesia gas scavenging system (Active adjustable flow)

You can connect the sample gas exhaust tube to the gas return port. Exhaust gas will be directed to the scavenging system.

10.4.3 Passive AGSS (Anesthetic Gas Scavenging System) (Fig. 10.4)

Passive Anesthesia Gas Scavenging System (AGSS) is using for operating room environments that do not operate an active gas extraction system for waste gas disposal.

The passive AGSS is contains both positive and negative pressure relief valves, to protect the breathing system.

Passive AGSS may be used with a non-recirculating ventilation system for waste gas disposal.

The tube connection from passive AGSS to the non-recirculating ventilation system should be an open connection, essentially at atmospheric pressure to an exhaust grill.

In passive AGSS, the waste gases proceed passively through the room ventilated exhaust gas of the OR.

Passive systems require that the patient must be protected from positive pressure buildup only.

10.5 Safety

10.5.1 Safety Valve for AGSS

Scavenging systems have safety features that prevent suction from being applied to the breathing circuit leading to negative pressure applied to the patient's lungs.

The anesthesia machines (Drager ZEUS), it has a valve to prevent anesthesia gas to return back to the machine, *it is called (Non-return valve to anesthesia gas scavenging system)* (Fig. 10.5).

Measuring levels of anesthetic agents in OR are important. The levels of both N_2O and halogenated agents in the OR can be measured by

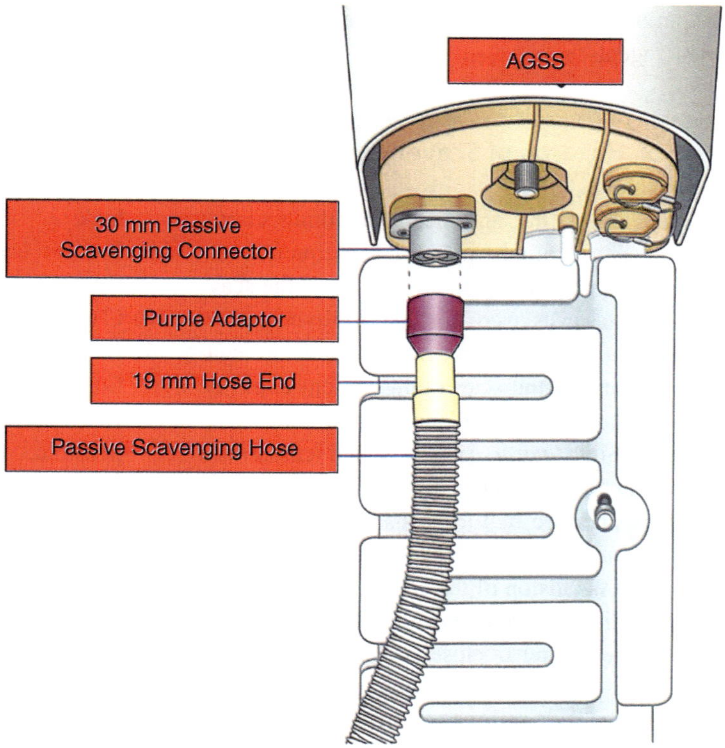

Fig. 10.4 Passive anesthesia gas scavenging system

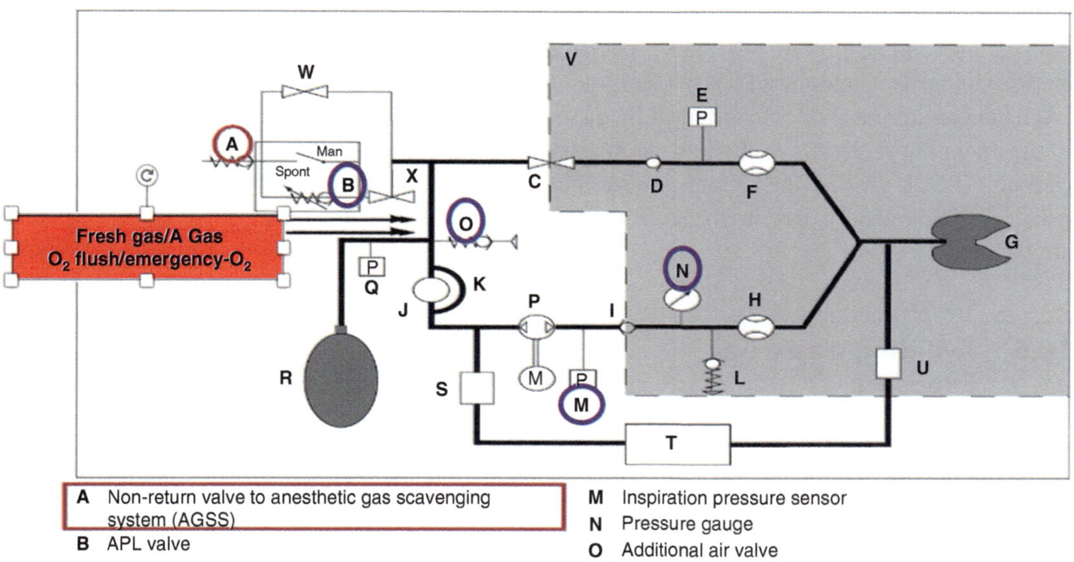

Fig. 10.5 Safety valve for AGSS

Infrared (IR) analyzers to trace levels of anesthetic agents.

10.5.2 Hazards of Scavenging

Scavenging of the anesthesia breathing circuit increases the complexity, and consequently the hazards, of administering anesthesia. If the scavenging interfaces were mistakenly bypassed or were to malfunction, excessive positive or negative pressure in the scavenging system could be directly transmitted to the breathing circuit.

This might cause cardiovascular embarrassment and barotrauma to the patient. Excessive negative pressure may be caused by unopposed vacuum and excessive positive pressure may be caused by occlusion of the connecting tubing.

In additional to occupational exposure for health care worker in close environment to anesthesia gas agents, barotrauma and ventilation dysfunction are a serious concern.

The effects of chronic exposure to volatile agents:

Some incidents have the potential to harm both patients and health care providers especially anesthesiologists, anesthesia providers, and PACU nurses are most directly affected by gases in the operating room and in the post-anesthesia care unit (PACU), where the patient continues to exhale physiologically gas in the surrounding atmosphere.

10.6 Avoiding Waste Gas Exposure

The following steps help to minimize gases exposure:

1. The scavenger system of the breathing system should be checked every day.
2. Tight mask fit is preferred during induction and recovery.
3. Prevent flow from breathing system into room air (while disconnecting or position the patient).
4. Avoid to washout anesthetics (into the breathing circuit) at the end of the anesthetic.
5. Do not spill liquid anesthetic agent.
6. Tight the vaporizers after filling.
7. Use low flows ventilation techniques.
8. Use cuffed tracheal tubes to minimize the leak.
9. Prevent leakage from Supraglottic Airway Devices (SAGD).
10. Check the machine regularly for leaks.
11. Disconnect nitrous oxide pipeline connection at wall at the end of the day.
12. Use total intravenous anesthesia (TIVA) if possible.

10.7 Scavenging System Troubleshooting Problems

10.7.1 High Pressures Scavenging System

It may result from a malfunction of pressure relief valve, the high pressures translate to increased circuit pressure and increased airway pressures, barotrauma may occur to the patient.

The patient has to be disconnected from the breathing circuit and ventilated by an alternative ventilation method. If the problem cannot be immediately corrected, a new anesthesia machine will need to be used.

10.7.2 Increased Circuit Pressures

- Check for the tube kinks.
- Check the vacuum control valve for proper adjustable (if it is there).
- Check the positive pressure release valve for proper functioning.

10.7.3 Decreased Circuit Pressures

- Check that the vacuum control valve if it is there for proper adjustable.
- Check the ventilator relief valve.

10.7.4 Overwhelmed Scavenging System

- Make sure the fresh gas flow is less than10 L/min.
- Check the vacuum control valve if it there (you may need to increase it).
- Ensure the gas disposal conduit is functioning.

10.8 Recommendations

- The scavenger system of the breathing system should be checked every day.
- Adequate precautions should be taken to ensure the safety supply of medical gases.
- Anesthesia providers must be aware of the sources of medical gas to ensure safety and an adequate supply when delivering to patients.
- All hospitals should have a documented maintenance schedule for the ventilation system in the Operating Room (OR), post-anesthesia care units (PACU), and the anesthesia machines.

10.9 Medical Gases

10.9.1 Introduction to Gas Cylinders and Medical Gases

Medical gases are used in all areas of a hospital. It constitutes an essential part of the operating theater, intensive care units, and for therapeutic treatment.

The most common medical gases are oxygen, nitrous oxide, and air, these gases are supplied via a large central source. Alternatively, they may be supplied via gas cylinders "E" size cylinders mounted on back of the anesthesia machine.

A waste anesthetic gas (WAG) scavenging system, medical suction system for surgical and anesthetic gases are provided centrally (Fig. 10.6).

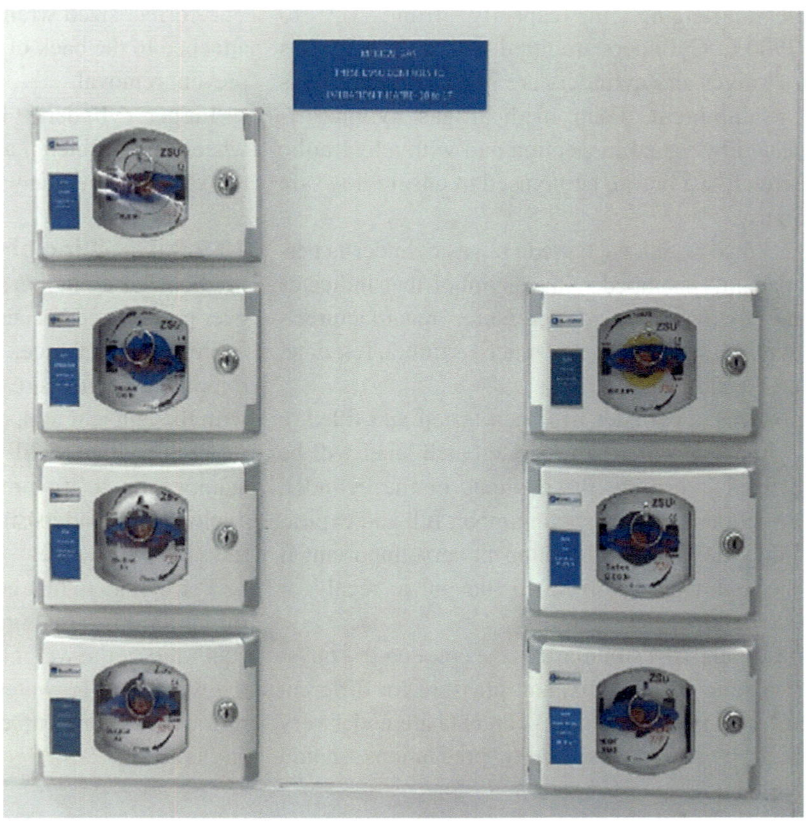

Fig. 10.6 Central gases control panel HMC-HGH

10.9.2 Medical Gas System Components

Each medical gas is supplied by a separate system. It is essential that all components of each system are gas specific to ensure that there is no possibility of cross-connection between systems. Indeed, a common configuration is designed to each system including the following components.

1. Sources.
2. Piping network.
3. Valves.
4. Warning and alarm systems.
5. Outlets and inlets.
6. Secondary equipment.

10.9.3 Medical Gas Supply and Storage

10.9.3.1 Introduction

Medical gases are stored in purpose-built cylinders, ranging in capacity from 1.2 to 7900 L. Cylinders are fitted with different types of valves and cylinders are made of steel alloys or aluminum. Each medical gas cylinder is tested by visual inspection and with a hydraulic stretch test before being used to ensure it is safe to use.

Once tested, each medical gas cylinder is permanently stamped with a symbol that indicates its contents, service pressure, manufacturer's symbol, serial number, owner's symbol, test date, and testing facility.

After a cylinder has been tested and filled, a cylinder label and a separate batch label will be affixed indicating the contents of the cylinder, directions for use, batch number, fill, and expiration date. This information is very important if the cylinder involved to be in a recall or accident.

Figure 10.7 summarizes the color codes, physical state in cylinders, and pressure for different medical gases. Cylinders contents are under very high pressures, and safety precautions should always be taken. Extreme temperatures and rapid temperature changes must also be avoided to prevent cylinder damage and/or leakage.

10.9.3.2 Valves

Common valves types include pin index valves (Fig. 10.2). The valve types on any given cylinder will typically vary according to the size.

Smaller cylinders (Type E cylinders), which are commonly used as backup on an anesthesia machine, usually have pin-indexed valves (Fig. 10.2).

Large cylinders, typically used to supply hospital pipelines, are usually fitted with bullnose valves.

The bullnose valve includes a non-interchangeable screw thread system, with a different number of threads per inch for each medical gas.

10.9.3.3 Cylinders Keys: (Opening/Closing)

Small cylinders (Type E) usually have a spindle, which may be opened or closed with a wrench. The correct sized wrench is usually permanently attached to the back of the anesthesia machine to prevent removal.

Larger cylinders (Type H) include a handwheel valve, which may be used to open or close the valves without any additional equipment.

10.9.3.4 Filling of Cylinder

Medical gas cylinders should not be overfilled or over pressurized because of the risk of accidental explosion or damage. It is important to keep in mind that the pressure inside a cylinder will vary with the ambient temperature

Each cylinder will have a service pressure stamped on it. To prevent damage or possible explosion, cylinders should never be filled above the service pressure.

For cylinders that contain liquefied gases, the filling limit is based on the filling density or percent ratio of the weight of a gas in the cylinder to the weight of the water in the cylinder. For both nitrous oxide and carbon dioxide, the filling density is 68%.

Gas	International Cylinder color	PSI at 21 Celsius	Physical state in cylinder	E-Cylinder capacity (liters)
Oxygen (O_2)	White	1900-2200	Gas	660
Carbon dioxide (CO_2)	Gray	838	Gas and liquid below 31°	1590
Nitrous oxide (N_2O)	Blue	745	Gas and liquid below 37°	1600
Air	White and black	1800	Gas	600

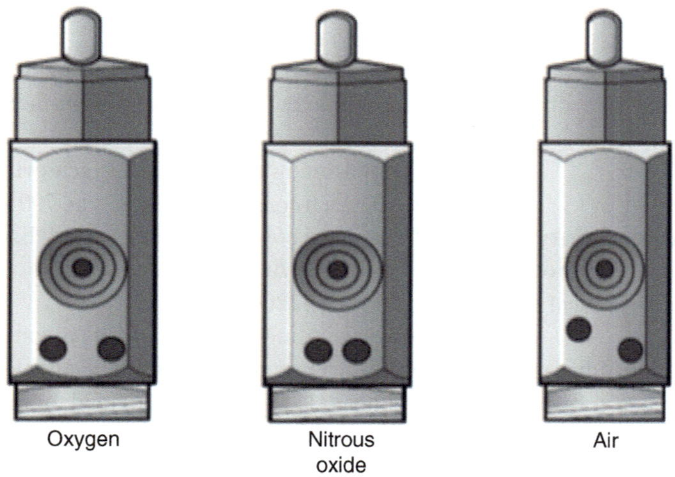

Fig. 10.7 PIN index system and physical properties for medical gas cylinders

Table 10.1 Types of medical gas cylinders

Gas	E-cylinder capacity[a] (L)	H-cylinder capacity[a] (L)	Pressure[a] (psig at 20°)	Color (USA)	Color (International)	Form
O_2	625–700	6000–8000	1800–2200	Green	White	Gas
Air	625–700	6000–8000	1800–2200	Yellow	White and black	Gas
N_2O	1590	15,900	745	Blue	Blue	Liquid
N_2	625–700	6000–8000	1800–2200	Black	Black	Gas

[a]Depending on the manufacturer

Types of Cylinders (Table 10.1)

Gas cylinders are usually made of light weight chrome molybdenum steel, aluminum or special alloy such as aluminum alloy used in MRI.

There are different types of gas cylinders available to use, however, the most common types used in anesthesia machine is E-type cylinder. These types have unique physical prosperities depending on the gas content, size, pressure limit, and volume limit.

Usually the E-Cylinder which used frequently in anesthesia machine is color coded according to gas content.

10.9.3.5 Safety Pressure Release Valves

All medical gas cylinders are fitted with a safety pressure release valve, which allows the gas inside to escape.

Types of safety release valves commonly used;

- Spring loaded pressure relief valves,
- Discs that rupture at a predefined pressure,
- Metallic plugs that melt at high temperatures.

Note: on cylinders with pin-indexed valves, the safety pressure release is located directly below the conical depression for the screw clamp. Care should, therefore, be taken not to damage this valve while mounting cylinders with pin-indexed valves onto the back of the anesthesia machine.

10.9.3.6 Medical Gas Cylinder Safety

- Medical gas cylinders should be properly stored and secured all the time to prevent damage or injury.
- Cylinders should never be dropped because a cracked pressurized cylinder can turn into a high-speed projectile missile.
- All cylinders should be stored away from open flame and in a dry, cool environment.
- All health care workers who are expected to handle medical gas cylinders should receive training and education about their proper use and storage.
- Medical gas cylinders should be always opened slowly to prevent rapid temperature rise from adiabatic expansion.
- Medical gas cylinders should be always kept closed when not in use.

Note

The medical gas cylinders are one of the simplest equipment used in the operating room, but it has the potential to be one of the most dangerous if not used and handled properly.

10.9.3.7 Calculating a Cylinder's Contents

It is possible to determine the contents of a medical gas cylinder that contains a compressed gas (such as oxygen or air) using Boyle's law (P1V1 = P2V2) where P1 stands for the atmospheric pressure, V1 the volume of gas at atmospheric pressure, P2 the pressure in the cylinder, and V2 the water capacity of the gas in compressed state. This is particularly important in remote location, emergencies, and during transport.

Example

If you have an O_2 cylinder with pressure meter pointing 550 PSI and you are about to transfer a patient who need 3 L/min oxygen supply in order to keep his saturation above 92%.

How many minutes this oxygen cylinder can provide oxygen with the above-mentioned parameters? the answer:

The maximum pressure for oxygen cylinder is 2200 psi which contains at this pressure 700 L of O_2.

To estimate how many liters, in O_2 cylinder we will use Boyle's law (P1V1 = P2V2) v2 = 550*700/2200 = 175 L.

Now according to our patient, he is consuming 3 L/min of O_2 consequently the available O_2 in the cylinder (175 L) will be provided for 58.3 min (175/3).

Note that there is simple equation available and online calculator to help with calculation which are useful in daily practice (http://www-users.med.cornell.edu/~spon/picu/calc/o2tankd.htm).

10.9.3.8 Medical Gas Pipeline Network and Manifold

The main oxygen supply in the operating room is the hospital pipeline. This system delivers oxygen at 55 pounds per square inch gauge (PSI) and comes from one of two sources:

1. A primary liquid oxygen tank (with either a manifold of compressed gas cylinders or a smaller secondary liquid oxygen tank as a backup).
2. Two banks of compressed gas cylinders (with a smaller bank of compressed gas cylinders as a backup).

All hospitals should always have at least a 2-day supply of oxygen on-hand, and a backup supply with at least a 1-day supply. (The total amount required will depend on the hospital capacity and specific needs).

The high-pressure oxygen source connects to the hospital pipeline through a two-stage pressure regulator. In hospitals where a manifold of oxygen cylinders is used, only one of the two oxygen banks will supply the main pipeline at any time. Once the first bank exhausted, the second bank will automatically switch over. This allows the finished cylinders to be changed out, without having to disrupt the whole system. The entire system is typically monitored by a centralized control station where visual indicators show the status of the two banks at all times.

10.9.3.9 Safety of Medical Gas Pipeline Network (Fig. 10.8)

All of the main hospital gas supplies and manifolds are typically physically located outside of the hospital. A network of supply pipelines conveys gas from the manifold to the required delivery points around the hospital campus. Safety standards for both oxygen and other positive pressure medical gases require the use of copper tubing to prevent the spontaneous combustion of organic oils. The supply networks are designed with pressure monitors and shut off valves throughout the system to allow isolation of specific areas for maintenance or emergency repairs. Supply lines typically have the contents and flow direction labeled at regular intervals.

10.9.3.10 Medical Gas Outlets

All hospital pipelines will end in terminal wall outlets. These color-coded outlets come in one of two varieties: (1) Diameter index safety system (DISS) outlets or (2) non-interchangeable quick coupling connectors.

DISS The DISS was developed to prevent accidental misconnections of different medical gases.

The connector system makes it physically impossible to connect the wrong hose to the wrong pipeline. Each connector is made up of a body, nipple, and nut. The body has two concentric bores, which match specific shoulders on the matching nipple. The diameters of the bores are different for each gas, making them non-interchangeable. Only appropriately matched parts will fit together and allow a complete connection.

Non-interchangeable Quick Connectors

Quick connectors allow flow meters, hoses, machines, and other pieces of equipment to be quickly connected/disconnected without using any tools or undue force. Each quick connector is made up of a pair of gas-specific male and female

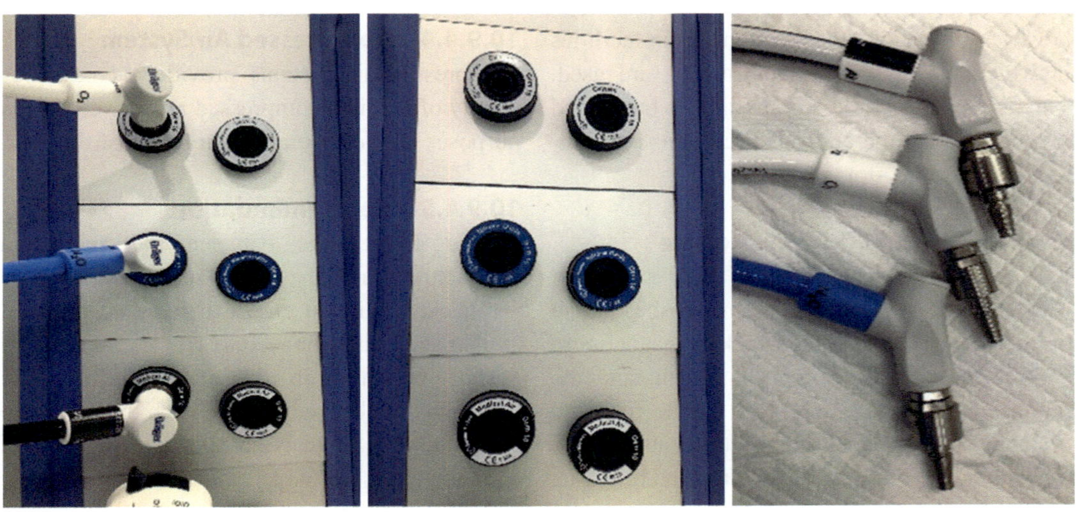

Fig. 10.8 (**a**) Medical gas outlets, (**b**) wall outlet sockets (**c**) Medical gas pipelines

parts. The two components are then locked together by a releasable spring mechanism. Different design prevents hoses from being placed into the wrong outlet. While quick connectors may be easier to use than DISS connections, however, they tend to leak with a higher frequency.

10.9.3.11 Pipeline Alarm Management System

The Gas Management System is a key component of every hospital. It is designed to provide an early warning indication for abnormality and to ensure optimum status of the central gas supply at all time.

10.9.4 Oxygen

Oxygen is an essential drug used by every anesthesiologist. Oxygen supply begins with the liquefaction of compressed air. Oxygen is separated from liquid air by taking advantage of the differences in the boiling points of oxygen and nitrogen. This enables evaporation of nitrogen first leaving liquid oxygen behind, which is later on evaporated and collected.

In the medical environment, oxygen can be supplied as either compressed gas from room temperature cylinders or as liquid oxygen from a cryogenic liquid system container. The system required to supply and store liquid oxygen is more expensive than regular oxygen cylinders; however, it is often more economical in facilities in which higher volumes of oxygen are used. This is because liquid storage is less bulky and less costly than the equivalent capacity of high-pressure gaseous storage.

10.9.4.1 Liquid Oxygen Storage Systems

The liquid oxygen storage system consists of one or more cryogenic storage tanks, one or more vaporizers, a pressure control system, and the piping necessary to support all of the requisite fill, vaporization, and supply functions. Liquid oxygen must remain under pressure and below its critical temperature of $-118\ ^\circ$ F to remain as a liquid. Because the temperature gradient between liquid oxygen and the surrounding environment is significant, keeping liquid oxygen well insulated from the surrounding heat is critically important.

Vaporizers attached to the system convert liquid oxygen into a gaseous state. Downstream, a pressure control manifold adjusts the gas pressure that is provided to the outgoing pipelines. Most cryogenic liquid systems include a backup system, which typically consists of another smaller sized liquid oxygen container or a separate manifold of oxygen cylinders. In the event of oxygen supply failure, anesthesia providers are called upon to ensuring patient safety.

10.9.4.2 Oxygen Concentrators

An oxygen concentrator provide oxygen from atmospheric air. It is used as the primary oxygen source in some remote locations. These devices work through the adsorption of atmospheric nitrogen by a molecule sieve. To ensure accurate delivery of oxygen, the oxygen output concentration should be carefully monitored when these devices are used.

10.9.4.3 The Dangers of Liquid Oxygen

As liquid oxygen is stored in medical gas cylinders at $-118\ ^\circ$ C, it can cause immediate damage of tissue on

Contact.

10.9.4.4 Compressed Air System

Compressed air systems provide a continuous supply of medical compressed air for ventilation purposes and for operating surgical instruments.

10.9.4.5 Recommendation

- The connections between the anesthesia machine and the wall supply should be checked daily to ensure here is no physical damage or misconnection.
- The pressures in the anesthesia machine should be checked prior to each theater list to ensure that there is an adequate quantity of medical gas available.
- Regular maintenance of pipeline, machines, and alarms.

- Make sure you know what is your hospital policy for oxygen supply failure and/or similar emergencies.

10.10 CO_2 Gas Analyzer

10.10.1 Gas Analyzers Troubleshooting Problems

CO_2 tracing wave appears on the machine does not appear.

Ensuring a proper CO2 tracing is part of the machine check out. We should identify any machine defect early but if no tracing appears during a procedure, we should check the following:

- First confirm that it is not a lack of patient ventilation.
- Check if the anesthesia machine was calibrated.
- Check if gas analyzer has been turned on and warm-up has completed.
- Check if the gas analyzer is not performing a temporary calibration.
- Check for sample line disconnect or obstruction.
- Anesthesia provider should confirm ETT placement.
- Check for a circuit disconnect.
- Check that the water trap is inserted properly and not full of water.
- Check for any recent aerosolized medication administration, when aerosolized medication is given through the ETT, the gas analyzer may have trouble identifying the various gases.

The common cause for inaccurate readings from the gas analyzer is condensation in the sample line or an incomplete connection to the machine (Kinked, fractured) in addition poorly connected sample lines can also cause faulty readings.

10.10.2 Troubleshooting Common Problems with CO2

Elevated CO_2 Wave on Capnography

- Examine inspiratory and expiratory flow valves.
- Check if an exhausted CO_2 absorber because commonly high inspired CO_2 is due to exhausted absorber and replace the CO_2 absorber.
- Faulty inspiratory or expiratory flow valve can increase CO_2, the valves can become incompetent if they are damaged, dried out, cracked, or get stuck.

10.11 Vacuum (Suction System)

Generally, a vacuum is a volume of space that has no matter in it. It results in a space having a much lower (negative) pressure than atmospheric pressure. Vacuums are essential in medical practice because they are used to create suction. Suction can then be used within the operating room to remove unwanted gases, liquids, and solid materials from both patient and the environment. Hospitals typically provide a vacuum to each patient care location via a pipeline system, which is capable of delivering a vacuum of close to 300 mm Hg at each terminus. Vacuum pipelines are typically constructed the same way medical gas supply lines are (copper tubing) but are usually larger in diameter. A vacuum is created placing two pumps in parallel with a reservoir between them to (1) even out the vacuum and (2) remove any debris from the system. Filters, before and after the wall connection, are important to prevent major leakage of harmful or contaminated materials into the central vacuum system.

In most modern hospitals, vacuum is available from wall outlets located throughout the building.

10.12 Maintenance of Suction Equipment

1. To ensure optimum performance of suction equipment, regular maintenance and inspection are important. Every hospital should have a maintenance program to minimize costly breakdowns and keep equipment operating at peak efficiency. Here is a suggested to make checklist for care of suction equipment after each patient use:
2. Thorough cleaning of reusable equipment and disposal of single-use components.
3. Careful inspection of the equipment, with special attention to filters.
4. Analysis of performance.
5. Adjustment and repair if necessary.
6. Re-cleaning.
7. Sterilization, if appropriate.
8. *biohazardous materials should be disposed according to local hospital guidelines.*
9. *any disposable parts of the suction system should be disposed properly and never ever to reused again.*
10. *personal protective equipment should be wearing during suction cleaning with contaminated materials.*
11. *Gloves, Face and Eye Protection.*
12. *Before start cleaning any electrical connection to suction system should be disconnected.*

Take-Home Message

Medical gases are a critical element of the practice of anesthesiology, but also a potential source of harm for patients and anesthesia providers alike. It is, therefore, critical that personnel who work in the operating room understand how to properly use, maintain, and store medical gases. Although the practice of anesthesiology is constantly changing, suctioning is an important part of daily patient care and in many cases can be a potentially life-saving procedure. A thorough understanding of the physics involved in creating suction, the factors affecting flow rate, and the clinical applications of negative pressure will make the procedure more effective and as safe as possible.

Scavenging system (waste gas) dispose all ventilated gases emitting from the patient and anesthesia machine.

It has a crucial rule in the operating room environment to prevent any pollution which could be hazardous.

The National Institute for Occupational Safety and Health (NIOSH) recommends limiting the room concentration of nitrous oxide to 25 ppm and halogenated agents to 2 ppm.

Scavenging system is integral part of anesthesia machine that it has to be familiar to anesthetists and anesthesia technicians. Also it should be monitored in between the cases frequently as well.

American Society of Anesthesia stressed that it is important by being a part of daily anesthesia machine checklist.

Further Reading

Al-Shaikh B. Essentials of anaesthetic equipment. 4th ed. Elsevier; 2013.

Ehrenwerth J, Eisenkraft J, Berry J. Anesthesia equipment: principles and applications. 2020.

Jesse Ehrenfeld MD, Sandberg W, Urman R. The MGH textbook of anesthetic equipment. 1st ed. Philadelphia, PA: Saunders; 2011.

Mackey DC, Butterworth JF, Wasnick JD. Clinical anesthesiology. 5th ed. McGraw-Hill Education, LLC; 2013.

Ronald D. Miller, anesthesia miller. 9th ed; 2020.

Complications and Emergencies in Operating Room

11

Wael Saleem, Ouissal Jouini, Abil Luez, and Nabil A. Shallik

Contents

W. Saleem (✉) · O. Jouini · A. Luez · N. A. Shallik
Department of Anesthesiology, ICU and Perioperative Medicine, Hamad Medical Corporation, Doha, Qatar
e-mail: wsaleem@hamad.qa; OAhmed8@hamad.qa; ALuez@hamad.qz; nshallik@hamad.qa

N. A. Shallik et al. (eds.), *Improving Anesthesia Technical Staff's Skills*,
https://doi.org/10.1007/978-3-030-88849-7_11

11.1 Introduction

It is always vital to prepare the patients preoperatively. Appropriate planning will prevent any unexpected complications and prepare well for complicated ones. Examining the patient's airway following various accredited guidelines will minimize any unanticipated difficult intubation or laryngeal spasms during airway management. Hemorrhage considered a critical complication and may end tragically if the concerned team is not well prepared with suitable monitoring tools and well functioned blood transfusion system. While managing cardiac arrhythmias would be challenging intraoperatively if the patient is not optimized pre-surgically, the anesthesia team will select a suitable anesthesia protocol, accordingly. Regional anaesthesia utilization is growing rapidly and the local anaesthesia toxicity has never dropped to zero incidence even with ultrasound modality utilization. By taking precautions towards these above points, cardiac arrest incidence will be avoided. The operating theatre is full of electric equipment and combustible substances. It is very crucial to have well-maintained devices and frequent check for any electric circuit problem. It is important to understand how to use and store combustible materials and how to operate devices such as LASER to prevent harm to patients and other health care providers.

11.2 Unanticipated Difficult Airway

Commonly happened with emergency cases which not well prepared and could happen with the elective cases as well. Once you encounter such a situation, please consider the following steps;

- Call for help
- Maintain oxygenation, and ensure monitoring SPO2, ETCO2, all the time.
- Maintain cricoid pressure (in case of a full stomach)
- Maintain patent airway consider the following;
  - Improve head position e.g., Jaw thrust and chin left, and maintain RAMP position and
  - use oropharyngeal airway (Guedel's pattern airway)
- Confirm the depth of both anesthesia and neuromuscular blockade.
- Request difficult airway trolley if needed
- Consider alternative airway management devices, e.g., Mac blade size, McCoy blade, Video-laryngoscopes, ETT different sizes, adjuncts (bougie, stylet), or fibroscopic intubation once needed.

In this critical situation, the anaesthesia technician should be aware of each step and acts on time when assisting the anaesthesiologist to make a good decision.

Difficult Airway Society (DAS) guidelines have been utilized in this chapter (Fig. 11.1).

These guidelines provide a sequential series of plans to be used when tracheal intubation fails and are designed to prioritize oxygenation while limiting the number of airway interventions in order to decrease trauma and complications. The principle that Anaesthesia team should have backup plans in place prior performing primary techniques still holds true.

Step 1 Face Mask ventilation and Tracheal intubation

- Optimize patient position.
- Maintain oxygenation.

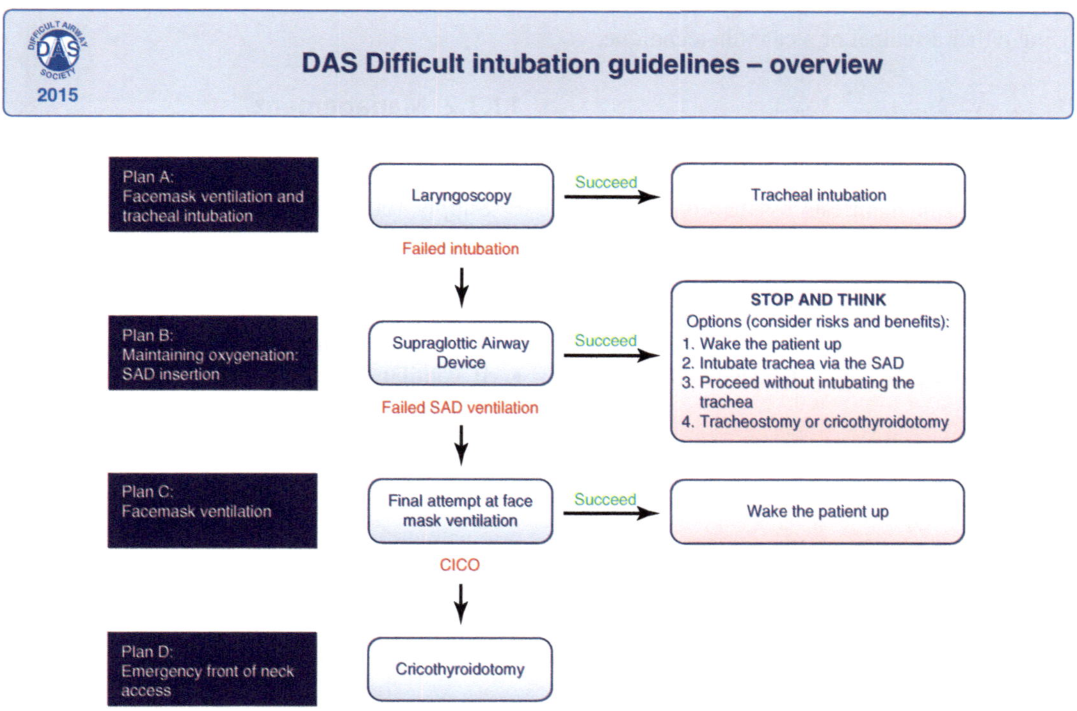

Fig. 11.1 Difficult Airway Society (DAS) intubation guidelines (with written permission from DAS Society)

- Adequate neuromuscular blocked.
- Try Direct/ video laryngoscopy (if available) intubation (Max 3 + 1 attempts).
- External laryngeal manipulation.
- Use bougie or stylet.
- Remove cricoid pressure.

Step 2 If step 1 failed

- Maintain oxygenation.
- Use the Laryngeal Mask, consider size and type changes if needed.
- Consider ETT intubation through SAD.
- Consider ETT intubation using fiberoptic if available.
- Maintain ventilation if possible.
- Wake up the patient if ventilation not possible.

Step 3 If step 2 failed

- If you can't maintain face mask oxygenation alone, use 2-person technique ventilation.
- If face mask ventilation is impossible, consider waking up the patient or proceeding to step 4.

Step 4 Cricothyroidotomy may be performed using either a scalpel or a cannula technique.

11.3 Bronchospasm

Bronchospasm manifests by the constriction of air passages of the lung by spasmodic contraction of the bronchial muscles. It occurs with or without a cause during general anaesthesia.

- Bronchospasm is characterized by the following:
  - Prolonged expiration,
  - Rise in $ETCO_2$ (shark-fin capnograph appearance) Fig. 11.2,
  - Wheeze,
  - Increased peak airway pressure,
  - Decreased tidal volume,

If not treated, it can cause hypoxia, hypotension, and increased morbidity and mortality.

11.3.1 Causes

- Patient causes.
  - Anaphylaxis reaction to antibiotics, neuromuscular blockers, blood products, and latex.
  - Aspiration or acute pulmonary oedema.
  - Asthma, chronic obstructive pulmonary disease (COPD).
  - Airway soiling (airway hyperactivity due to secretion, regurgitation, or aspiration).
  - Upper respiratory tract infection (URTI).
- Mechanical causes.

11.3.2 Management

- Call for help.
- Supply 100% oxygen and deepen anaesthesia level.
- Perform manual ventilation.
- Stop stimulants and exclude all potential precipitant mentioned above.
- If ventilation through ETT difficult/impossible, check tube position and exclude blocked/

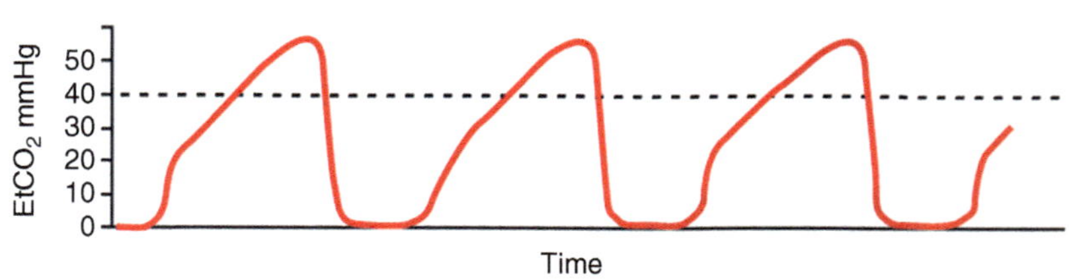

Fig. 11.2 $ETCO_2$ (shark-fin appearance) in bronchospasm

misplaced tube. If non-intubated patient, consider aspiration.

- self-inflating bag is a confirmative step for breathing circuit occlusion.
  - Mild bronchospasm usually responds to the above steps; however, severe bronchospasm may require further management.

11.3.3 Medication

While excluding the potential causes above, consider immediately to provide the following medication in sequence and titrate to response:

- In the initial step;
  - Consider Salbutamol; start as inhaler (6–8 puffs) repeat as needed. Use as nebulizer 5 mg repeat as needed or as intravenous 250 mcg slowly, then 5 mcg/min up to 20 mcg/min.
  - Practical trick for salbutamol nebulization: you can put Salbutamol inhaler container inside 50 ml syringe. By pushing the plunger of the syringe, you can give an accurate dose of the drug after removing the $ETCO_2$ sample line to prevent the machine to aspirate the drug (Fig. 11.3).
- If no improvement, consider.
  - Ipratropium 0.5 mg nebulized/6 h.
  - Magnesium Sulphate: 50 mg/kg over 20 min (max 2 gm).
  - Hydrocortisone 200 mg IV/ 6 h.
  - Aminophylline: 5 mg/kg IV over 20 min then 0.5 mg/kg/h infusion.
  - In serious condition; Epinephrine: Nebulized: 5mls 1:1000/ IV 10 mcg-100 mcg titrate to response/ IM- 0.5–1.0 mg if no IV access.
  - For paediatric patients, adjust the dosage.
- Continuous reassess of the patient condition, and if no improvement considers pulmonary oedema/embolus and/or pneumothorax, treat accordingly.
- Request chest X-ray and consider transferring to ICU for further management.

11.4 Aspiration Under Anaesthesia

Pulmonary aspiration is defined by the inhalation of oropharyngeal or gastric contents into the larynx and the respiratory tract.

This is due to the reduction in the laryngeal protective reflexes level.

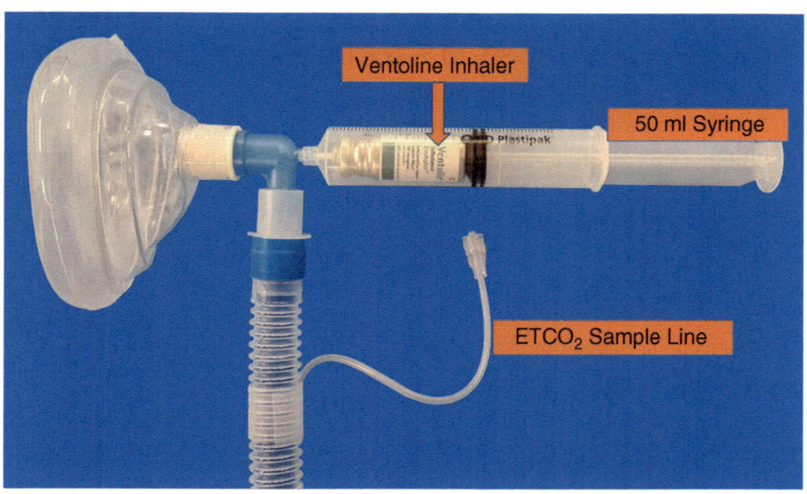

Fig. 11.3 Injection of Salbutamol inhaler through 50 ml syringe and connected to anaesthesia circuit instead of $ETCO_2$ sample line by using Luer lock

- Aspiration of solid matter can cause hypoxia by physical obstruction,
- Aspiration of acidic gastric fluid can cause a pneumonitis which lead to progressive dyspnoea, hypoxia, bronchial wheeze, and patchy collapse, consolidation on chest X-ray or all.

11.4.1 Risk Factors

Patients of increased risk of aspiration with the induction of anaesthesia:

- Full stomach (emergency surgery, inadequate fasting time).
- Patient with increased intraabdominal pressure (obesity, pregnancy, hiatus hernia, regurgitation).
- Patient with gastrointestinal pathology.
- Surgical factors; laparoscopy, trendelenburg position.
- Anaesthesia factors; light anaesthesia, supraglottic airways, Positive Pressure Ventilation (PPV), difficult airway.

11.4.2 During Aspiration

- Call for help.
- Place the patient head down and lateral position.
- Use Suction Assisted Laryngoscopy Airway Decontamination (SALAD) technique in case of vomiting during intubation (Fig. 11.4).
- Secure the airway and positive pressure ventilation (PPV) after active suction of the airway.
- The patient may need to be shifted to ICU for further management when the airway is affected.

11.4.3 Recommendations

- Appropriate assessment for aspiration risk before surgery.

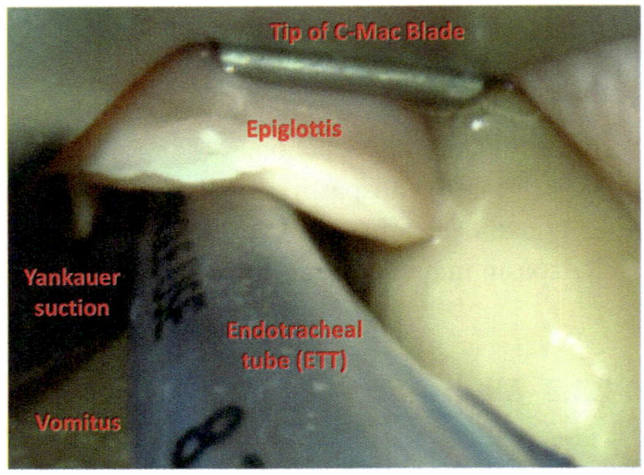

Fig. 11.4 Technique Suction Assisted Laryngoscopy Airway Decontamination (SALAD) Intubation

- Prepare for rapid sequence induction and intubation and appropriate cricoid force applied.
- The equipment and skills to identify and handle regurgitation and aspiration should be ready.
- Blood clot may cause a flat capnography trace occurs when blood has been near the airway.

11.5 Cardiovascular Complications

11.5.1 Sinus Bradycardia: It Is Defined as HR < 60 Beats/Min with Regular Rhythm (Ratio of *P* to QRS 1:1; and Normal QRS)

11.5.1.1 Causes

Hypoxia; hypothermia; vasovagal stimulation; endotracheal suctioning; increased intracranial pressure; neuraxial anaesthesia; or medications.

- Hemodynamic stable: If the patient is stable during severe sinus bradycardia (e.g., <40 bpm), give.
  - IV glycopyrrolate in 0.2 mg increments (up to 1 mg) to avoid tachycardia in patients with ischemic heart disease.

- Or give small incremental doses of atropine 0.2 mg.

- Hemodynamic instable (HR < 40 beats/min) with hypotension.
  - Ephedrine 10 to 20 mg (up to 50 to 60 mg). Avoid it in patients with ischemic heart and/or tachycardia. Instead, use one of the following: epinephrine, isoproterenol, dopamine, and dobutamine.
  - Consider continuous infusion of a positive chronotropic agent in persistent bradycardia, (Algorithm 1).

11.5.2 Atrial Tachycardia: It Is Defined as HR > 100 Beats/Min with Regular Rhythm

11.5.2.1 Causes

- Sympathetic stimulation: painful stimulus due to inadequate anaesthetic depth.
- Others: fever, hypercarbia, and hypovolemia.

- Hemodynamic stable.
  - Esmolol infusion (e.g., 50–300 mcg/min) if post-anaesthesia care unit (PACU) monitored setting is available. Alternately;
  - Metoprolol or labetalol: use as small bolus doses of metoprolol 1–5 mg or labetalol 5–10 mg. Labetalol should be titrated in small doses in patients with asthma, chronic obstructive lung disease, heart failure, or hyperadrenergic states such as cocaine or methamphetamine overdose.
  - Deepening anaesthesia and adding opioids expected to slow a rapid HR.
- Hemodynamic instable and/or narrow QRS complex or Wide QRS complex.

Table 11.1 Common medications used for arrhythmias intraoperatively

Medication	Recommended dosage (IV)
Adenosine	IV bolus: Rapid dose 6 mg; double the dose of no effect within 2 min, and repeat 12 mg if no response within 1–2 min
Amiodarone	IV bolus: 150 mg over 10 min Infusion: 0.1 mg/min for 6 h, then 0.5 mg/min for the next 18 h
Diltiazem	IV bolus: 0.25 mg/kg over two mins Infusion: 5–15 mg/h
Esmolol	IV bolus: 1 mg/kg Infusion: 150 mcg/kg/min
Verapamil	IV bolus: 0.07–0.15 mg/kg over 3 min. Repeat every 15–30 min if needed Infusion: 0.005 mg/kg/min

  - Further management refer to (Algorithm 2).
- Common medications used for intraoperative arrhythmias (Table 11.1).

11.5.3 Ventricular Tachycardia

Have wide QRS complex (>120 ms) and need immediate treatment, please consider the;

- "H"; Hypoxia, hypovolemia, hypothermia, hypo/hyperkalaemia, H ion (acidosis).
- "T's"; tension pneumothorax, cardiac tamponade, toxins, pulmonary or coronary thrombosis.

11.5.3.1 Treatment

Please refer to (Algorithms 2 and 3) and (Table 11.1).

11.5.4 Cardiac Arrest

Immediate Cardiopulmonary resuscitation (see Asystole) (Algorithm 3).

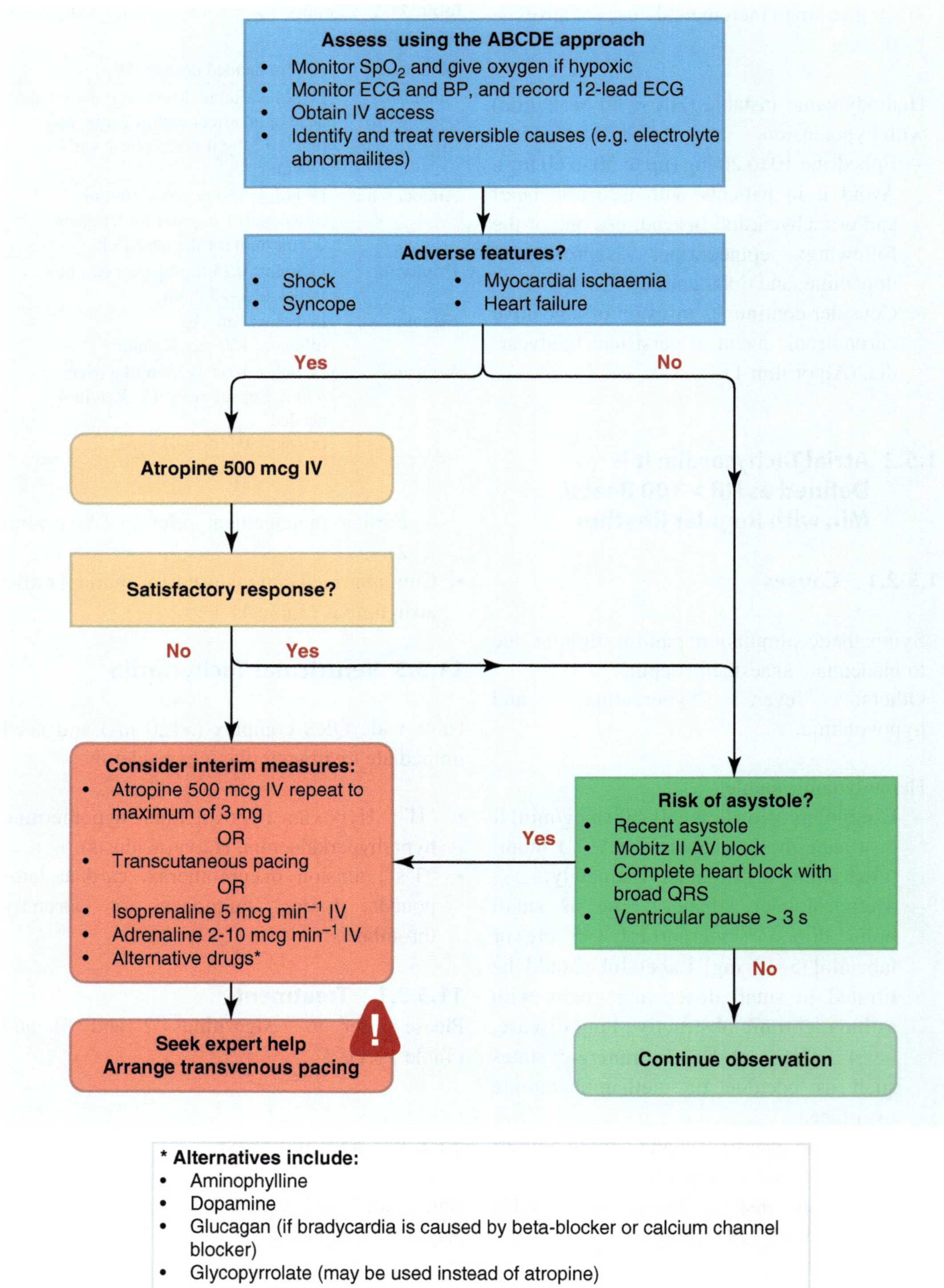

Algorithm 1 *IV* intravenous, *ECG* electrocardiogram. With written permission from Resuscitation Council UK Guidelines for Peri-arrest arrhythmias management

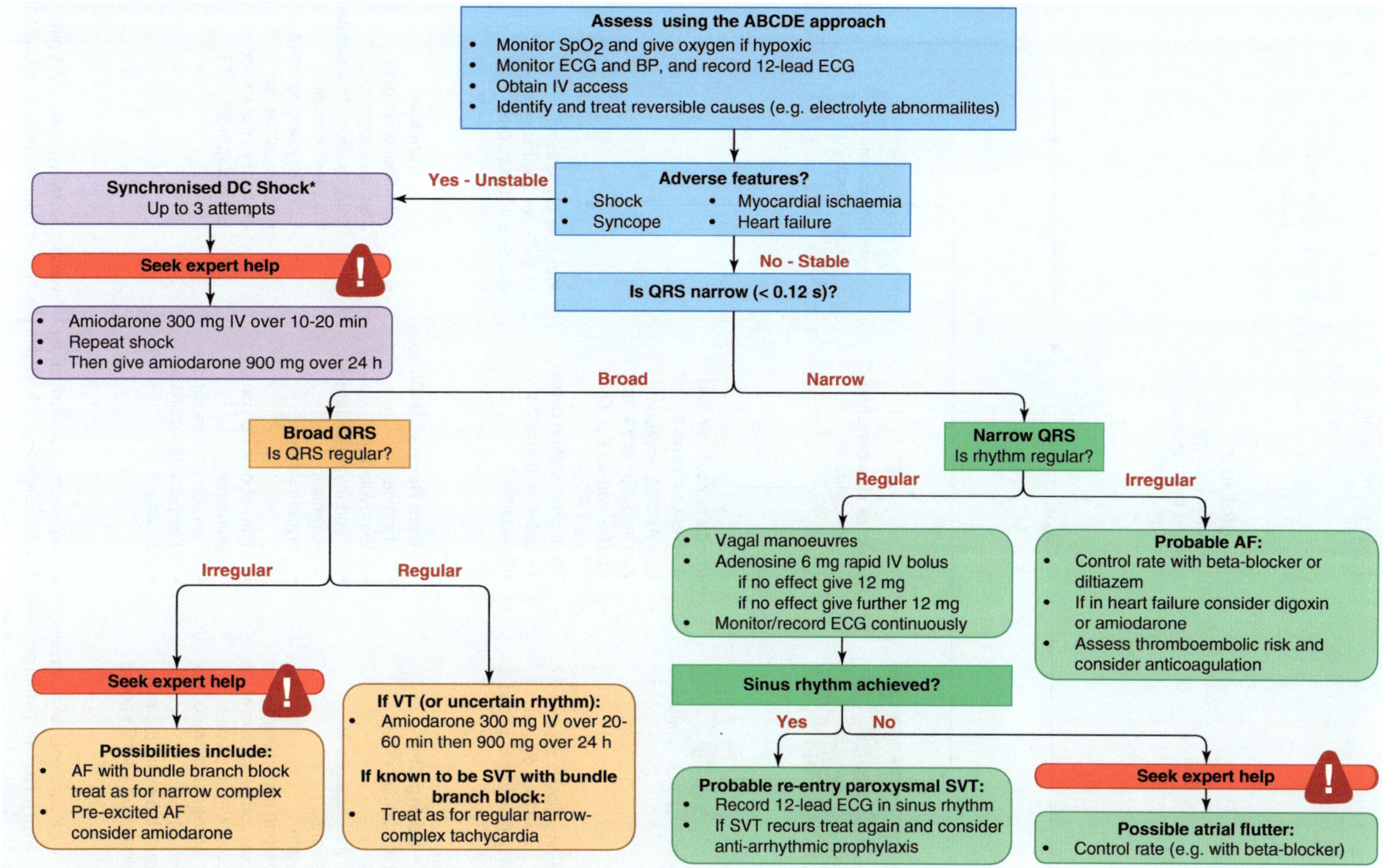

*Conscious patients require sedation or general anaesthesia for cardioversion

Algorithm 2 *IV* intravenous, *ECG* electrocardiogram, *AF* atrial fibrillation, *SVT* supraventricular tachycardia, *VT* ventricular tachycardia. With written permission from Resuscitation Council UK Guidelines for Peri-arrest arrhythmias management

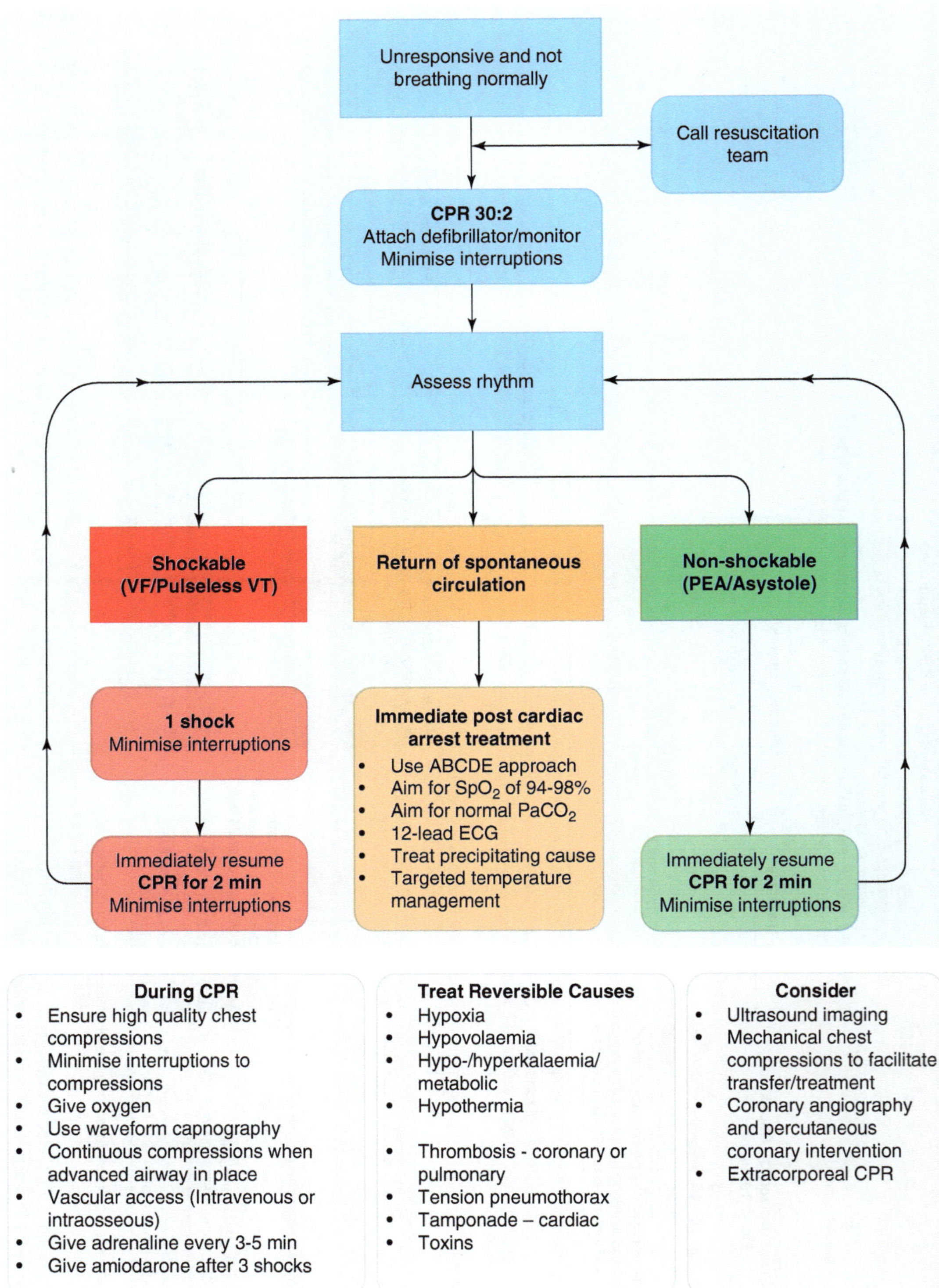

Algorithm 3 *CPR* cardiopulmonary resuscitation, *VF* ventricular fibrillation, *VT* ventricular tachycardia, *PEA* pulseless electrical activity, $PaTCO_2$ partial pressure of carbon dioxide. With written permission from Resuscitation Council UK Guidelines for Adult Advance life support

11.5.4.1 Recommendation

- Exclude risk factors intraoperatively that may contribute to the occurrence of the arrhythmias.
- Consult seniors immediately including cardiologist if needed.

11.6 Intraoperative Haemorrhage

Intraoperative haemorrhage is defined as a blood loss exceeding 1000 ml or becomes massive when exceeding 25% of the total blood volume. Elective patient with high risk of intraoperative bleeding should be prepared prior to the operation and it is out of the scope of discussion in this chapter.

11.6.1 Management

Once the surgeon reports uncontrolled bleeding and or the volume of bleeding exceed 1000 ml, then

- Call for help.
- Reduce intravenous /inhalation anaesthetics.
- Make sure the inspired oxygen fraction is high enough and avoid hyperoxia [PaO_2 > 26.7 kPa (200 mmHg)].
- Check IV access, insert cannula with larger gauge, e.g., 14G immediately.
- Use vasopressors when low blood pressure is noted.
- Insertion of arterial line, urinary catheter, Central Venous Catheter (CVC).
- Perform ABG and act accordingly.
- Monitoring invasive BP, CVP, temperature.
- Coordinate with surgeons' team to control bleeding (pressure, tourniquet).
- Call blood bank and activate major haemorrhage protocol or Massive Transfusion Protocol (MTP) (Hb 5 or less with ongoing bleeding) O negative or specific group should be used.
- If large blood loss for every 8 Unit of Packed red blood cells (PRBC) delivered, give 2 Unit of fresh frozen plasma (FFP).
- If more than 10 U of PRBC are delivered, give 10 units of platelets, preferably at the end of the procedure.
- With prolonged PTT, give FFP 15 ml/kg to prevent haemostatic failure.
- If fibrinogen is low, give 2 U of cryoprecipitate.
- Communicate how quickly blood is required.
- Active patient warming.
- Use rapid infusion and fluid warming equipment using Level 1 infusion set or any alternative sets (Fig. 11.5).
- Consider antifibrinolytics agents.
- Replace calcium and consider giving tranexamic acid.
- Maintain regular laboratory tests check: ABGs, clotting screen, electrolytes.

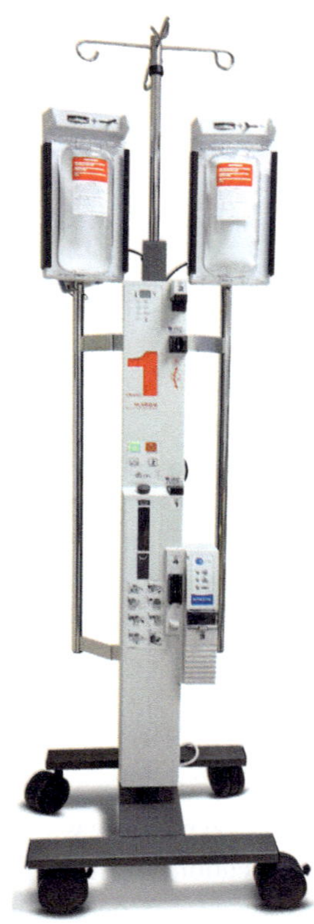

Fig. 11.5 Level 1® H-1200 fast flow fluid warmer with integrated air detector/clamp

11.7 Blood Transfusion and Complications

Early recognition of symptoms to blood transfusion would help significantly to reduce morbidity and mortality rate. Some complications have high mortality rate such as the following:

- hemolytic reaction due to ABO incompatibility occurs within an hour following transfusion,
- graft-vs-host disease (GVHD);
- circulatory overload;
- acute lung injury.

Other complications such as

- Febrile nonhemolytic reactions;
- Chill-rigour reactions;
- Allergic reactions;
- Oxygen saturation fluctuation;
- Delayed haemolytic transfusion reaction;
- Infections.

11.7.1 Symptoms

Might be observed on the affected patient, depending on the severity

- Feeling of discomfort, dyspnoea, facial flushing, and anxiety.
- Fever, chills, and lumber pain.
- Shock; tachycardia, hypotension, cold, clammy skin, nausea and vomiting, jaundice.

11.7.2 Management

- Stop the transfusion.
- Call for help.
- Use 100% O_2.
- Treat according to the signs and symptoms.
  - Maintain blood pressure with fluids + vasoactive medication (if needed);
  - Bronchospasm; bronchodilators, e.g., Salbutamol;
  - Maintain normothermic avoid hypo/hyperthermic temperatures;
  - Proceed to anaphylaxis algorithm if anaphylactic shock (epinephrine infusion 0.1 mcg/kg/min give antihistaminic);
  - Treat coagulopathy if needed;
  - Maintain urine output (diuretic therapy: furosemide, mannitol).
- Take blood and urine samples for analysis.
- Return all products to blood bank.

11.8 Anaphylaxis: Allergic Reaction During Anaesthesia

During anaesthesia muscle relaxants, latex, antibiotics, and colloids are considered as common causes of anaphylactic reactions. This immediate hypersensitivity reactions can be immune-mediated (allergic) or non-immune mediated (anaphylactoid reactions). Vigilance and rapid recognize of clinical manifestations are important to treat these reactions.

11.8.1 Diagnosis

- Skin signs (rash, urticaria, angioedema).
- Airways reactions (bronchospasm and laryngeal oedema).
- Hypotension/cardiovascular collapse/tachycardia.
- Nausea and vomiting in awake patient.

11.8.2 Management

- Discontinue the triggers, e.g., antibiotics.
- Call for help.
- Monitor vital signs, SPO_2.
- Ventilate with 100% O_2 and intubate if the airway is compromised.
- Give IV fluids:20 ml/kg.
- Consider placing the patient in supine in the Trendelenburg position.
- IV Epinephrine bolus: 1 mcg/kg _IM Epinephrine bolus 500 mcg. If the patient developed bradycardia and or hypotension, then give 1mg Epinephrine IV.

- Dosage titration should always be applied based on your clinical outcome.
- Start Epinephrine infusion 0.15 mcg/kg/min or Vasopressin 0.4–1 units/kg IV, up to 40 units maximum.
- Consider Norepinephrine IV infusion if there is persistent hypotension 0.1 mcg/kg/min.
- Insertion arterial line for monitoring and repeated ABG reading.
- Collect blood sample for mast cell Tryptase level.

11.8.3 Additional Therapy

Consider to add the following agents;

- Diphenhydramine bolus (1 mg/kg IV, maximum dose 50 mg).
- Hydrocortisone (5 mg/kg IV).
- Ranitidine (1 mg/kg IV).
- Aminophylline (5 mg/kg IV) and Salbutamol inhaler if resistant bronchospasm.
- ABG if acidosis: Sodium bicarbonate (0.5–1 mmol/kg IV).
- In case of cardiac arrest, follow the advanced cardiac life support protocol.
- Transfer to Intensive Care Unit.

11.9 Total Spinal Anaesthesia

It is a complication of spinal/epidural anaesthesia involving the spread of local anaesthesia (LA) cranially causing loss of consciousness. If the spread of LA is reaching cranially above T4 is called high spinal anaesthesia.

11.9.1 Manifestations

Cardio-respiratory	Hypotension
	Bradycardia
	Apnoea
	Reduced oxygen saturation
	Cardiac arrest (asystole)
Neurological	Nausea and anxiety
	High sensory level block > T1
	Slurred speech
	Loss of consciousness (a cranial nerve involvement).

11.9.2 Causes

- Higher dose (higher dose leads to higher risk).
- Baricity (cephalad spread is easier to control with hyperbaric solution).
- Body morphology (higher BMI or abdominal girth, e.g., pregnancy) can reduce thecal volume and increase the risk of high block).
- Abnormality of the spinal canal.
- Body Position (following spinal anaesthesia).
- Effects of the speed of injection.
- Excessive barbotage.
- Do not inject during a contraction in pregnancy/cough/Valsalva as this can increase the cephalad spread of local anaesthetic.

11.9.3 Management

Once TSA is recognized immediately;

1. Call for help.
2. Put face mask and deliver high oxygen.
3. Put the patient position in reverse Trendelenburg/head up.
4. Assess the patient ABCD (Airway, Breathing, Circulation, Disability).
5. In case of loss of consciousness, secure patient airway.
6. If bradycardia occurs start vagolytics, e.g., Atropine, Glycopyrrolate.
7. Start fluid bolus as needed if the patient is hypotensive add vasopressors, e.g., Ephedrine, Phenylephrine as needed. If no response, then consider diluted adrenaline (10mcg/ml minimum dilution) to be titrated.
8. If the patient lost consciousness, then intubate and ventilate.

11.10 Local Anaesthetic Systemic Toxicity (LAST)

Local Anaesthetic Systemic Toxicity (LAST) is a life-threatening that may occur following the administration of local anaesthetic drugs through a variety of routes. Neurological symptoms are the most common and first symptoms to appear, however, 20% of the reported cases present with cardiovascular disorder only.

11.10.1 Signs

- Perioral paraesthesia.
- Audio-visual disturbance.
- Taste disturbance (dysgeusia).
- Confusion.
- Reduced level of consciousness.
- Convulsion.
- Coma.
- Respiratory arrest.
- Cardiac arrest.

11.10.2 Management

- Stop drug injection.
- Call for help.
- Secure the airway, intubate if necessary and ventilate with 100% O_2.
- Start Cardiopulmonary Resuscitation (CPR) if required and follow ACLS protocol.
- Intravenous lipid emulsion therapy should be initiated simultaneously as; 20% Intralipid IV (1. 5 mg/kg bolus over 1 min (100 ml in adult) and start infusion of 15 ml/kg/h (1000 ml/h in adult). If not responding at 5 min, then give another bolus dose and double infusion rate 30mg/kg/h (allow 3 bolus doses each 5 min) (Fig. 11.6).
- Treat the following if occurs;
  - Convulsions (Midazolam 5–10 mg/ Thiopentone 50 mg/Propofol 50–100 mg).
  - Treat arrhythmia as needed, avoid lidocaine to treat arrhythmia.
- Maintain hemodynamic stability and reassess the patients following each bolus/infusion set of intralipid.
- If the patient has an episode of LAST with CVS features, then the patients should be monitored for at least 6 h, while with only CNS signs, it requires the patient monitoring for a minimum of 2 h.

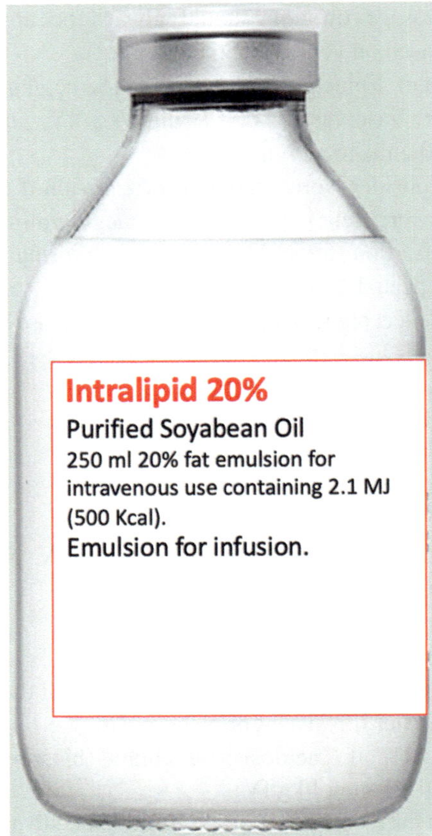

Fig. 11.6 Intravenous lipid emulsion 20%

11.11 Malignant Hyperthermia

Malignant Hyperthermia (MH) is a clinical condition of hypermetabolism involving the skeletal muscle. The abnormality in the ryanodine receptor caused an accumulation of calcium in the skeletal muscle, resulting in a substantial metabolic reaction.

11.11.1 The Early Clinical Signs Are as Follows

- Elevated $ETCO_2$ (metabolic and respiratory acidosis) despite of adequate ventilation.
- Tachycardia, Tachypnoea.
- Muscle/Masseter spasm (rigidity or trismus).
- Hyperkalaemia.

11.11.2 The Late Clinical Signs Are as Follows

- Temperature rise (late sign).
- Myoglobinuria.
- Multiple organ failure.

11.11.3 Management

- Call for help.
- Request the pre-prepared MH trolley (if available Fig. 11.7).
- Hyperventilate with 100% oxygen.
- Cease the volatile agents, change the soda lime, circuit and/or machine if possible.
- Maintain anaesthesia using TIVA (e.g.) + ND (non-depolarizing neuromuscular blocking drug).
- Prepare DANTROLEN (2–3 mg/kg bolus dose, then 1 mg/kg PRN).
- Actively cool the patient, but avoid vasoconstriction; use cold IV fluids, cold peritoneal lavage, extracorporeal heat exchange when needed.
- Assist for the insertion of arterial line, CVC, urine catheter, monitor core temperature and coagulation.
- Use sodium bicarbonate for acidosis.
- Initiate sodium bicarbonate, glucose and insulin, and IV calcium chloride in hyperkalaemia.

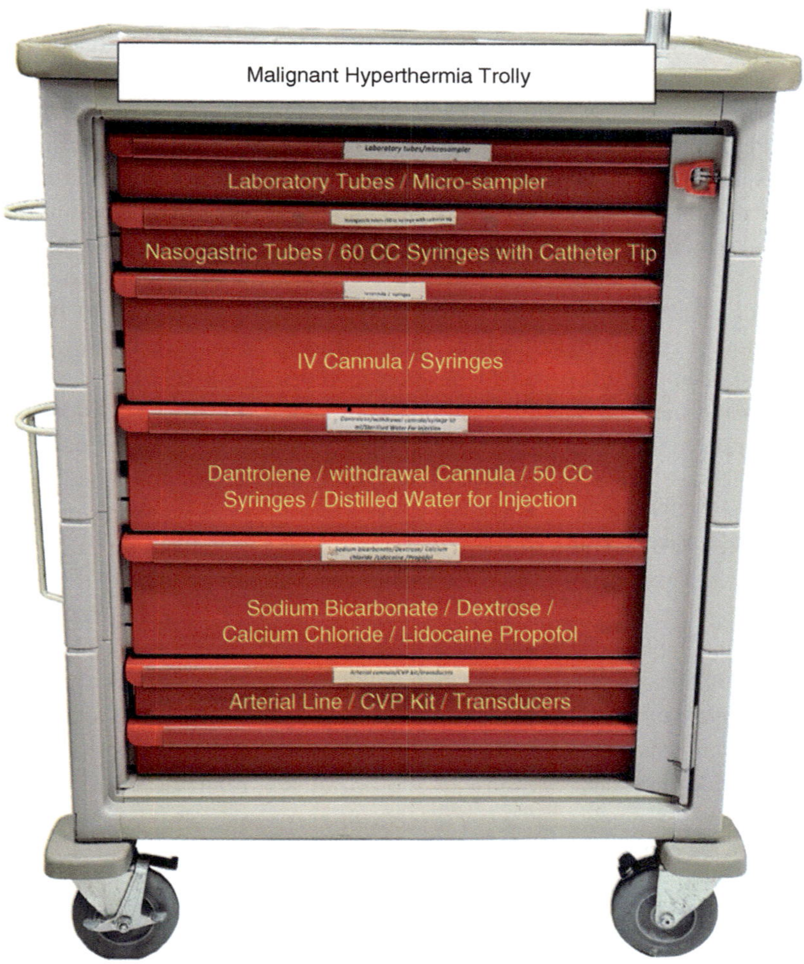
Malignant Hyperthermia Trolly
Laboratory Tubes / Micro-sampler
Nasogastric Tubes / 60 CC Syringes with Catheter Tip
IV Cannula / Syringes
Dantrolene / withdrawal Cannula / 50 CC Syringes / Distilled Water for Injection
Sodium Bicarbonate / Dextrose / Calcium Chloride / Lidocaine Propofol
Arterial Line / CVP Kit / Transducers

Fig. 11.7 Malignant hyperthermia trolley

- Initiate Myoglobinaemia if urine output <3 ml/kg/h, and urine pH < 7.0).
- If the patient developed disseminated intravascular coagulation, infuse fresh frozen plasma, cryoprecipitate, and platelets.
- If there are signs of cardiac arrhythmia, start procainamide, magnesium, amiodarone (avoid calcium channel blockers interact with dantrolene).
- Admit the patient to ICU for follow up and management.

11.12 Patient Positioning

The main target to place a patient on a certain position is to provide the surgeon with adequate exposure of the operative site. It is a responsibility that is shared by the operating room team.

The team should assess:

- Procedure length.
- Surgeon's preference of position.
- Patient s risk factors (age, weight, skin condition, mobility, and airway).

All positions can cause cardiovascular and pulmonary physiologic changes, nerve injury, and skin injury. Ideal patient position involves balancing between surgical comfort against the risks related to patient position.

11.12.1 Objectives of Appropriate Position

- Maintain patient s airway.
- Avoid pressure on the chest cavity.
- maintain circulation.
- Prevent nerve damage.
- provide adequate exposure of the operative site.
- provide comfort and safety to the patient.

11.12.2 Types of Position

11.12.2.1 Supine

Arms should be abducted <90°.

The arms, sacrum, and occiput should be poisoning and padded with gel or viscoelastic material to avoid pressure and injury.

11.12.2.2 Trendelenburg Position: (Fig. 11.8a)

Increase intracranial and intraocular pressure. Prolonged Trendelenburg position can cause oedema of the face and airway obstruction. Brachial plexus injury is not uncommon and precaution should be applied. Avoid this position in patients with major cardiovascular diseases.

11.12.2.3 Reverse Trendelenburg: (Fig. 11.8b)

The cardiovascular effect may be similar to the effects of the sitting position. Therefore, gradual increase in the position is highly advisable.

Lateral decubitus position: patient should be supported with rolls or bolsters to avoid rolling to prone or supine position. The head should be supported in a neutral position. Use chest support (axillary roll) to avoid compression of neurovascular structures.

11.12.2.4 Flexed Lateral Decubitus Position (Fig. 11.8c)

Table should be flexed at the iliac crest to minimize compression of the vena cave and thoracic structures.

11.12.2.5 Prone Position: (Fig. 11.8d)

To avoid abdominal compression the torso should be supported on rolls or bolsters. Breast and genitalia should be not compressed. Neck should be on the neutral position. Eyes and nose should be free from pressure and checked regularly during surgery.

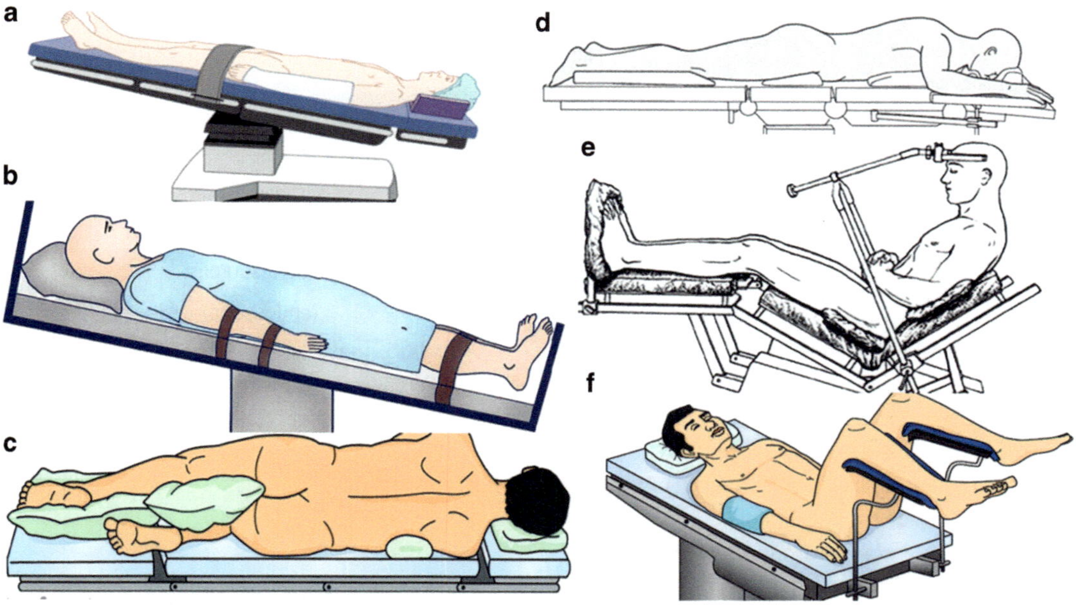

Fig. 11.8 Intra operative Patient Positioning, (**a**) Trendelenburg position (**b**) Reverse Trendelenburg (**c**) Flexed lateral decubitus position (**d**) Prone position (**e**) Sitting position (**f**) Lithotomy position

11.12.2.6 Sitting Position: (Fig. 11.8e)

The most important physiologic changes are cardiovascular effects (decrease of cardiac preload, stroke volume, and mean arterial pressure). Maintain MAP within 20%of baseline preoperative resting value and >70 mmHg. Therefore, gradual increase in the position is highly advisable.

11.12.2.7 Lithotomy Position: (Fig. 11.8f)

Legs should be positioned without hyperextension or flexion to avoid nerve injury. The legs should be raised into position simultaneously by two attendants and taken out of the lithotomy position in the same time.

11.13 Operating Room Fire Safety

Fires in operating room are rare but preventable. Fire requires three components: an oxidizer (oxygen, nitrous dioxide), an ignition source (electrocautery, lasers), and a fuel (flammable prepping agents, drapes, PPE). Whenever these three items are in close contact, fire will occur (Fig. 11.9).

11.13.1 Fire Occurring in OR Environment

When a fire occurs in OR, commonly electrical equipment is involved. Immediately unplug safely the equipment and remove it from OR. If impossible extinguishing the device in the room.

11.13.2 Fire Occurring on the Patient

- Extinguishing the flames.
- Removing burning material from the patient.
- Use CO_2 extinguisher to put out the fire.
- Immediately discontinued all gases (especially oxygen and nitrous oxide).
- Fire occurs on the patient airway.
- Discontinue all gases and remove the endotracheal tube.
- Remove any residually burning items.
- Pour saline or water into the airway.
- Reintubate patient and ventilate with medical air if no sever damage or keep mask ventilation if applicable. Tracheostomy is needed is sever airway damage OPERATING ROOM'S FIRE. Algorithm adopted from Anaesthesia Patient Safety Foundation (Fig. 11.10).

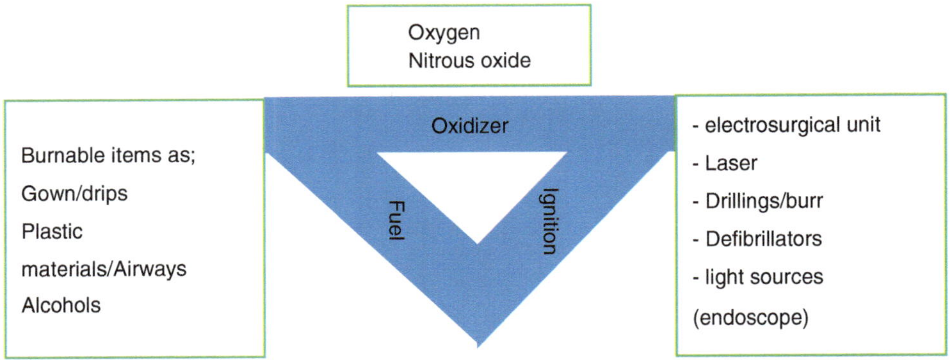

Fig. 11.9 Three components of fire inside OR

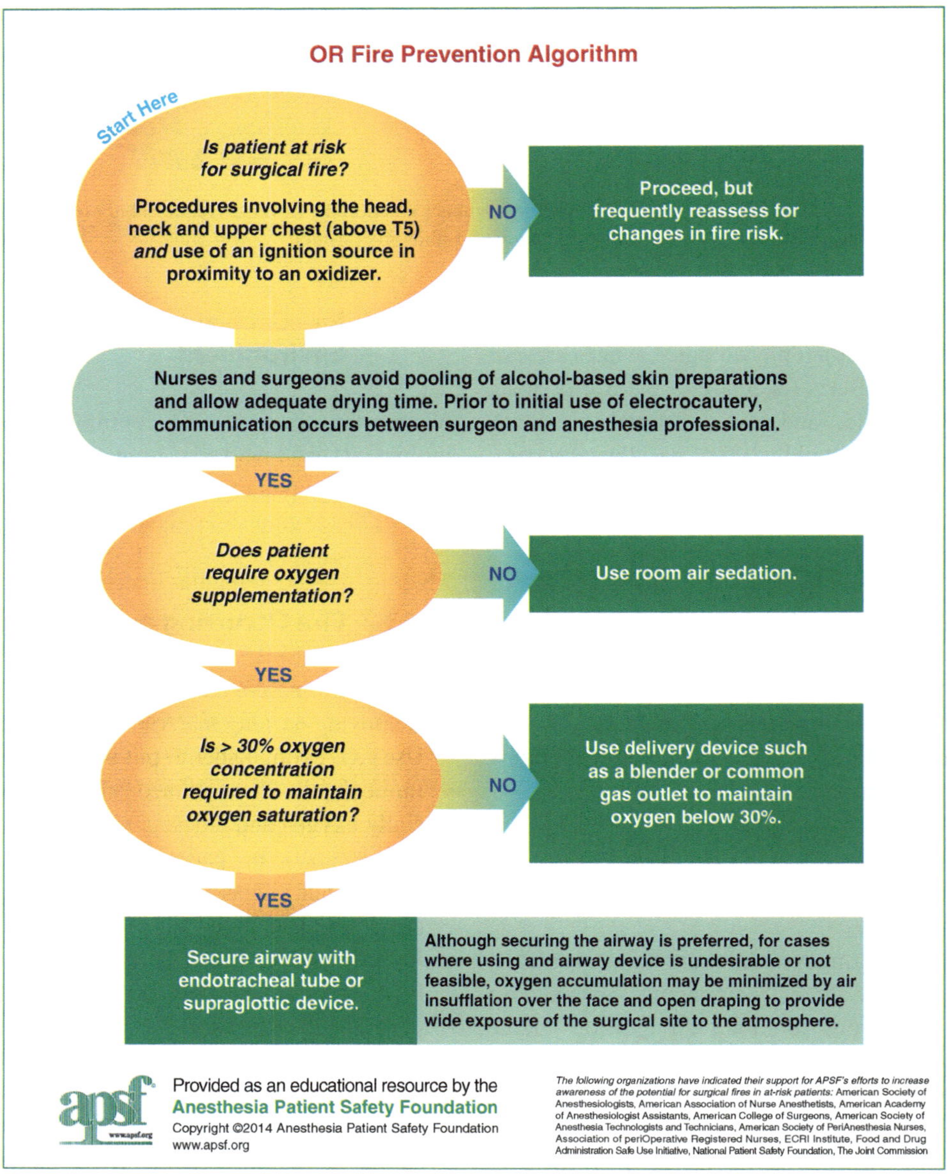

Fig. 11.10 Operating room's fire. (With written permission from Anaesthesia Patient Safety Foundation (APSF))

11.14 Laser and Operating Room Safety

Laser is commonly used nowadays during surgery and has both pros and cons.

11.14.1 Pros

- Decrease in postoperative pain and surgical site infections.
- Improved wound healing.
- Precise cutting.
- Reduction in blood loss.

11.14.2 Cons

It may lead to fire and damage to the eyes both physiologic and biological hazards (e.g., LASER plume) Fig. 11.11. Therefore, efficient preparation during LASER use is mandatory; such as covering reflective surfaces, donning proper LPE, LASER plume management, and prevention electrical hazards.

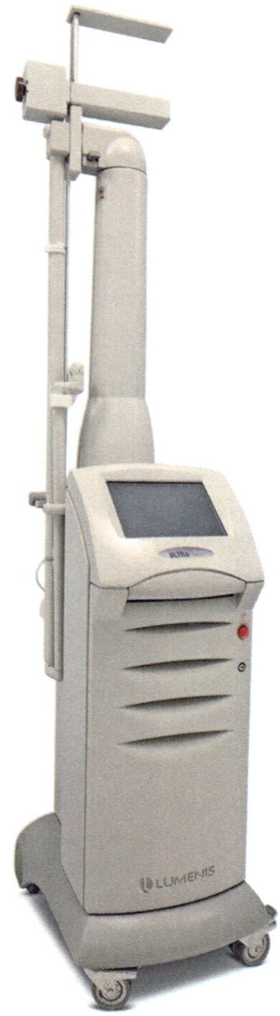

Fig. 11.11 LASER machine

11.14.3 Measures Taken by Anaesthesia Provider in Case of Airway Fire

- The ET tube cuff should be inflated with saline (in case of rupture saline will help for extinguishing airway fires).
- The anaesthesia provider should remove immediately the ET tube and turn off the anaesthetic gases to the patient.
- All flammable and burning material should be removed from the airway.
- Water should be poured into the patient's airway.
- When the airway fire is extinguished, the anaesthesia provider should re-establish ventilation by mask.

11.15 Conclusion and Recommendations

Enhancing our knowledge and skills will improve the preparedness for surgical cases of any kind of clinical condition. This in return will help to learn how to manage and avoid such complications.

It is not uncommon to find Anaesthesia technician working solo in several countries across the globe due to the lack of MD Anaesthesiologist. Therefore, the input in this chapter will provide a fast concise information to act properly and safely once needed.

Suggested Readings

Anesthesia Patient Safety Foundation: prevention and management of operating room fires (Video). 2010. https://www.apsf.org/videos/or-fire-safety-video/. Accessed 30 June 2020.

Beck-Schimmer B, Bonvini JM. Bronchoaspiration: incidence, consequences and management. Eur J Anaesthesiol. 2011;28:78–84.

Bux J. Transfusion-related acute lung injury (TRALI): a serious adverse event of blood transfusion. Vox Sang. 2005;89:1–10.

Cook T, Frerk C. 4th National Audit Project (NAP 4): major complications of airway management in the United Kingdom Report and Findings—Chapter 19. Aspiration of gastric contents and of blood, 2011 March the Royal College of Anesthetists and The Difficult Airway Society.

Cook TM, Counsell D, Wildsmith JA. Major complications of central neuraxial block: report on the Third National Audit Project of the Royal College of Anaesthetists. Br J Anaesth. 2009;102:179–90.

Fatalities reported to FDA following blood collection and transfusion: annual summary for fiscal year 2018. Silver Spring, MD: US Food and Drug Administration; 2018.

Frerk C, Mitchell VS, McNarry AF, et al. Difficult Airway Society intubation guidelines working group, Difficult Airway Society 2015 guidelines for management of unanticipated difficult intubation in adults. BJA: Br J Anaesth. 2015;115:827–48. https://doi.org/10.1093/bja/aev371.

Guarney H, Brown A, Litman RS. Malignant hyperthermia and muscular dystrophies. Anesth Analg. 2009;109:1043–8.

Harper NJ, Dixon T, Dugué P, et al. Working Party of the Association of Anaesthetists of Great Britain and Ireland. Suspected anaphylactic reactions associated with anaesthesia. Anaesthesia. 2009;64:199–211.

Hopkins PM. Malignant hyperthermia: pharmacology of triggering. Br J Anaesth. 2011;107:48–56.

Kaur H, Katyal N, Yelam A, Kumar K, Srivastava H, Govindarajan R. Malignant hyperthermia. Mo Med. 2019;116:154–9.

Kumeta Y, Hattori A, Mimura M, Kishikawa K, Namiki A. A survey of perioperative bronchospasm in 105 patients with reactive airway disease. Masui. 1995;44:396–401.

Laser use and safety. ECRI Institute. Available at www.ceeducation.org/Documents/3-Lasers/ECRI-SurgAn17.pdf. Accessed 19 Oct 2018.

McEwen DR. Intraoperative positioning of surgical patients. AORN J. 1996;63:1059–63.

Neal JM, Barrington MJ, Fettiplace MR, et al. The third American Society of Regional Anesthesia and Pain Medicine practice advisory on local anesthetic systemic toxicity: executive summary 2017. Reg Anesth Pain Med. 2018;43:113–23.

Nolan TE, Gallup DG. Massive transfusion: a current review. Obstet Gynecol Surv. 1991;46:289–95.

Nolan JP, Hazinski MF, Aicken R, et al. Part I. Executive summary: 2015 international consensus on cardiopulmonary resuscitation and emergency cardiovascular care science with treatment recommendations. Resuscitation. 2015;95:e1–e32.

Olsson GL. Bronchospasm during anaesthesia. A computer-aided incidence study of 136,929 patients. Acta Anaesthesiol Scand. 1987;31:244–52.

Soar J, Callaway CW, Aibiki M, et al. Part 4: advanced life support: 2015 international consensus on cardiopulmonary resuscitation and emergency cardiovascular care science with treatment recommendations. Resuscitation. 2015a;95:e71–e122.

Soar J, Nolan JP, Bottiger BW, et al. European resuscitation council guidelines for resuscitation 2015 section 3 adult advanced life support. Resuscitation. 2015b;95:99–146.

Surgical fires: decreasing incidence relies on continued prevention efforts. Pennsylvania Patient Safety Advisory. 2018. Available at: http://patientsafety.pa.gov/ADVISORIES/Pages/201806_SurgicalFires.aspx. Accessed 20 Apr 2020.

Watson DS. New recommendations for prevention of surgical fires. AORN J. 2010;91:463–9.

Vascular Access: From Cannulation to Decannulation

12

Nissar Shaikh, Arshad Chanda, Adel Ganaw,
Mohammad Sameer, Jazib Hassan,
Muhmmad Waqas Farooqi,
and Mohammed Mohsin A. M. Haji

Contents

All figures are compiled by the authors.

N. Shaikh (✉)
Department of Anesthesia, ICU and Perioperative Medicine, Hamad Medical Corporation, Doha, Qatar

Surgical Intensive Care, Hamad Medical Corporation, Doha, Qatar
e-mail: smaheboob@hamad.qa

A. Chanda · A. Ganaw · M. Sameer · J. Hassan
M. W. Farooqi · M. M. A. M. Haji
Department of Anesthesia, ICU and Perioperative Medicine, Hamad Medical Corporation, Doha, Qatar
e-mail: achanda@hamad.qa; Aganaw@hamad.qa; msameer@hamad.qa; Jhassan1@hamad.qa; Mfarooqui@hamad.qa; Mhaji@hamad.qa

N. A. Shallik et al. (eds.), *Improving Anesthesia Technical Staff's Skills*,
https://doi.org/10.1007/978-3-030-88849-7_12

12.1 Introduction

Vascular access is one of the most common procedures done in many setups like the scene of medical emergencies, ambulances, and numerous hospital facilities. It is done in hospitals on both outpatient and inpatients basis. It is an important modality to deliver intravenous therapy in the acute care of the patients. It is one of the core skills performed by various health care workers like physicians, nurses, and technicians depending upon their training and privileges. The vascular access can range from minimally invasive like procedures like phlebotomy in a lab to highly invasive like central line and arterial line insertion in intensive care units (ICU).

12.2 Vascular Access Can Be Divided into the Following Categories

12.2.1 Phlebotomy

It is also called venipuncture; it is a one-time procedure in which a metallic needle is inserted in the vein (usually upper limb) to draw blood for investigations.

12.2.2 Peripheral Intravenous (IV) Cannulation

It is temporary venous access and is usually done in inpatients. It is the insertion of a sterile, PVC tube called a cannula into a blood vessel. It is used to deliver various medications, fluids, blood, and blood products. They can last up to 3–7 days. When performed properly, peripheral IV placement is a safe procedure with little serious risk.

12.2.3 Central Venous Access (CVC)

This is a more invasive procedure in which the central veins (jugular, subclavian, and femoral) are catheterised. They are accessed by using flexible PVC catheters, left in the body for intermediate duration (usually for 1–2 weeks). These are used to deliver highly irritant medication like a chemotherapy agent, electrolytes, long-term IV feeding, blood transfusion, haemodialysis, etc. They are also used for monitoring purposes like to assess the central venous pressure (CVP) and cardiac output etc.

12.2.4 Arterial Vascular Access

It is also an invasive procedure wherein a cannula or catheter is inserted in arteries like radial, brachial, femoral arteries, etc. They are accessed for monitoring purposes like continuous BP, Cardiac output, and diagnostic purposes like repeated arterial blood gas analysis (ABG), and therapeutic purposes like selective thrombolysis, stenting, and embolisation.

12.2.5 Interosseous Cannulation (IO)

Intraosseous cannulation is a type of vascular access wherein a needle is introduced into the medullar cavity of the long bones. Interosseous cannulation is an emergency procedure. It is done in the critically ill or injured patients in whom the peripheral or central venous access is difficult or delayed. Nowadays, it is usually used in the prehospital setup. It can be done by less skilled health care providers and needs less practice when compared to the peripheral and central line placement.

12.3 The Peripheral Venous Access

Peripheral IV cannulation also called peripheral line insertion is usually done in the superficial veins of the upper limb, less often in the lower limbs (avoided because of the high rate of complications), and very rarely in scalp veins (usually in neonates). These IV cannulations are either done under anatomical landmark guidance or by visual and palpatory methods. Anatomical landmark has been the standard practice until the advent of point of care ultrasound (POCUS) which is real-time imaging. Ultrasound (US) guided IV cannulation is done in difficult access e.g. like obesity or multiple failed attempts. But the US-guided IV cannulation needs training and there is a steep learning curve.

12.3.1 The Anatomy of the Accessible Superficial Veins for Peripheral IV Cannulation

There are many sites in the body where the superficial peripheral vein can be cannulated. The selection of the site is based on various factors like vascular assessment (ease of accessibility), size of the vein dictates the catheter gauge, indication for IV cannulation, duration of therapy, and patient preferences. Identifying access sites by the anatomical landmark method may be more difficult in obese patients, children, patients in shock, repeated cannulation for chemotherapy, intravenous drug abuse, and dark skin [1].

The advantages of the peripherally inserted IV cannula are ease of insertion, less expertise, and equipment needed, less pain than central access, faster especially in a situation like cardiac arrest or shock, can be inserted repeatedly, safer as no complications of the central line like pneumothorax, hemithorax, infections, and economical.

A brief discussion will be done about the anatomical landmarks of the commonly accessed superficial peripheral veins. Ideally preferred veins should be a straight, non-branched, adequate length to match the cannula length, and distal in the extremity.

12.3.2 Different Sites for Peripheral IV Cannulation

12.3.2.1 Upper Extremity Veins [2, 3]

The venous drainage starts from the metacarpal veins on the dorsum of the hand which forms the dorsal venous arch. They are the most accessible sites because they are easily visible and palpable. The arch drains in the cephalic and basilic veins of the forearm.

In the antecubital fossa, these two veins are connected by the median cubital and median antebrachial veins. They are usually large and can be easily cannulated. These veins are not a primary choice during elective cannulation but are a very useful option during an emergent IV access. There is an increased risk of arterial puncture and nerve injury.

12.3.2.2 Neck Veins [2, 3]

The external jugular vein drains into the subclavian vein. It is a large vein that becomes more prominent in Trendelenburg's position or during the Valsalva manoeuvre. These two manoeuvres are adopted to distend the veins to ease the cannulation in severe volume-depleted condition [2].

12.3.2.3 Lower Extremity Veins [2, 3]

Like the upper extremities, the dorsal venous plexus of the foot continues proximally as great and small saphenous veins in the leg. The greater saphenous vein at the level of the medial malleolus and the dorsal metatarsal veins on the dorsum of the foot is often accessible [3]. However, lower extremity sites should be used only if veins in the arm cannot be cannulated.

12.3.2.4 Scalp Veins [2, 3]

The superficial temporal veins are the most accessed in the scalp. The frontal, occipital, or posterior auricular veins are the other options. But they are not accessible in neonates or infants (Fig. 12.1).

The non-dominant upper extremity is commonly chosen, because of comfort, reduced risk of dislodgement, and lower incidence of thrombosis or thrombophlebitis.

12.3.3 Indications for Peripheral IV Cannulation

When any invasive procedure is planned always consider the indication and contraindications of the procedure.

There are many indications for peripheral IV cannulation; they can be divided into diagnostic and therapeutic indications. These are few indi-

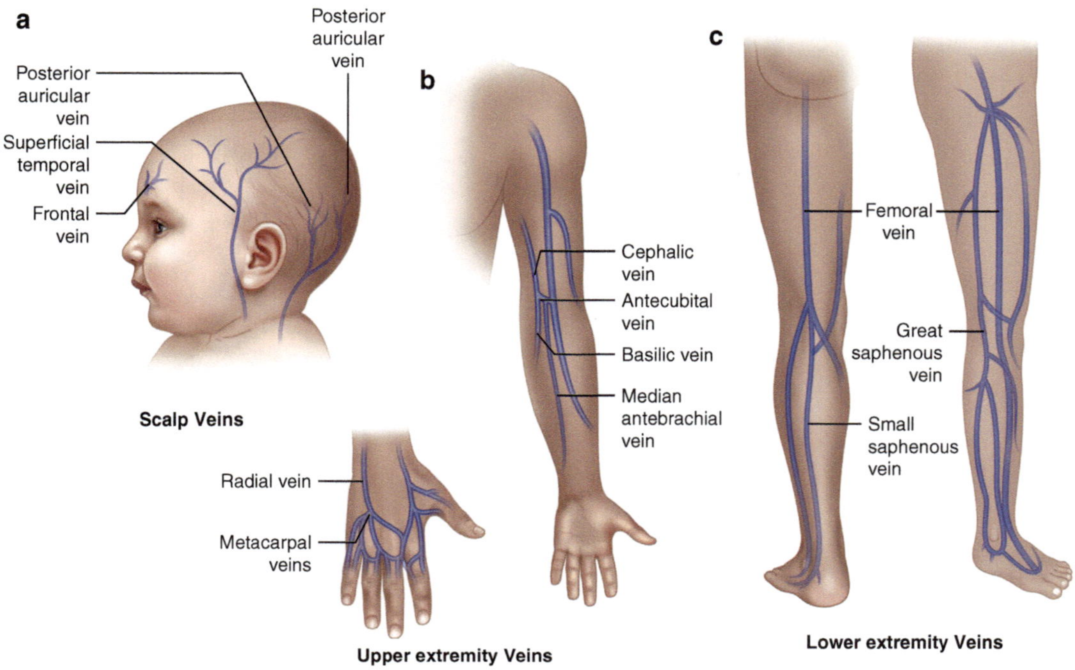

Fig. 12.1 (**a**) Scalp veins. (**b**) Upper extremity veins. (**c**) Lower extremity veins

cations listed in the following but they are not limited to these.

Diagnostic Indications It includes repeated blood sampling but peripheral IV cannulas (once used for delivering medications) are not ideal to draw blood for investigations, administration of IV contrast agents for computed tomography (CT), magnetic resonance imaging (MRI), or nuclear imaging, etc.

Therapeutic Indications These indications are the administration of fluid, medications (especially for rapid onset of action or increased bioavailability), chemotherapeutic agents, peripheral parenteral nutrition, blood, or blood products.

Contraindications of the Peripheral IV Cannulation There are no absolute contraindications other than a patient's refusal. The relative contraindications can be site-specific like local infection, injury to the area of the venous access, or burns.

Some contraindications are medications related as they can cause tissue necrosis (in case of extravasation) thrombosis, and intense pain on injection. Those medications are chemotherapeutic agents, vasopressors in high concentration, medications with highly acidic and highly alkaline (pH < 5 or pH > 9), Osmolality >600 mOsm/L. They can be given through a peripheral vein in emergencies with careful monitoring and in higher dilutions.

12.3.4 Types of IV Cannulas

There are various types of IV cannulas available worldwide (Fig. 12.2): There are different sizes and they are sized according to the French gauge. The higher the gauge, the lesser the diameter of the cannula. They are colour coded according to the diameter. Various types of the commercially available cannula can be winged or non-winged, ported or non-ported, and the closed or open system. The closed system will have a self-activating safety mechanism to prevent needle stick injuries and blood splatter.

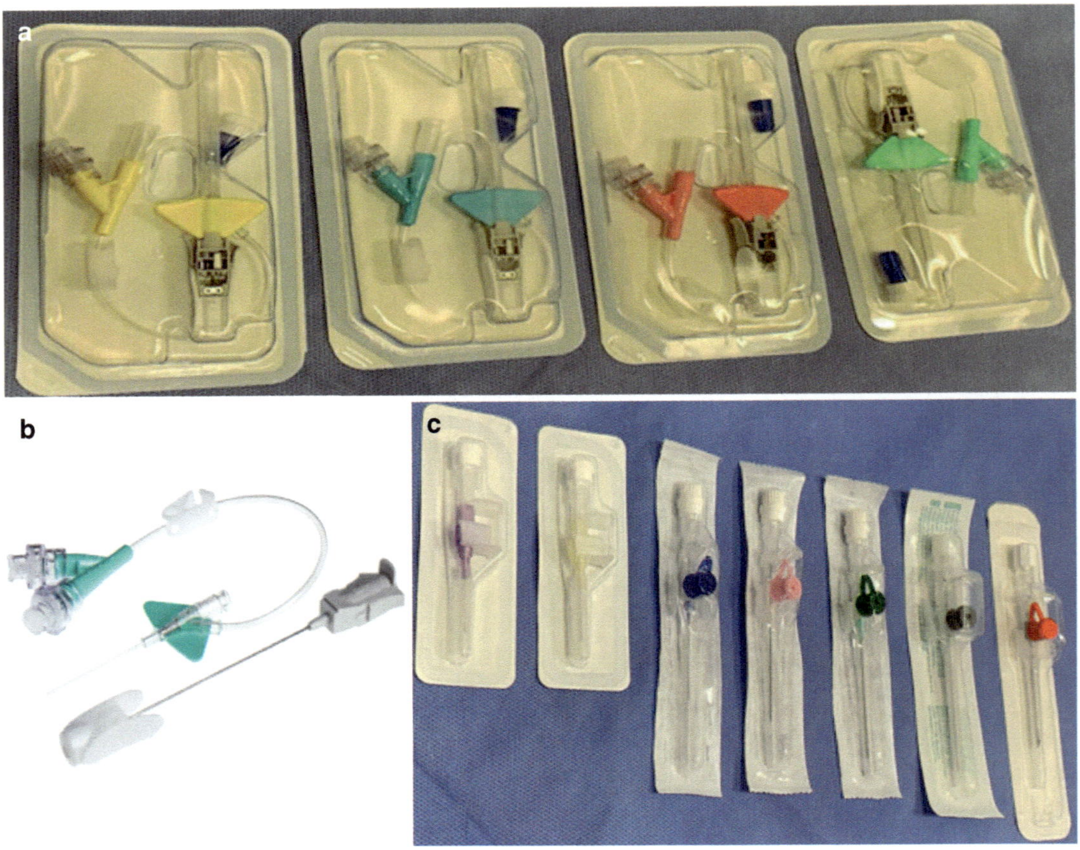

Fig. 12.2 Types of IV cannulas. (**a**) Winged non-ported, (**b**) Winged, non-ported, and closed system with the needle outside the catheter, (**c**) Winged and ported but the non-closed system

12.3.5 Part of the Typical IV Cannula

The parts of a typical IV cannula are labelled in Fig. 12.3 and they are self-explanatory.

12.3.5.1 Size of the Peripheral IV Cannulas and Their Flow Rate (Table 12.1)

Peripheral IV catheters range from the smallest 26 to the largest 14 gauges. As the gauge increases, the diameter decreases.

The diameter and the length of the cannula determine the flow rate of the fluids through the peripheral IV cannula. The larger the diameter and the shorter the length; the more rapid is the flow. It follows Poiseuille's law ($V = \prod p\ r4/8\ \acute{\eta}$ l), which states that flow is directly related to the pressure driving the fluid and to the internal radius of the catheter raised to the fourth power, and inversely related to the length of the catheter and to the viscosity of the fluid [4].

While choosing the cannula the smallest gauge and appropriate length should be selected. Smaller the size less the trauma and phlebitis. 20G catheters are usually used in routine medical practice. They are appropriate for medication administration and infusion of moderate volumes of IV fluids. If larger volume and rapid infusion of fluids are needed, then an 18G catheter or greater gauge cannula is indicated. The risk of dislodgement is less with longer catheters.

Catheter length is longer for the US-guided cannulation because they must travel a longer distance before piercing the veins.

The performance and complications of venous access placement without the use of ultrasound guidance will be discussed in the following section.

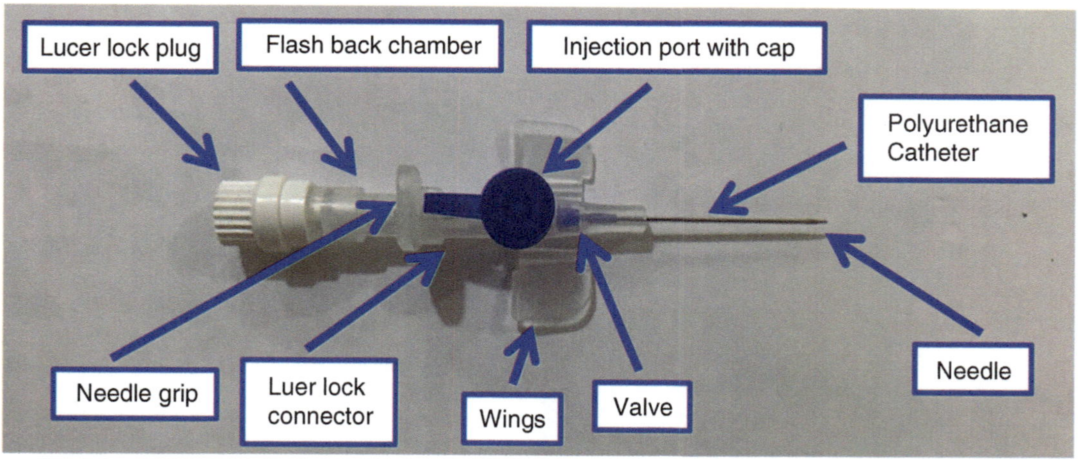

Fig. 12.3 Part of the IV typical IV cannula

Table 12.1 The gauge, colour code, and flow rates through the cannulas. The flow rates are approximate values. Companies specify the flow rates of their cannulas on the back of the IV cannula pack

Colour Code	Gauge	External dia mm	Length mm	Flow rate mL/ hr
Orange	14G	2.1	45	240
Grey	16G	1.8	45	180
Green	18G	1.3	45	90
Pink	20G	1.1	32	60
Blue	22G	0.9	25	36
Yellow	24G	0.7	19	20
Violet	26G	0.6	19	13

12.3.6 Performance of Peripheral IV Cannulation

Step for performing IV cannulations starts with the discussion with the patient about the plan for cannulation, its indications, procedure, and complications. Informed consent is usually obtained (usually it is implied consent in the general consent). Assessment of the veins and site selection, preparation of the patient, and equipment. Perform the cannulation, secure it, and check for complications. Remove the IV cannula if no more indicated.

12.3.6.1 Equipment for Peripheral IV Cannulation

Equipment required for intravenous (IV) cannulation include the (Fig. 12.4) IV Cannula of appropriate size at least two cannulas each of two different sizes, tourniquet, nonsterile gloves, connective tubing. The antiseptic solution preferably 2% chlorhexidine in 70% isopropyl alcohol for skin preparation, 2 × 2 in. gauze and vacuum collection tubes and adaptor. Saline flush and or heparin lock (avoid in patients with coagulopathy and HIT). EMLA cream for paediatrics patients, local anaesthetic solution 1% Lidocaine, and an

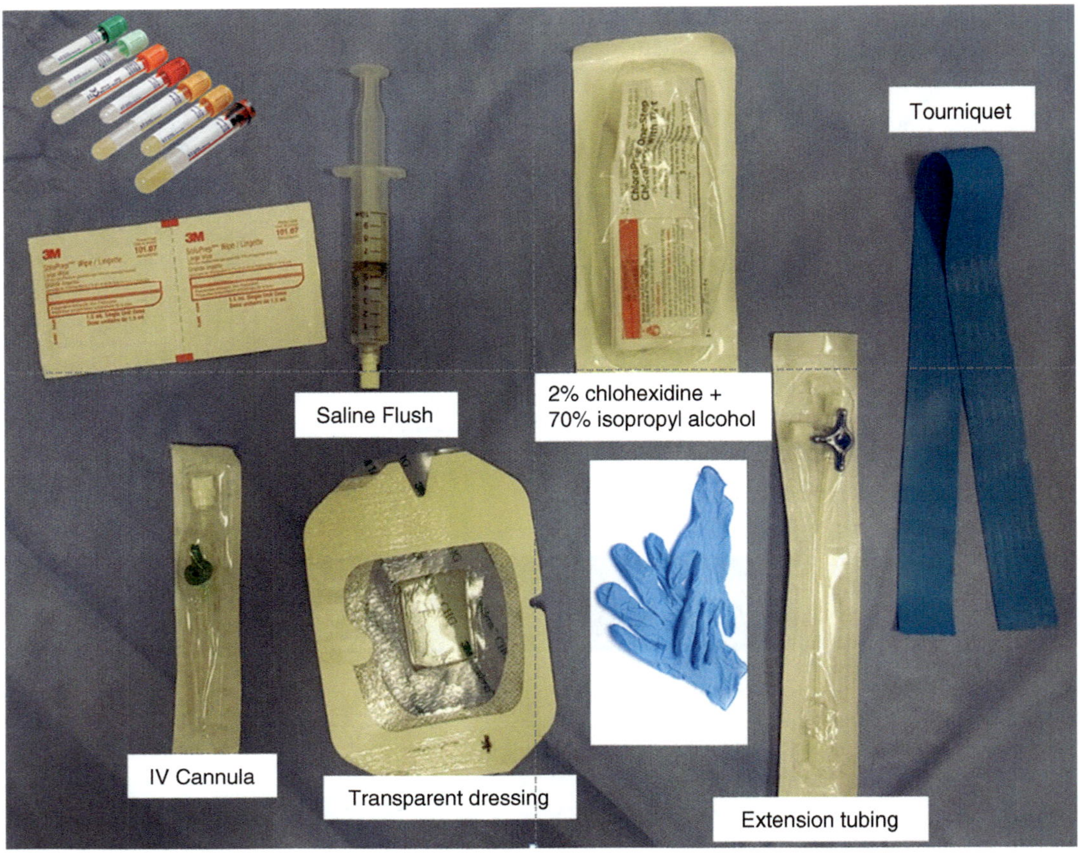

Fig. 12.4 Equipment required for intravenous (IV) cannulation

Insulin syringe with a 26 to 30-gauge needle (required only for thick gauge cannulations like 14 G in adults). Transparent dressing and tape to secure the cannula, sharp disposal box. Ultrasound Machine with Vascular probe.

Other equipment and materials needed are infusion pump, fluid warmers, and pressure infusers. A splint to reduce movement and decrease the risk of dislodgment of the catheter if placed over a joint.

12.3.7 Assessment of the Veins and Site Selection

12.3.7.1 Ideal Site for IV Cannulation Is

There is no ideal site for cannulation as such. Site selection depends on the clinical circumstances, indication for cannulation (therapeutic or diagnostic, and expected duration of therapy).

During trauma resuscitation, the larger veins of the antecubital fossa for peripheral IV catheters are ideal as they are large and in adults can accommodate cannulas as big as 14G.

It is preferable to select a site with the following considerations like patients' preferences, medical history of the patient, condition of the veins, expected duration of I.V. therapy, age, size, general condition.

Select a vein that is easy to access, larger the vein easier it is to cannulate, select a nondominant limb if possible as it allows daily activities, and reduces inconvenience in complications like extravasation. Avoid lower extremities because of the high risk of thrombosis and infection. Avoid cannulating through the infected areas and areas with burns as it can cause systemic infection, cannulation area near joints because it increases the risk of kinging, dislodgment, and restricts the movement of the limb, avoid cannulation near arteries, and nerves (potential risk of injury). The selection of the vein also depends on the type of I.V. medications or IV fluids to be infused. Always try to start distally in the extremity; if started with the proximal one and failed, a successful attempt in the distal site can cause extravasation of medication and hematoma formation, this also saves the proximal sites for subsequent cannulation, if needed. Finally, the skill of the performing health care worker also matters.

Avoid cannulation in the below a phlebitic area, sclerosed or thrombosed veins, areas of skin inflammation, disease, bruising, or breakdown due to the risk of introducing a systemic infection. Avoid cannulating an arm with an arteriovenous shunt or fistula, post-radical mastectomy or lymph node dissection as it exacerbates the impaired lymphatic drainage. Avoid cannulation in the veins below a previous I.V. extravasation or infiltration, especially if a hematoma is formed. Veins over the joints especially the wrist and antecubital fossa have nerves and arteries in the proximity, and it is preventing movement. It may also increase the risk of catheter dislodgement and kinking.

The superficial veins of the lower extremity related to the deep veins which can lead to Thrombophlebitis, deep vein thrombosis (DVT), and embolism. Catheters in the lower extremity should be moved as soon as the patient is stable. Avoid cannulation in the injured extremity as it may interfere with surgery, etc.

Placement of the peripheral IV cannula in a limb with a significant motor and/or sensory deficit (paralysed limb) is relatively contraindicated by some. This is because of the concern that the paralysed extremities are increased risk of developing deep vein thrombosis [5]. There may a delay in the detection of fluid or medication infiltration due to loss of sensation and patients cannot complain about it. These limbs can be cannulated in emergency and then decannulated once a suitable IV access is secured but needs close monitoring.

12.3.7.2 Prepare the Patient

Explaining the procedure is mandatory. It must be explained that IV cannulation is a painful procedure. Some patients tolerate it very well (adults) but some are apprehensive, especially the children.

If the cannulation is an elective procedure take time to explain to the patient the reason for venous cannulation, the amount of pain inflicted during the procedure. Try to quantify the pain inflicted with cannulation (e.g. it will be like an insect bite, pinprick, or a thorn prick). Approximately how long the catheter will be insitu depending on the planned treatment. The benefits and risks. Any alternatives if the patient wants to avoid cannulation. Consider the patients' preferences if not hampering the clinical indications and benefits.

12.3.7.3 Preparation for the Procedure

It is very important for successful cannulation. At first respect patient privacy. Both the patient and the person inserting the cannula should be comfortable. Anxiety in patients can cause vasoconstriction of veins due to the sympathetic nervous system stimulation [6]. Place the patient in a reclining or supine position. The extremity on which the venipuncture is being performed should be below the heart level to engorge the veins. Keep the patient warm as cold can cause vasoconstriction of superficial veins due to the sympathetic nervous system stimulation [6]. Clip the hair around the cannulation site but do not shave as it increases the risk of infection from the abrasions. It also helps in dressing adherence. Topical anaesthetic especially the EMLA Cream 5% needs enough time at least 60 min to be effective [7].

12.3.7.4 Perform the Cannulation

After explaining the procedure, positioning the patient, making the patient comfortable, arranging the equipment, and help if needed, the actual procedure of cannulation starts.

Select the vein and try to dilate (engorge) it. There are several methods to dilated veins. Proximal compression by using a rubber tourniquet tied proximal to the venipuncture site (approximately 5–10 cm). It impedes venous return and venous dilation [8]. Tourniquet pressures enough to cause venous compression but less than arterial pressure to maintain the blood flow. The vein should feel spongy and non-pulsatile on palpation; veins that feel hard are more likely to be thrombosed, and pulsatile flow indicates an artery. Positioning the cannulation site below the heart levels to fill the veins. Gentle stroking or tapping the vein can cause some venous distension. Active clenching and relaxing the first alternating by the patient. Warm fomentation can elevate skin temperatures can cause venous dilation.

12.3.7.5 Infection Control Measures

The procedure should be a completely sterile technique. The infection prevention principle must be followed to protect both the patient and the healthcare provider from infection. It starts with hand washing, donning clean gloves, and protective eyewear. Prepare the skin puncture site with 2% Chlorhexidine in 70% Isopropyl alcohol and don touch the cleaned area.

12.3.7.6 Analgesia

Analgesia is not routinely required for IV cannulation [9]. Though it alleviates the pain from venipuncture, but involves another injection causing pain and distorts the puncture site anatomy.

Analgesia for I.V cannulation can be divided into Topical and Parenteral (injected). These methods have their advantages and disadvantages. The topical agents are preferred but they some time to achieve optimal effect.

Parenteral (Injected)

Intradermal local anaesthetics with 1% Lidocaine is the most common method of anaesthetising a puncture site. It gives rapid anaesthesia and increases the success rate of IV cannulation catheter placement [10]. Never use anaesthetics that contain epinephrine as it can cause the vein to constrict and skin necrosis.

Topical

Several topical anaesthetics can be used to reduce the pain of venipuncture:

1. *Vapocoolant sprays* (Fig. 12.5e): Topical vapocoolant sprays (e.g. Ethyl chloride, Fluorohydrocarbon, and Alkane mixtures). can produce immediate skin anaesthesia. They act by cooling the skin surface immediately before IV placement. Their effect depends on the site, blood flow, subcutaneous fat, etc.
2. *EMLA Cream 5% (the eutectic mixture of local anaesthetics)* (Fig. 12.5a): It is a eutectic mixture of Lidocaine and prilocaine(50:50). It is one of the commonest and famous agents in practice. It must be applied at least an hour to attain a peak effect effect [7]. 1 to 2 g/10 cm^2

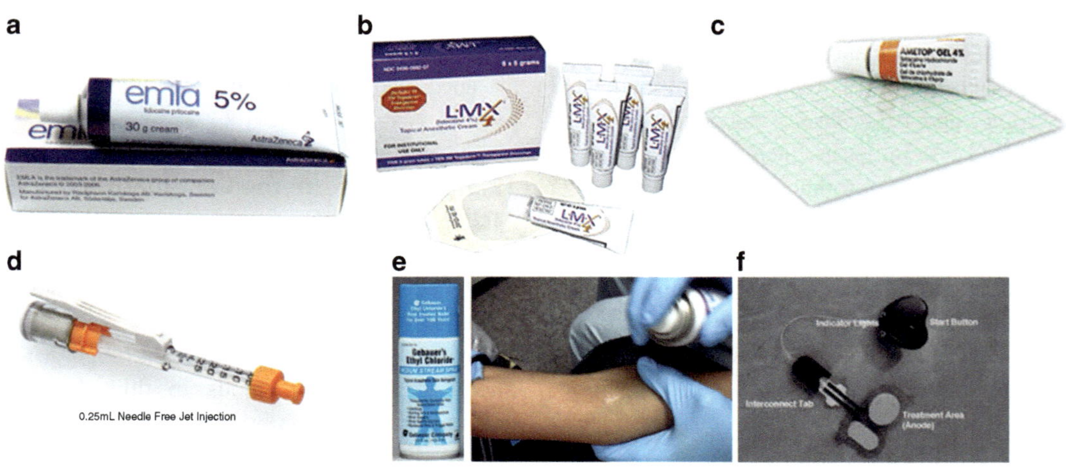

Fig. 12.5 Analgesics used before peripheral IV cannulation. (**c**) Tetracaine hydrochloride gel 4%.(**d**) The J-tip needle free injection. (**e**) Topical vapocoolant. (**f**) Iontophoresis system

of skin and then covered with an occlusive dressing. It is safe but can cause methemoglobinemia in some patients because of the Prilocaine [11].

3. *Tetracaine* (Fig. 12.5c): It is an Ester anaesthetic. Over 4% cream or 5% gel can be used. 5% liposomal encapsulated cream (LET). Its efficacy and time of onset are like EMLA [12].
4. *LMX lidocaine* (Fig. 12.5b): It is a topical preparation of Lidocaine which is encapsulated in liposomes, liposomes act as phospholipid-based carriers that promote passage of the anaesthetic through intact skin. It takes 30 min to have an optimal effect [13].

Methods that Can Enhance the Effect of Topical Local Anaesthetics Are as Follows

- *Iontophoresis* (Fig. 12.1f): It is a method of delivering local anaesthesia to the skin using a mild electrical current. This small electrical current moves ionised lidocaine through intact skin. It decreases the time for optimal effect from 1 h to 10 to 20 min. Its disadvantage is it can cause minor skin irritation and blistering [14].
- *Sonophoresis*: It uses low-frequency ultrasound to facilitate skin penetration of a local anaesthetic. It also hastens the time to attain the optimal effect. First, apply 15–20 s of ultrasound followed by a local anaesthetic application for 5 min. Its disadvantage is that it requires an ultrasound machine which is expensive equipment [15].
- *LASER*: An Erbium yttrium-aluminium-garnet (Er: YAG) LASER can be used to remove the stratum corneum. This will improve the penetration of local anaesthetic. It was used only for research with some positive results. It is very expensive [16].

12.3.8 How to Make the Vein Accessible for Cannulation

12.3.8.1 Tourniquet

As explained above.

12.3.8.2 Venodilator

Nitroglycerin ointment has been topically applied to the venipuncture site and left for 2–3 min. It causes venous dilation makes it easy to puncture the vein. No hypotension was noted with the use of Nitroglycerine [17].

12.3.8.3 Tools to Assist Vein Location

There are situations when veins are visible or palpable. This is usually seen in patients who are morbidly obese, hospitalised for a long time, on chemotherapy, paediatric age group, patients in shock, etc.

12.3.8.4 There Are Several Devices Available Commercially

They work on various principles like [18] transillumination uses a light frequency that causes deoxygenated venous blood to appear darker than surrounding tissues. Infrared light, which reflects off tissue surrounding the veins, but not the vein itself. Ultrasound can be used to identify veins larger than 2 mm.

More details regarding the vein viewer.

Vein Viewing Devices

Difficult Venous Access as mention earlier in the chapter is frequently encountered in neonates, paediatrics, elderly, and dark-skinned patients. They are also a challenging task in patients who are obese, hypotensive, multiple injuries, intravenous drug abusers, post-chemotherapy, etc. Difficult venous access causes distress due to multiple punctures, pain, fear, and delay in carrying out the treatment [19].

With the advances and improvements in technology, the development of vein viewing devices came into existence. These devices ease of viewing the peripheral veins; they provide a clear and detailed view of the veins. The details like their pattern, bifurcations, valves, assess the refill, and flushing of veins in real time. It is rendered incorporation of the technologies like Infrared light absorption, transillumination, and ultrasound guidance. These devices significantly reduce the number of cannulation attempts, time taken for cannulation, patients, and healthcare satisfaction [19, 20].

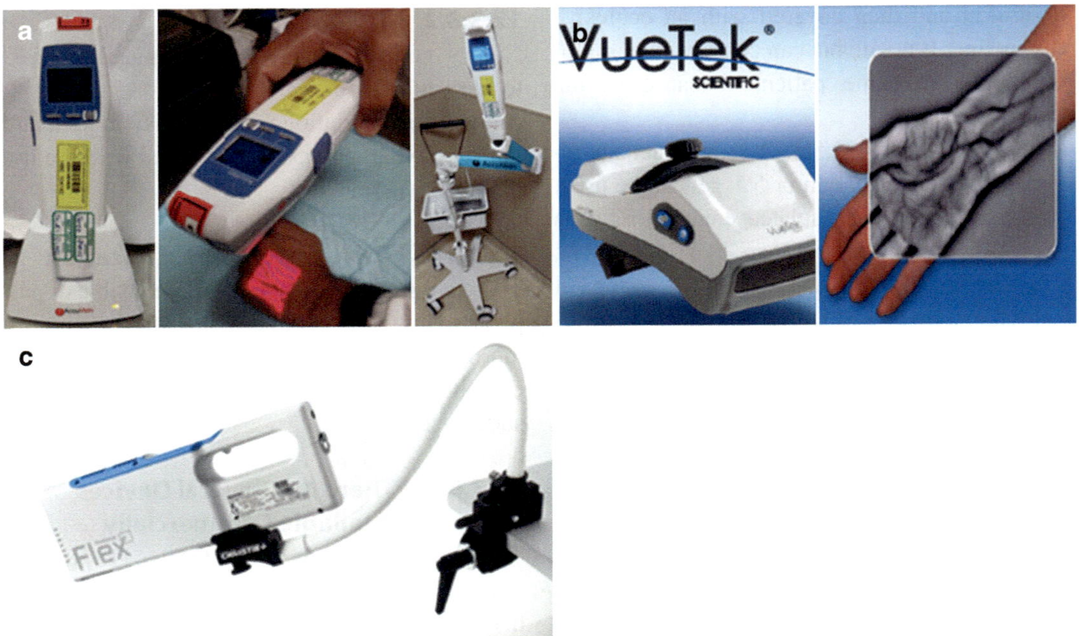

Fig. 12.6 Examples of the infrared vein viewing devices. (**a**) Accuvein, (**b**) Veinsite, (**c**) VeinViewer

Various devices are available commercially for vein visualisation. The transilluminators, near-infrared, and infrared devices.

Devices Using Near-Infrared (NIR) Imaging Technology

These devices use near-infrared light without any radiation (Fig. 12.6). These are invisible infrared laser and a visible red laser. When they are projected on the skin, haemoglobin in the veins absorbs the near-infrared light but it is reflected by the surrounding tissues. It helps in identifying the vein by vein mapping. It is a real-time visual map of the subcutaneous veins. These are small, lightweight, battery-operated, portable, and noncontact devices. They have to be held at a distance of about 7 in. above the skin surface. The device can map subcutaneous veins up to a depth of about 10 mm. They can also be mounted on a wheeled stand or headwear to operate hands-free.

AccuVein, Veinsite, and VeinViewer are a few commercially viable infrared vein viewing devices.

Transillumination Method

In these devices, vein pattern visualisation is facilitated by illuminating the skin surface by using LEDs (Fig. 12.7). De-oxygenated blood in veins absorbs the light and appears as dark lines which help in easier visualisation of veins. These devices help in identifying veins in all age groups, different skin tones, and different sized patients.

Veinsite and Wee-Sight are some commercially available transilluminator type of devices.

The devices like Viensite keep the vein from rolling out of the field but requires patient contact and they cannot work effectively with the ambient light. The infrared devices do not need patient contact and they work in light or dark conditions but require practical training [21].

12.3.8.5 Catheter Insertion

The classical technique of IV cannulation starts with explaining the patient about the procedure, selecting an appropriate vein, visualise and palpate the vein, tie the tourniquet 10–15 cm proximal to the puncture site. Sterilise the skin and once sterilised do not touch the puncture site with unsterile hands. A local anaesthetic may be injected. IV catheter should be held in the dominant hand between the thumb and forefingers. Stabilise the vein by holding the area with the non-dominant hand. Avoid wobbling movement

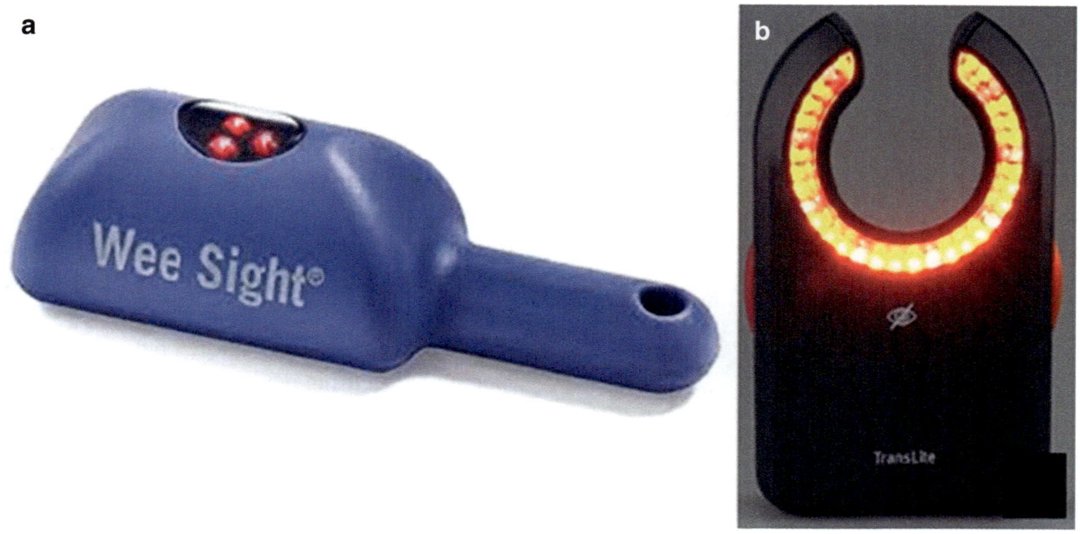

Fig. 12.7 Examples of the transilluminator type of vein viewing devices. (**a**) Wee-Sight, (**b**) Veinsite

of the vein during insertion by gently pulling the vein with the thumb. Puncture the skin at an angle of 15–30°. Once the flashback of blood is seen in the flashback chamber push the needle another 2 to 3 mm to ensure that the catheter tip in in the lumen of the vein. Hold the needle and advance the catheter into the vein (do not pull out the need from the catheter). The non-dominant hand to continue the pull the vein gently to maintain the straight path and prevent movement of the vein. The catheter traverses the path of the vein without resistance and pain if it is in the lumen of the vessel. A properly placed IV catheter there be no swelling and will have a steady flow of the blood. Once it is confirmed that the catheter is in the vein remove the needle. Untie and remove the tourniquet. Secure the catheter with a sterile dressing and attach the appropriate IV set up. Once the fluids and medicine are started and there is a steady flow with pain or swelling once confirms that the catheter is in the vein. Upon completion of the procedure, all sharp objects should be disposed of in the sharp bins and the soiled gauge and the underpad in the appropriate bins (Fig. 12.6).

12.3.8.6 Troubleshooting

The catheter cannot advance, the needle entered the vein, but the catheter is outside the lumen. Advance the needle 2–3 mm and then advance the catheter. The catheter is advanced too far and pierced the posterior wall. Here you must withdraw the needle 2–3 mm and pull back the catheter until you see a flashback of the blood. Then advance the catheter. The catheter is in the lumen of the vein but cannot be advanced. This is because of the tortuous path of the vein or a valve. If this is suspected, a saline stylet can be used. The saline stylet is a saline-filled syringe attached to the catheter. Saline is gently pushed through ensuring there is no swelling while doing so the catheter so slowly advanced till the hilt. A maximum of 2 attempts should be given if not successful just abandon the site and try at a different site (Fig. 12.8).

Swelling and extra-venous placement: Remove the catheter and apply pressure and try a different site above the current site.

Arterial cannulation. Inadvertent arterial cannulation does occur usually seen in the wrist and antecubital area. It is identified by the pulsatile jets of bright red blood. If the patient is in ICU and the transducer is attached will show an arterial waveform. If it happens, immediately remove the catheter and apply pressure for approximately 10 min and more if the patient is in a hypocaogulable state. Check the pulses distal to the puncture site and look for a capillary refill and SpO_2 for

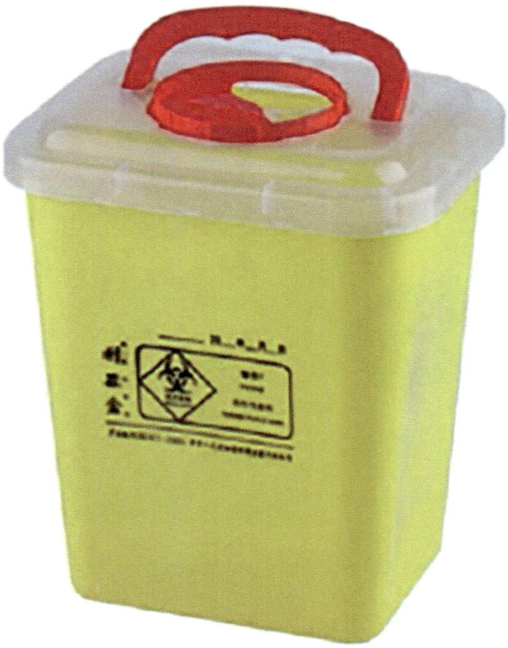

Fig. 12.8 A sharp disposal bin

some time to rule out the arterial block. Use of ultrasound, in the past two decades ultrasound is being used to perform many medical procedures under time images. We will discuss this in more detail in the ultrasound-guided IV cannulation.

12.3.8.7 Care of the IV Catheter Post-insertion

Securing and Dressing

Post-insertion secure the catheter with a sterile, transparent dressing. It will prevent the dislodgement of the catheter during movement of the limb. Movement can also increase the risk of thrombophlebitis and extravasation of IV fluids and medications.

Peripheral IV catheter can be secured by many different methods. It can be secured with ordinary sticking tape which is very cheap and easily available. Tapes are prone to be moved from one patient to another which can increase the risk of infection. Commercially available adhesive dressings are also used (Tegaderm, Opsite). They are a bit expensive and not easily available in third world countries. Curl the tubing to the side to avoid dislodgment if there is a pull on the line.

Transparent dressing allows the health care provider to observe the insertion site for swelling, infiltration, phlebitis infection without removing the dressing [22]. They waterproof as well. Do not stretch the plastic dressing as they can tear, become non-adhesive, and can cause itching.

Other methods are suture but very rare. Specific IV securing devices have been shown to reduce complications and increase catheter dwell time.

In children and if the IV catheter is placed over a joint place a splint to secure the catheter.

Maintaining Patency

Loss of patency is a common problem of the peripheral IV catheters. It is usually seen when the catheter is used for intermittent injections. Periodic flushing with isotonic saline can help to maintain their patency. 2–10 mL of isotonic saline after an IV medication and or every 4 – 12 h is the common practice. Heparin flush also called as "heparin lock" has been used but in use for peripheral IV catheters. These heparin locks can cause heparin-related complications [23].

Monitoring the Peripheral IV Access Site

Health care workers should periodically assess the catheter to check for proper placement (dislodgements). Extravasation usually manifests as swelling and pain at the site and slowing of the infusion rate, frequent high-pressure alarm by the infusion pumps. Patency, a kink, or a clot may have formed within the catheter. These can be detected if IV fluids no longer infuse via gravity or the catheter cannot be flushed. Avoid forceful flushing of thrombosed catheters as it can dislodge a clot into the circulation. Phlebitis can be manifest as redness, oedema, pain, and tenderness. Sometimes fever and sepsis. If any of these conditions are observed, immediately remove the catheter.

12.4 Complications of Peripheral IV Cannulas

Complications are rare but can occur. Complications are more common in catheters placed in emergency circumstances. The most common complications are haematoma formation, extravasation of IV fluids, Phlebitis, bruising, thrombophlebitis, and bloodstream infections are rare but can happen.

Less commonly compilations are skin necrosis, venous air embolism, nerve injury, arterial injury, compartment syndrome, septic discitis, pneumocephalus, tendon injury, and venous aneurysm formation.

12.4.1 Ultrasound-Guided Peripheral IV Cannulation [24]

Ultrasound (US) is being used commonly in many medical procedures. The use of ultrasound for peripheral IV cannulation is also rapidly gaining popularity with the health care worker. Ultrasound is preferred for access of veins that are >7 mm deep to the surface. Its use has been shown to reduce the number of unsuccessful attempts and complications. It also increases patient satisfaction as it decreases patient stress and pain. US guidance helps to choose an appropriate vein, know the depth of the vein, the diameter of the vein, course of the vein (straight of tortuous), length of the veins, junctions, and valves in the course of the vein, patency of the vein, check the adjacent structures like nerves and arteries, dynamic ultrasound guidance allows for real-time needle visualisation during puncture of the vessel.

US guide will reduce the risk of complications like hematoma, inadvertent puncture arteries, or, nerves, unsuccessful cannulation, time to successful cannulation, and costs of the procedure.

12.4.2 Equipment

The equipment required are an ultrasound machine, a High-frequency (5–15 MHz) linear transducer, the vascular probe (Fig. 12.9a), The "hockey-stick" 10–15 MHz transducer, it is a very high-resolution linear transducer, it gives a greater degree of needle and vein visibility, ultrasound gel (sonogel), sterile probe cover.

Ultrasound images of the veins the vein appears as black anechoic, they are easily compressible with light pressure, oval-shaped, thin-walled, non-pulsatile, application of limb tourniquets usually distends the veins and doppler will give a humming sound.

Arteries are circular, thick-walled, less easily compressible, and pulsatile. The Doppler will give a whoosh sound.

12.4.3 Ultrasound Views

12.4.3.1 There Are Three Views in the Ultrasound Imaging

The transverse view or short axis or out of plain.

The longitudinal views also called a long axis or in plain.

The oblique view—some operator uses it.

12.4.3.2 Transverse View (Fig. 12.9b, d)

Also called as or short axis or out of plain. The probe is placed at a 90-degree angle to the course of the vein. The cross-section of the vein is seen in this view. This view helps in localisation and visualisation of the vein.

The short axis is also preferred for puncturing the vein, the distinction between the vein and the adjacent artery is easy with the compression. The trajectory of the needle can easily be corrected. Ideally, the needle should enter the vein ate 12 "O" Clock position. The time to successful cannulation may be less with the short axis view.

12.4.3.3 Drawbacks of the Short Access Views

Visualisation of the needle tip throughout the process of needle insertion is difficult especially in inexperienced hands as it needs probe manipulation. This may result in perforation of the posterior wall and or injury to the adjacent nerve or artery.

12.4.3.4 The Longitudinal View (Fig. 12.9c, f)

This view is also called a long axis or in plain. It provides further information about the vein morphology, the diameter of the vein, and the presence of valves. It is difficult to maintain the centre of the vessel during procedures as the US beam is very thin. It is always advised to do both the short and long views before attempting cannulation. Viewing in both the plains will give detailed information about the local anatomy, condition of the vein, and increases the success rate and reduces the rate of complications.

12.4.4 Figure 12.9: Ultrasound Vascular (Linear Probe) and Mages of Peripheral IV Cannulation

12.4.4.1 The Dynamic Vs the Static Ultrasound

The "Dynamic" is also known as "real-time" ultrasound guidance which is preferred during the cannulation where the vein is continuously viewed during the procedure.

The "static" ultrasound guidance is just viewing the vein once and marking the landmarks. The subsequent venipuncture is done blindly. It is

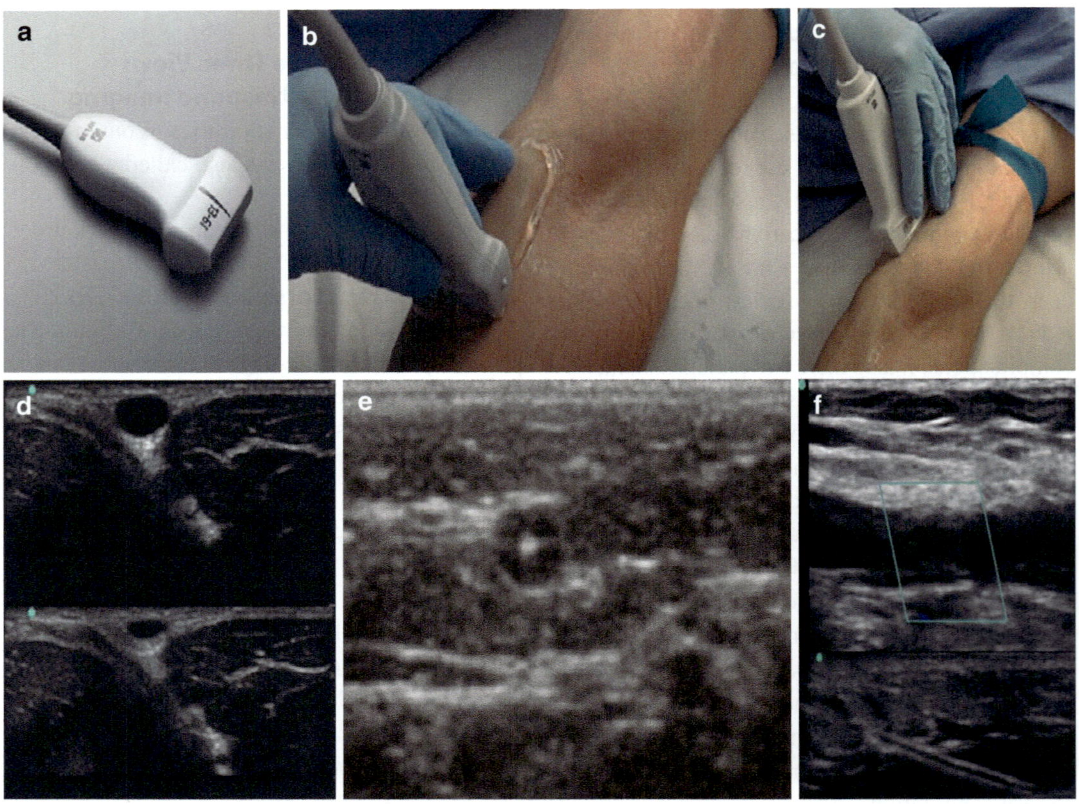

Fig. 12.9 Ultrasound vascular probe and images of the peripheral vein: (**a**) Linear high frequency. (**b**) Probe placement out of plain. (**c**) Probe placement in plain. (**d**) View of the vein out of plain (**e**) The vein in the out of plain with the bright shiny needle tip in the centre. (**f**) The vein in the plain with the bright shiny needle seen in its length

not preferred as this has similar complications as with non-use of ultrasound.

12.4.4.2 Limitations of Ultrasound for Peripheral IV Cannulations

The benefits vary depending upon the age of the patients, lack of cooperation during the procedure, the small size of the child's extremity. In neonate's ultrasound has no role for peripheral venous access. The anatomic site, quality of the ultrasound device, needles, comorbid clinical conditions like morbid obesity, drug abuse, post-chemotherapy, and operator training, and experience also limit the successful cannulation by the US guide.

Intraosseous (IO) Access

Intraosseous (IO) access can be used for fluid resuscitation, drug delivery, blood transfusion, and sampling for laboratory evaluation. The Intraosseous (IO) will give access to the medullary cavity which then ends in the and venous channels that drains the long bones. There is an extensive network of vessels in the bone marrow that is non-collapsible and it drains into the central venous canal which drains into the central venous circulation. The intraosseous route is as effective as the peripheral venous access; the fluids and medications can reach the central circulation within seconds. It can be done in all age groups and is a relatively safe procedure. It can be accessed by a manually operated needle or a battery-operated intraosseous needle driver.

The proximal tibia is the most common site accessed but the distal femur, distal tibia, and medial malleolus in the lower extremity and the proximal humerus, distal radius, and ulna in the upper extremities are the other accessible sites. The clavicles, manubrium sternum, and anterior inferior iliac spine can also be accessed in the axial skeleton.

Indications for Intraosseous Access For resuscitation in cardiac arrest, shock hypovolemic (haemorrhagic and non-haemorrhagic), anaphylactic, septic, and cardiogenic shock. Peripheral or central venous access is not easily accessible or unable to be obtained quickly in an emergency. It has been used extensively during mass causalities or military combats.

Contraindications for Intraosseous Access Difficulty in identifying anatomical landmarks, bone trauma at or proximal to the insertion site which can cause extravasation of infusate and development of compartment syndrome, limbs with the prosthesis in the like knee replacement, tibial nail, humeral plate or previous sternotomy, cellulitis overlying the site of insertion or osteomyelitis of bone to be accessed are other contraindications. If inferior vena cava or an ipsilateral vascular injury is suspected, then the bone below it should be avoided for intraosseous access. Osteogenesis imperfecta may end up fractures, Fractured bone, Crush injuries or loss of skin integrity, previous attempt on the same leg bone, Cardiac diseases with right-to-left intracardiac shunt, e.g., Tetralogy of Fallot as may increase the risk of cerebral fat and bone marrow emboli complications.

Equipment for Intraosseous Access There are three different types of devices used for intraosseous access:

Manual Insertion Needles *This device comes with a* trocar, a needle with a handle, an adjustable flange for depth marking.

Battery-Powered Driver (EZIO) It is battery-operated motorised device.

Impact-Driven Devices: Bone Injection Gun It comes in two sizes, i.e., the adult and the paediatrics. It is used for the manubrium injection.

Complications of Intraosseous Access Through and through penetration of the bone, failure to enter the medullary cavity and extravasation or subperiosteal infusion, osteomyelitis, epiphyseal plate injury, injury to the structures in the vicinity, local infection, skin necrosis, pain, compartment syndrome, fat, and bone microemboli can occur but rare.

What Can Be Injected Through the Intraosseous Access Any intravenous (IV) medications and fluids can be administered by an IO route in an emergent situation. Colloids, crystalloids, blood products, antibiotics, vasopressors, inotropes, contrast agents, steroids, sodium bicarbonate, dextrose, heparin, hyperosmolar fluids, sedatives, and analgesics can all be given via an IO route.

12.5 Central Venous Lines (Fig. 12.10)

A central venous line is a catheter that is placed in a large midline vein and whose tip is in the superior vena cava, in the right atrium, or the inferior vena cava. Central lines are now one of the important procedures in the management of critically ill patients or patients undergoing major surgeries.

12.5.1 Indications for Central Venous Line Insertion [25]

They can be diagnostic, therapeutic, short term, or long term.

Indications for hemodynamic monitoring like central venous pressure (CVP), cardiac parameter via pulmonary artery catheter or PiCCO, central venous oxyhaemoglobin saturation ($ScvO_2$).

Peripherally incompatible infusions: Infusions that cause phlebitis when infused through peripheral lines like vasoactive drugs, electrolytes especially potassium and hypertonic saline, chemotherapy, parenteral nutrition, inadequate peripheral venous access. Extracorporeal therapies like Haemodialysis, Continuous renal replacement therapy (CRRT), Veno-venous (VV), Veno-arterial (VA), Extra Corporeal Membrane Oxygenation (ECMO), plasmapheresis. Device placement like pacemakers/defibrillators, vena cava filters, catheter-directed therapies like venous thrombolytic therapy/venous angioplasty/venous stenting.

Remember that when central lines are inserted for fluid resuscitation then a large bore haemodialysis catheter is needed.

12.5.2 Contraindication for Central Venous Lines

There are no absolute contraindications for central venous. The relative contraindications are uncooperative awake patient, obstructed vein due to thrombosis or stenosis, severe coagulopathy-especially avoid subclavian should be avoided as it is non-compressible. The infected site, trauma, or suspected proximal vascular injury. In the cervical spine avoid Internal jugular veins (IJV), clavicle fracture avoids the subclavian line, pelvic fracture avoids femoral. Previous radiation therapy (avoid IJV) or burned site. Inexperienced and the unsupervised operator are also important contraindications.

*The common anatomic sites for central venous line access are (*Fig. 12.10a*) are* internal jugulars, subclavian, and femoral.

12.5.3 Selection of the Central Venous Line Site

The site selection for the central venous line depends on various factors like the urgency of insertion, femoral line is of choice because it will not interfere with resuscitation like intubation or cardiopulmonary resuscitation (CPR), coagulation status is unknown.

Indication for central venous access is pacemaker insertion then right IJV is the choice, for temporary dialysis IJV or femoral, avoid subclavian as they may be needed for long-term dialysis lines. Co-morbidities like anticoagulation IJV or Femoral are preferable as they are easily compressible, pulmonary pathology like post-pneumonectomy avoid IJV and subclavian.

The duration of the therapy like long-term haemodialysis and chemo port best is subclavian (Fig. 12.8). Finally, operator training and expertise also matter.

Each site has its advantages and disadvantages. The anatomic site chosen for central catheter placement influences the risk for and type of complications, including catheter-associated infection.

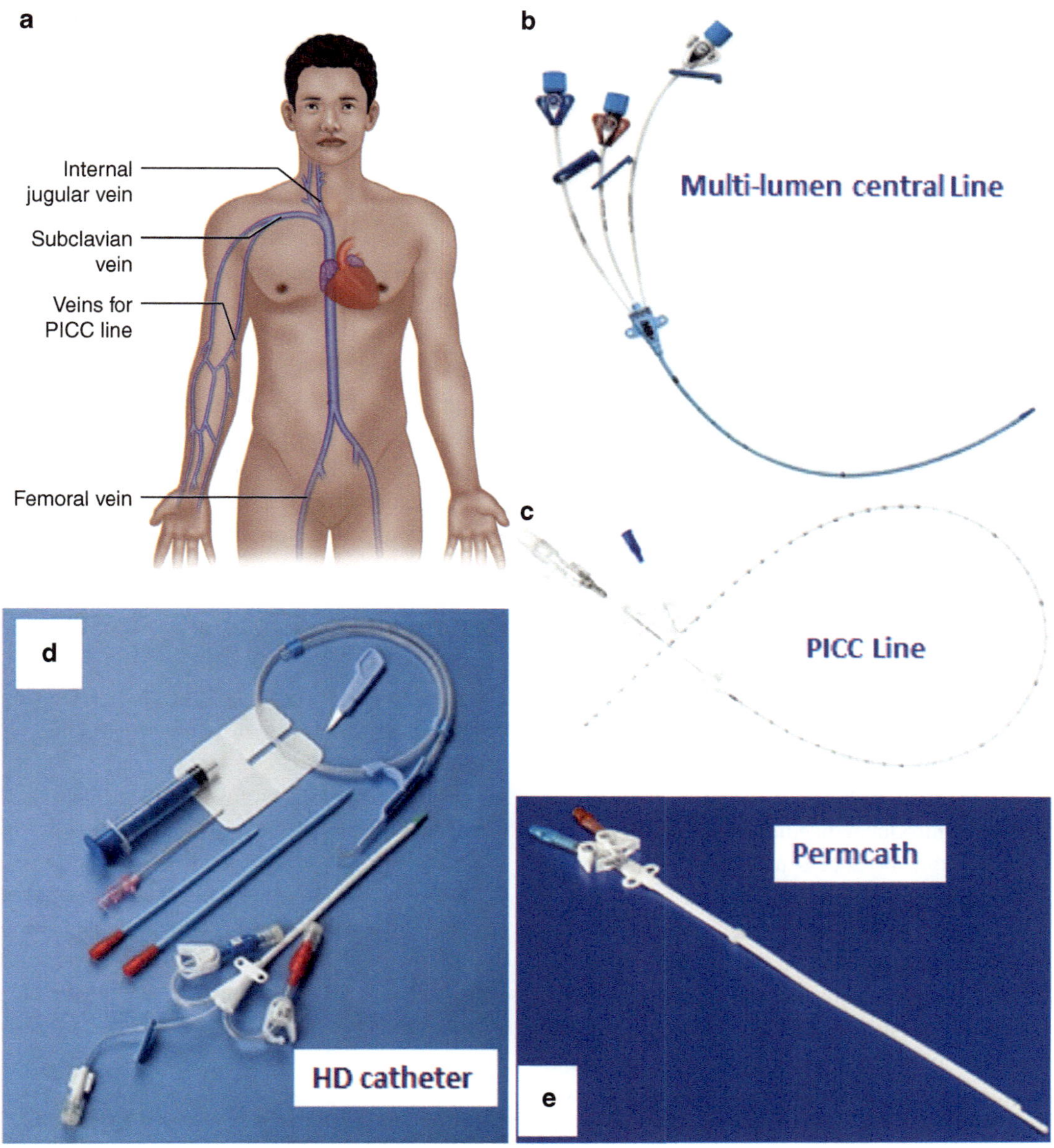

Fig. 12.10 Sites for central insertion (**a**) and different types of central lines, (**b**) Triple lumen central line, (**c**) Peripherally Inserted Central Line, (**d**) Haemodilaysis catheter (**e**) Perm Cath

12.5.4 Complications of the Central Venous Cannulation [26]

Complication can be immediate like the failure of the procedure, pneumothorax, haemothorax, retroperitoneal haematoma, arterial puncture, local haematoma, guidewire-induced arrhythmia, thoracic duct injury, guidewire embolism, air embolism, arrhythmias, cardiac perforation, and catheter malposition.

Early post-insertion complications are catheter blockage, chylothorax, and catheter knotting.

Late post-insertion complications are central line-related bloodstream infection, catheter fracture, vascular erosion, vessel stenosis, thrombosis, and osteomyelitis of clavicle (subclavian access).

12.5.5 The Technique of Central Line Insertion

The preparation starts with the indication for line, checking the coagulation status, looking for contraindications, US assessment of the sites and selecting a site and patency of the target vein, informed consent, positioning the patient—the patient is positioned to make the vein easily accessible, but the patient is comfortable and cardiopulmonary stability is not compromised. Hook the patient to monitor like continuous cardiac rhythm and pulse oximetry and start supplemental oxygen if indicated, appropriate sedation and analgesia, arrange for help if needed before starting the procedure, prepare the equipment and devices, procedural time-out to verify the patient, procedure, site, and technique to be conducted. Always take steps to adopt a sterile technique like surgical antiseptic hand wash, long-sleeved sterile gown, surgical mask, gloves, and head covering, prepare the skin with A chlorhexidine-alcohol skin antiseptic, and drape the patient head to toe. Use dynamic ultrasound, infiltrating the skin with a local anaesthetic, cannulating the vein via standard introducer needle, inserting the guidewire through the access needle, confirmation of the intravenous guidewire via ultrasound, keep monitoring the patient for arrhythmias induced by the guidewire, remove the needle while controlling the guidewire and then making a single small stab incision in the skin at the puncture site adjacent to the guidewire. Advance the tissue dilator over the guidewire, then remove the tissue dilator, thread the catheter over the guidewire, remove the guidewire, aspirate blood from each hub and flush with saline, secure the catheter with suture. Sterile dressing to be applied. Transparent dressing is widely used because of the ease of monitoring and for the local signs of infection, fluid accumulation, etc. These dressing should be replaced if they are soiled with blood, damped because of sweat or fluids. Sometimes these transparent dressing are chlorhexidine gluconate-impregnated sponge (CHGIS) which reduces catheter-related infections.

Confirm the position of the tip of the catheter with chest radiography, US or by the fluoroscope if inserted in OR. Check for immediate complications like pneumothorax, hemothorax [27].

12.5.6 Central Line Care [28]

The two most important steps in the management of central venous catheters are the prevention of catheter-related infections and thrombosis.

Catheter-related infections can be prevented by minimising the duration of stay in situ, remove the line if not needed, regular site inspections, change of the dressing according to the need and guidelines. Strict aseptic precautions when handling catheters. Prevention of catheter block by Use of catheter lock solutions and sometimes thrombolysis can restore lumen patency.

12.5.7 Catheter Removal

The most important complications noticed during the catheter removal are bleeding and air embolism.

Bleeding can be margined by application of firm pressure at least 3 min after removal and application of sterile pressure dressing.

Prevention of air embolism by positioning the patients in the supine or Trendelenburg position (if tolerated) before removing the line and Valsalva manoeuvre or remove the catheter during exhalation.

12.6 Peripherally Inserted Central Catheters (PICCs) [29]

PICC line (Fig. 12.10c) is a variety of central venous catheters. They are long catheters that are placed in the upper extremity veins, namely the basilic, cephalic, medial cubital, or the brachial vein. So they start peripherally in the arm vein and terminate in the thorax. These lines are inserted in the upper extremities only. As they have traversed a long course their length is usually 50–72 cm. They can be single or multi-lumen up to three lumens. They can be used for medium term that can be between several weeks and

6 months but the optimal dwell time is unknown. PICCs lines are considered to be a safe alternative to centrally inserted Central lines. Hence, it is a reliable form of IV access.

Advantages of PICC Lines These liens are less invasive as the insertion technique does not require implantation or tunneling, the low rate of mechanical complications like pneumothorax and haemothorax. It can be inserted in hypocoagulable conditions as the site is accessible for direct compression. Ease of insertion as it needs less expertise when compared to the centrally inserted central lines. Safety factors like lower rates of infections, long indwelling time, and ease of removal [30]. The procedure time is comparatively shorter and found to have a high rate of acceptance and patient satisfaction [31].

Indications for PICC Line Insertion These lines are inserted in patients who need long-term IV medication administration like antibiotics, vasoactive drugs, chemotherapeutic agents, total parenteral nutrition, frequent blood sampling, difficult peripheral venous such as obesity, diabetes, long-term hospitalisation. These lines can also be used in patient patients who have contraindications for centrally inserted central lines like coagulopathy, neck, or chest abnormalities. Remember that these lines are not good for fluid resuscitation.

Contraindications for PICC Line Insertion Contraindication for any central like holds good for PICC line insertion as well. There are no absolute contraindications. There are some relative contraindications like infection at the site of insertion, conditions like trauma and radiation distorting the anatomy, mastectomy and axillary lymph node dissection, Burns having a raw area and a source of infection at the entry point, history of venous thrombosis which can be ruled out by compression ultrasound. A special concern that needs attention is that patients with chronic kidney disease (CKD) are candidates for dialysis catheter placement hence their veins should be preserved from thrombosis and stenosis. Arm veins less than 3–4 mm will not accommodate the catheter, threading of the catheter will difficult and traumatic and more prone to thrombosis. The condition which increases the intrathoracic pressure persistent cough and vomiting can cause catheter malposition, vessel erosion, or cardiac tamponade [32].

Complications of PICC Lines Bloodstream Infection though less when compared to the centrally inserted central lines, catheter malposition can cause venous thrombosis and arrhythmias, migration can cause venous thrombosis, vessel wall erosion, and cardiac tamponade. Mechanical dysfunction like sharing or fracture of the catheter can cause catheter embolisation, phlebitis, infiltration, air embolism if accidentally left open to the air, etc.

Prevention of PICC Line Complication These precautions and practices can prevent complications for any vascular access. Appropriate training for the staff for insertion and maintenance of lines, the strict hand-washing policy before and after handling the line, use of chlorhexidine cleansing of the ports/hubs before any injections, adopt international and local policies for the exit site care like the type of dressing, frequency of changes of dressing, change of administration sets at specified intervals, reduce the dwell time by removal of the PICC lines as soon as possible if they are no longer nedded [33].

12.7 Arterial Line Access [34]

It is the placement of a catheter into the lumen of an artery to continuously record the blood pressure and for frequent arterial blood sampling for ABG analysis for high-risk surgical and critically ill patients. They are also called arterial cannulas or A-lines. An arterial line insertion is common in the intensive care units and operating room.

12.7.1 Sites of Insertion (Fig. 12.11a)

The radial artery is the most common site of insertion followed by the ulnar artery, brachial artery, femoral artery, dorsalis pedis artery, posterior tibial artery, and the superficial temporal artery.

12.7.2 Indications for Arterial Cannulation

In intensive care settings and intra-operative for continuous (beat to beat or minute to minute) blood pressure monitoring. Especially when vasoactive medications are being administered to help titration of these medications. Frequent arterial blood sampling for ABGs and cardiac output (cardiac parameters monitoring). The other indications are VA ECMO, cardiac catheterisation, radiological interventional procedures, exchange transfusions, and plasmapheresis.

12.7.3 Contraindications for Arterial Line Insertion

Peripheral or distal arterial insufficiency, peripheral vascular disease, anatomic variants like lack of collateral circulation, infection, and burns at the site of insertion, coagulation disorders, and surgical intervention at the site of Insertion are few contraindications.

Types of the arterial line are Catheter-over-needle technique (Fig. 12.11c), Catheter-over-wire technique (Seldinger) (Fig. 12.11b), Catheter-over-wire technique (modified Seldinger) (Fig. 12.11d).

12.7.4 Allen Test

Allen test is performed before radial artery cannulation is done. It is tested to evaluate the adequacy of the collateral circulation of the palmar arches of the hand. The palmar arch is supplied by both the radial artery and the ulnar artery. If any injury to the radial or the ulnar artery, the collateral circulation takes care of the perfusion of the hand.

It is a bedside procedure. Elevates the hand of the patient and ask to clinch the first for 30 s.

The examiner applies simultaneous pressure to the ulnar and radial arteries to occlude the flow of blood into the palmar arch. Then ask the patient to open the hand, it will appear blanched.

Release the pressure over the ulnar artery and observe the time of the return of perfusion and colour.

12.7.4.1 Interpretation of the Allen Test [35]

Colour returns to the hand within 5 s—Allen test is negative (normal), colour returns to the palm more than 5 s, the test result is positive (abnormal).

According to another view, Allen test results may be divided into the following three categories:

Return of perfusion to the hand in less than 7 s is normal, the return of perfusion in 8–14 s is equivocal and the return of perfusion in more than 14 s is abnormal.

12.7.5 Equipment for Arterial Line Insertion

Arterial line depending upon the site selected. It includes an ultrasound probe—5–13 MHz linear array vascular probe, sterile ultrasound probe cover and sterile lubrication, chlorhexidine and Alcohol skin preparation solution, sterile gloves, sterile gauze (4 × 4 cm), sterile towels, 1% Lidocaine without Epinephrine in a 3–5-mL syringe with a 25–27-gauge needle, a 5-mL syringe with the heparinised flush, nonabsorbable suture (3–0 to 4–0), sterile dressing, three-way stopcock, pressure transducer kit along with the pressure tubing and arm board of appropriate size for the patient (e.g., neonate, paediatrics, adult).

12.7.6 Complications of Arterial Cannulation

Complications may be general or unique to the site of arterial catheterisation. They are usually pain and swelling, the temporary arterial spasm

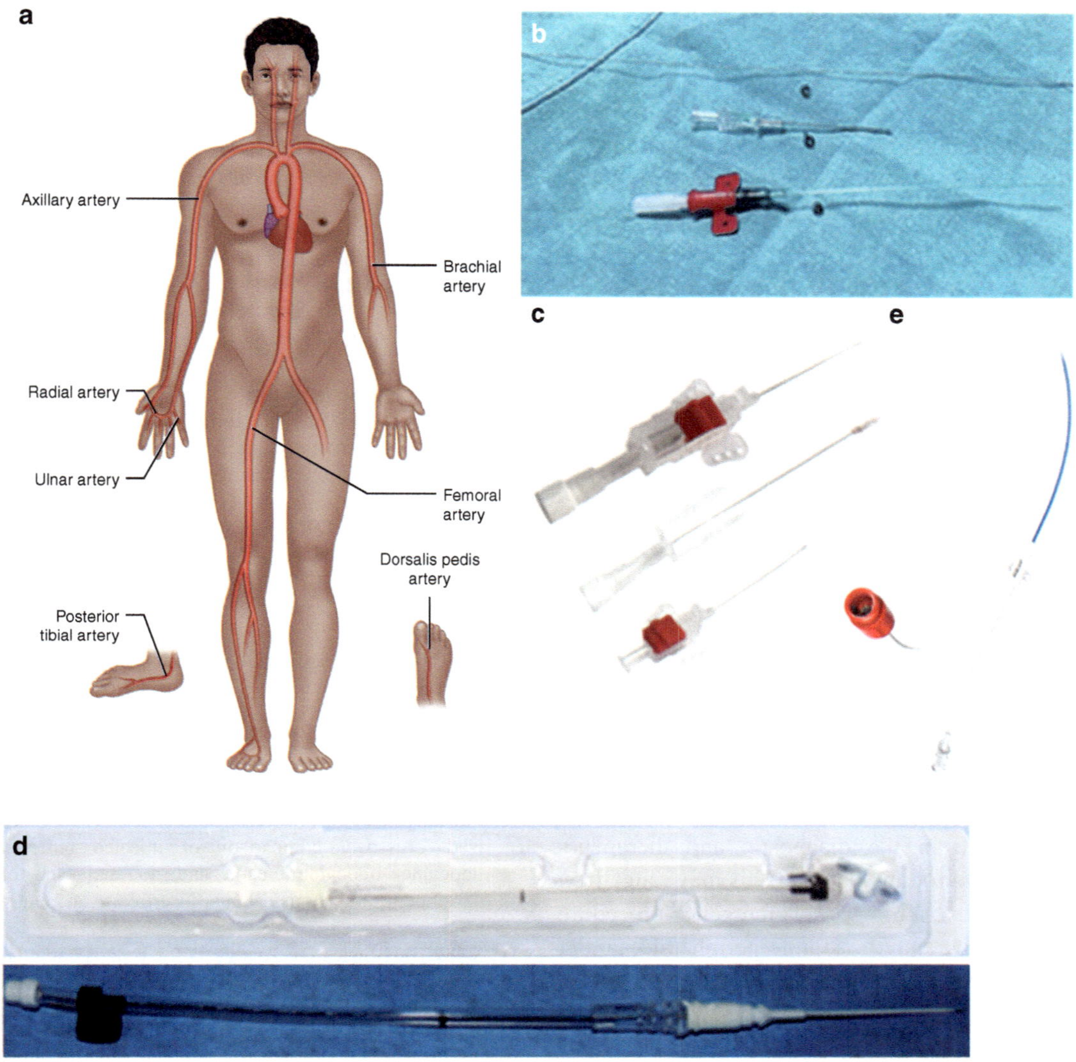

Fig. 12.11 (**a**) Sites for arterial insertion and different types of arterial lines - Catheter-over-wire technique (Seldinger) (**b**), Catheter-over-needle technique (**c**), Catheter-over-wire technique (modified Seldinger) (**d**), Pulse induced Continuous Cardiac Output (PiCCO) line (**e**). (Courtesy: https://clinicalgate.com/analysis-and-monitoring-of-gas-exchange/)

is usually seen in radial and ulnar artery, hematoma/bleeding, thrombosis, cerebral embolisation, ischemic damage of the limbs, compartment syndrome, carpal tunnel syndrome, localised catheter-site infection, line-related bloodstream infection, but it is rare, pseudoaneurysm formation, stenosis, arteriovenous fistula, air embolism, paralysis of the median nerve, femoral artery dissection, and retroperitoneal haematoma.

12.7.7 Care of Arterial Lines

A sterile transparent dressing should be applied and replaced if it becomes damp, loose, or soiled. Arterial catheters are not routinely changed if inserted in a sterile condition. Arterial catheters should be removed if not indicated anymore. Femoral catheters have a higher risk of infection and should not be left longer than 5 days. All disposable or reusable transducers are replaced at 96-h intervals.

12.8 Removal of an Arterial Catheter

Arterial catheters should be removed if not indicated anymore. Check the coagulation profile before the removal of the arterial catheter. Extended compression times (5–10 min) will be needed if any coagulation abnormality or therapeutic anticoagulation. Always check the catheter for its integrity if any fragmentation seeks urgent surgical opinion. Five minutes of pressure for the radial artery and 10 min of pressure for the femoral artery site is needed. Bigger diameter catheters need a longer duration of compression. Always check for the pulse at the puncture site and pulses distal 15 min after the removal line for haematoma or signs of ischemia in the limbs. The hip joint should not flex for at least 2 h after the removal of the femoral catheter.

12.9 Conclusion

Vascular access is one of the initial and important steps both in the diagnostic and therapeutic approaches for any patient. This may range from an elective to a life-saving emergency procedure. The elective may be simple peripheral cannulation in a ward or central venous line and arterial line in an operation theatre for complex surgical procedures. In an emergency these can range from the intraosseous cannulation, wide bore peripheral cannulas, central line, the arterial line to hemodialysis lines. The health care provider should be well versed in anatomy, equipment, and complications. They should be aware of the indications and contraindications like coagulopathy, cervical spine injury, etc. for central line insertion. The patients should be carefully monitored for post-insertion complications like line-related infection, thrombosis, ischaemia, etc. One the line is not in use I should be promptly removed. Training and revalidation of the competencies for vascular have a significant role in successful cannulation with a decreased rate o complications.

References

1. Lamperti M, Pittiruti M. II. Difficult peripheral veins: turn on the lights. Br J Anaesth. 2013;110(6):888–91.
2. Liu SW, Zane RD. Peripheral intravenous access. In: Roberts JR, Hedges JR, editors. Clinical procedures in emergency medicine. 4th ed. Philadelphia: Saunders; 2004. p. 401.
3. Beecham GB, Tackling G. Peripheral line placement. [Updated 2020 Jan 5]. In: StatPearls [Internet]. Treasure Island, FL: StatPearls Publishing; 2020.
4. Reddick AD, Ronald J, Morrison WG. Intravenous fluid resuscitation: was Poiseuille right? Emerg Med J. 2011;28:201.
5. Saseedharan S, Bhargava S. Upper extremity deep vein thrombosis. Int J Crit Illn Inj Sci. 2012;2:21.
6. Pang CC. Autonomic control of the venous system in health and disease: effects of drugs. Pharmacol Ther. 2001;90:179.
7. Hsu DC, Stack AM, Wiley JF. Clinical use of topical anesthetics in children. UpToDate. 2020. Retrieved September 5, 2020, from https://www.uptodate.com/contents/Clinical-use-of-topical-anesthetics-in children
8. Roberge RJ. Venodilatation techniques to enhance venepuncture and intravenous cannulation. J Emerg Med. 2004;27:69.
9. Sado DM, Deakin CD. Local anaesthesia for venous cannulation and arterial blood gas sampling: are doctors using it? J R Soc Med. 2005;98:158.
10. McNaughton C, Zhou C, Robert L, et al. A randomized, crossover comparison of injected buffered lidocaine, lidocaine cream, and no analgesia for peripheral intravenous cannula insertion. Ann Emerg Med. 2009;54:214.
11. Selby IR, Bowles BJ. Analgesia for venous cannulation: a comparison of EMLA (5 minutes application), lignocaine, ethyl chloride, and nothing. J R Soc Med. 1995;88(5):264–7.
12. Arendts G, Stevens M, Fry M. Topical anaesthesia and intravenous cannulation success in paediatric patients: a randomized double-blind trial. Br J Anaesth. 2008;100:521–4.
13. Oni G, Brown S, Kenkel J. Comparison of five commonly-available, lidocaine-containing topical anesthetics and their effect on serum levels of lidocaine and its metabolite monoethylglycinexylidide (MEGX). Aesthet Surg J. 2012;32(4):495–503.
14. Galinkin JL, Rose JB, Harris K, Watcha MF. Lidocaine iontophoresis versus eutectic mixture of local anesthetics (EMLA) for IV placement in children. Anesth Analg. 2002;94(6):1484–8. https://doi.org/10.1097/00000539-200206000-00020.
15. Kim DK, Choi SW, Kwak YH. The effect of SonoPrep® on EMLA® cream application for pain relief prior to intravenous cannulation. Eur J Pediatr. 2012;171(6):985–8. https://doi.org/10.1007/s00431-012-1696-6.

16. Singer AJ, Regev R, Weeks R, Tlockowski DS. Laser-assisted anesthesia prior to intravenous cannulation in volunteers: a randomized, controlled trial. Acad Emerg Med. 2005;12:804.
17. Roberge RJ, Kelly M, Evans TC, et al. Facilitated intravenous access through local application of nitroglycerin ointment. Ann Emerg Med. 1987;16:546.
18. Mbamalu D, Banerjee A. Methods of obtaining peripheral venous access in difficult situations. Postgrad Med J. 1999;75:459–62.
19. Gopalakrishnan S, Abhinaav R, Akshaya Sapthasri M, Anusha V, Nivetha S. Near-infrared based real-time peripheral superficies venous imaging solution for difficult venous access. Int J Recent Technol Eng (IJRTE). 2019;8(3):6416–25.
20. Juric S, Flis V, et al. Towards a low-cost mobile subcutaneous vein detection solution using near-infrared spectroscopy. Sci World J. 2014;2014:365902.
21. Cantor-Peled G, Halak M, Ovadia-Blechman Z. Peripheral vein locating techniques. Imag Med. 2016;8(3):83–8.
22. Karpanen TJ, Casey AL, Das I, et al. Transparent film intravenous line dressing incorporating a chlorhexidine gluconate gel pad: a clinical staff evaluation. J Assoc Vascul Access. 2016;21(3):133–8.
23. Goode CJ, Titler M, Rakel B, et al. A meta-analysis of effects of heparin flush and saline flush: quality and cost implications. Nurs Res. 1991;40:324.
24. Blanco P. Ultrasound-guided peripheral venous cannulation in critically ill patients: a practical guideline. The Ultras J. 2019;11:27. https://doi.org/10.1186/s13089-019-0144-5.
25. American Society of Anesthesiologists Task Force on Central Venous Access, Rupp SM, Apfelbaum JL, et al. Practice guidelines for central venous access: a report by the American Society of Anesthesiologists Task Force on Central Venous Access. Anesthesiology. 2012;116:539.
26. McGee DC, Gould MK. Preventing complications of central venous catheterization. N Engl J Med. 2003;348(12):1123–33.
27. Chui J, Saeed R, Jakobowski L, et al. Is routine chest X-ray after ultrasound-guided central venous catheter insertion choosing wisely?: a population-based retrospective study of 6,875 patients. Chest. 2018; 154:148.
28. Practice Guidelines for Central Venous Access 2020: an Updated Report by the American Society of Anesthesiologists Task Force on Central Venous Access. Anesthesiology. 2020;132(1):8–43.
29. Al Raiy B, Fakih MG, Bryan-Nomides N, et al. Peripherally inserted central venous catheters in the acute care setting: a safe alternative to high-risk short-term central venous catheters. Am J Infect Control. 2010;38:149.
30. Velissaris D, Karamouzos V, Lagadinou M, Pierrakos C, Marangos M. Peripheral inserted central catheter use and related infections in clinical practice: a literature update. J Clin Med Res. 2019;11(4):237–46.
31. Duwadi S, Zhao Q, Budal BS. Peripherally inserted central catheters in critically ill patients - complications and its prevention: a review. Int J Nurs Sci. 2018;6(1):99–105. https://doi.org/10.1016/j.ijnss.2018.12.007.
32. Linenberger ML. Catheter-related thrombosis: risks, diagnosis, and management. J Natl Compr Cancer Netw. 2006;4(9):889–901.
33. ESPEN. Guidelines on Parenteral Nutrition: central venous catheters (access, care, diagnosis and therapy of complications).
34. Eiting E, Kim HT. Arterial puncture and cannulation. In: Roberts JR, Custalow CB, Thomsen TW, et al., editors. Roberts and Hedges' clinical procedures in emergency medicine and acute care. 7th ed. Philadelphia: Elsevier; 2019. p. 377–93.
35. Grisham J, Stankus JL. Arterial puncture and cannulation. In: Reichman EF, editor. Reichman's emergency medicine procedures. 3rd ed. New York: McGraw-Hill; 2019. p. 623–34.

Hypothermia and Its Management

13

Ruggero Corso and Davide Cattano

Contents

13.1 Introduction

Humans are a homeothermic species, like other mammals. Homeothermic organisms are able to maintain a constant core temperature irrespective of changes to ambient temperatures: a characteristic known as normothermia. The suggested rationale for this is that enzymes function optimally at a core body temperature of around 36.8 °C (98.2 °F); (range 36.0–38°C, 96.2–100.4°F). Consequently, core body temperature is acknowledged as a vital sign. The human thermoregulatory system actively maintains normothermia, but the anesthetic-induced inhibition of

R. Corso (✉)
Department of Surgery, Anesthesia and Intensive Care Section, G.B. Morgagni Hospital, Forlì, Italy

D. Cattano
Department of Anesthesiology, McGovern Medical School, UTHealth Houston, Houston, TX, USA

Department of Otorhinolaryngology, McGovern Medical School, UTHealth Houston, Houston, TX, USA

Anesthesia Clinic, Memorial Hermann Hospital-TMC, Houston, TX, USA

School of Dentistry, Department of Oral and Maxillofacial Surgery, UTHealth Houston, Houston, TX, USA
e-mail: davide.cattano@uth.tmc.edu

N. A. Shallik et al. (eds.), *Improving Anesthesia Technical Staff's Skills*,
https://doi.org/10.1007/978-3-030-88849-7_13

thermoregulatory control, coupled with a cool or hot environment, make normothermia common place during surgery. Conventionally, perioperative hypothermia refers to a drop in core body temperature to below 36 °C (96.8 °F) during surgery or under anesthesia. Fifty to 90% incidence of hypothermia in surgical patients during the perioperative period has been reported; an estimated 70% of patients are hypothermic on admission to the Postanesthesia Care Unit (PACU). On the opposite end of the scale, an increase in body temperature to above 38 °C (100.4 F) is referred as hyperthermia. Standard measures are implemented to control and manage body temperature due to physiological changes which occur during hypothermia or hyperthermia, as well the increased pathophysiological risk of infection and other conditions. The primary focus of the chapter will be on perioperative hypothermia.

13.2 Mechanisms

In the normal non-anesthetized patient, the hypothalamus—the thermostat of the body—hormonally regulates core temperature based on information received from thermoreceptors in the hypothalamus, spinal cord, abdominal organs, and other central locations. Thermoreceptors in the skin communicate with the hypothalamus peripherally. Based on core and peripheral temperature information, the hypothalmus regulate body temperature through various methods. Shivering is a first-line response to raising body temperature, however, it is costly to the body due to increased oxygen and caloric consumption. Shivering may be insufficient and so heat is shunted to the core by means of vasoconstriction. Vasoconstriction caused by hypothermia decreases blood flow, meaning less oxygen and nutrients for tissues, a reduced immune response and increased risk of infection. Increased oxygen demand and decreased blood flow due to shivering and hypothermia can potentially lead to myocardial infarction and death. The induction of regional, neuraxial, or general anesthesia impairs the body's thermoregulatory processes by shutting down the normal response of the body's thermoregulator, the hypothalamus.

Intraoperative hypothermia develops in a characteristic three-phase pattern:

1. During the initial hour after induction of general anesthesia or activation of a neuraxial block, core temperature decreases rapidly due to redistribution from the core to peripheral tissues. This initial rapid reduction in core temperature is primarily due to anesthetic-induced vasodilation, caused by impaired central thermoregulatory control rather than direct peripheral effects of anesthetics.
2. Redistribution hypothermia is typically followed by a slower, linear reduction in core temperature which occurs when heat loss exceeds metabolic heat production. Heat is usually dissipated into the environment by radiation and convection. Normally, only small amounts of heat are lost via conduction and evaporation. Unknown amounts of heat are lost through surgical incisions, however, the amount may be substantial when incisions are large, especially during open abdominal surgery. The rate at which temperature decreases is a result of the difference between metabolic heat production and heat loss, which in turn depends on ambient temperature, the extent of surgical exposure of skin or body cavities, and whether the patient is insulated or actively warmed.
3. Once patients become sufficiently hypothermic for their body to activate thermoregulatory vasoconstriction (typically at approximately 34.5 °C during general anesthesia), core temperature plateaus and does not decrease any further, regardless of incision size or the duration of surgery. A plateau in core temperature may also be a result of a passive process if heat production is balanced against heat loss. Once activated, arteriovenous shunt vasoconstriction effectively retains metabolic heat in the core tissues, thus preventing further decreases in core hypothermia. However, heat loss from peripheral tissues continues. Consequently, body heat content continues to decrease even though core temperature remains constant.

Hyperthermia in the perioperative period could be related to an iatrogenic source (pharmacological or overheating) and is a likely manifestation of infection, a reaction to drugs or the environment (heat stroke). Here we refrain from discussing the mechanisms and details of hyperthermia, which will be covered on another occasion.

13.3 Risk Factors

Extremes in age, low body weight, chronic or systemic health conditions, and poor nutritional status are all patient factors associated with an increased risk of perioperative hypothermia. Neonates and patients over the age of 70 years are particularly vulnerable. Higher body mass indices reduce the risk of hypothermia. Patients with diabetes, peripheral vascular disease, hypothyroidism, and other endocrine disorders, cardiac conditions, arthritis, paralysis, hypoglycemia, intoxication, and head or spinal cord injuries are at a greater risk of hypothermia. Risk factors for surgery include the following:

- low core temperature before surgery,
- preoperative fasting and fluid deprivation prior to anesthesia,
- cool IV or irrigation fluid administration,
- large body surface area exposure,
- evaporative heat loss caused by the use of volatile solutions for skin preparation,
- large open cavity or abdominal surgery,
- lengthier surgery and exposure to anesthesia,
- burn injuries and extensive blood loss.

Patients' risk of hypothermia can also be increased by environmental factors, like cool ambient temperatures and airflow in the OR, minimal cover in surgery and cool temperatures or drafts during patient transport.

13.4 Risks Associated with Hypothermia

Numerous physiological changes occur in patients with perioperative hypothermia. Metabolic changes, peripheral vasoconstriction, altered tissue perfusion, and inhibited enzymatic reactions of the coagulation cascade increase the likelihood of adverse effects in patients which range from discomfort to increased morbidity and mortality. Patients experiencing hypothermia are at a high risk of:

1. cardiac arrhythmias, ischemia, and arrest;
2. impairments in immune function and increased risk of infections;
3. longer intensive care stays;
4. prolonged overall hospital stays;
5. increased intraoperative blood loss and blood transfusions;
6. increased mortality.

It is interesting to note that hypothermia-induced coagulopathy is often missed in routine laboratory tests as they are run at 37 °C; results would certainly not be reported as normal if they were temperature-adjusted. The prolonged effect of drugs is another consequence which is often overlooked. Even mild hypothermia prolongs the action of drugs used during anesthesia, neuromuscular blocking agents (NMBAs) in particular. Hypothermia also decreases the minimum alveolar concentration of volatile inhalation anesthetic agents necessary to prevent movement in response to a surgical stimulus. Consequences include delayed reversal or neuromuscular blockade and delayed emergence.

Regular patient monitoring coupled with interventions to maintain or restore normothermia feature in guidelines and recommended best practices. Maintaining ambient room temperature at ≥24 ° C (75.2 °F), the active warming of hypothermic patients and preoperative warming are all recommended prevention strategies.

13.5 How to Measure It

Temperature measurement is of critical importance for maintaining normothermia or in selected cases, monitoring and maintaining hypothermia (rarely hyperthermia).

Typically in the operating room, skin, nasopharynx, esophageal, or bladder temperature is checked. Temperature can also be measured by special catheters inserted in the vascular system (i.e. a pulmonary catheter or central line catheter). The temperature measurement is referred as outer core (skin) or inner core (bladder/esophageal), with other, in between measurements. Nasopharyngeal measurement, when accessible (not possible during head and neck surgeries) is preferred as it is easy to access and reliable.

Different types of probes are designed for measuring temperature, and typically consist of a sensor, wiring, and a connector for the temperature cable that connects to the monitor. Esophageal probes are often paired with an esophageal precordial stethoscope (outer chamber, distal cuff) or are designed to measure temperature only, in which case the wire is covered by a special sleeve that is self-lubricating in the presence of moisture. Bladder probes are present in special Foley catheters: the wire and sensor end inside the tip of the urinary catheter which then measures the temperature in the bladder. Recently new sensors such as the Tcore™ monitoring system (Drägerwerk AG & Co. KGaA, Lübeck, Germany) have aroused interest in non-invasive skin measurement systems, however, more evidences are needed before adoption in clinical practice.

13.6 How to Prevent It

Temperature management mostly relies on the mechanisms responsible for the early and late phases of body temperature redistribution, direct and indirect loss as well other conditions (exposure, humidity, ambient temperature, fluid, etc.). Therefore, it is fundamental for the anesthesiologist or anesthesia technician to consider all these factors in order to determine the best management plan.

Protocols, standardized procedures, and equipment are all fundamental for further reducing the risk of hypothermia.

The anesthesia technician plays a key role in providing, maintaining, retrieving, reprocessing, restocking equipment, temperature measuring devices, and disposable parts.

The most effective methods are based on convection air blowers (i.e. forced-air warming system, FAWS, like the Bear Hugger, 3M, Air Mistral, Stryker) or intravenous fluid warmers (Figs. 13.1, 13.2, 13.3, and 13.4); non-air based systems include the Hot Dog warming and Augustine systems; water or fluid mattresses, or induction mattresses are used in other systems. The modification of ambient temperature and/or (albeit rarely) humidity is also used in temperature management.

Fluid warmer systems can be simple (warming of existing intravenous tubing lines) or complex (requiring external pressure bags, inflatable system, rotating pumps). There are different

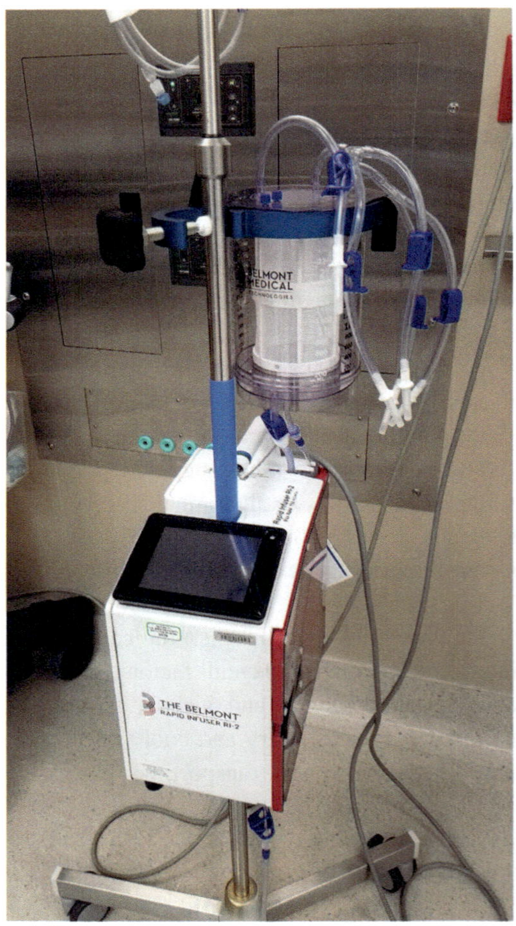

Fig. 13.1 Belmont Infusion system. This system consists of several components that are reusable and disposable. Requires priming with a primer solution (electrolyte solution, colloid or blood product)

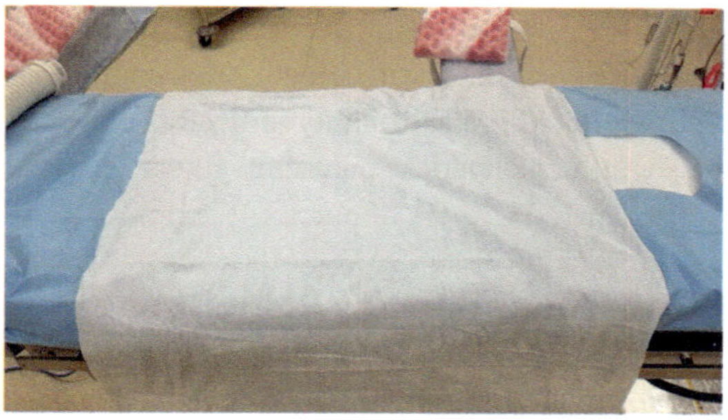

Fig. 13.2 Conduction system blanket. Underbody blanket. Other types of blanket can also be used with air flow blowing systems

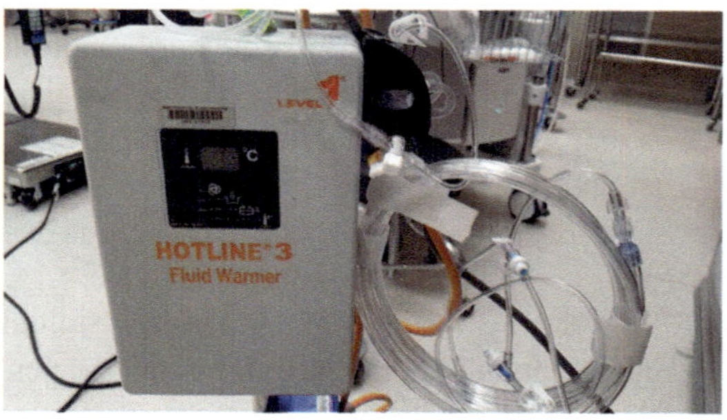

Fig. 13.3 Level 1 infusion system. Fluid warmer. One of the systems used to warm infusion fluids through dedicated tubing for infusions

complex systems available for intravenous fluid warming that can provide high flows of infusion, yet the following are typically used in OR, especially in trauma cases or for surgeries presenting a high risk of bleeding: Level 1 (Smith Medical), Belmont System (Belmont Med Tech) or the more recent Thermacor (Smisson-Cartledge).

Certain temperature control systems are used not only for warming but also for cooling (primary treatment and management of hyperthermia or therapeutic hypothermia). Cooling blankets (circulating cold water or similar) may be used or a cooling effect may be actively created using a heat/cool pump exchanger (like a refrigerator) in situations and clinical conditions in which cooling is paramount (malignant hyperthermia, neuroleptic syndrome, high fever, heat stroke, cardiac surgery, cardiac arrest, and neuroprotection).

Another important aspect of temperature control in anesthesia and intensive care management is the use of the low flow gas anesthesia technique, carbon dioxide absorbents, closed-recirculating ventilation circuits, humidifying filters, and active heat-induced vaporizers for moisture. Without going into detail, heat is preserved, reducing the dry-high flow of circulating fresh gases in the ventilator-anesthesia systems. In contrast, the very techniques avoided to warm patients are used to cool them, however, the efficiency of operating in this manner is questionable. It is also important to stress the management of temperature control before and after surgery. A subject warmed prior to general anesthesia induction or exposure to lower operating theater temperature has more heat reserve. In fact, literature highlights that the preoperative prevention of

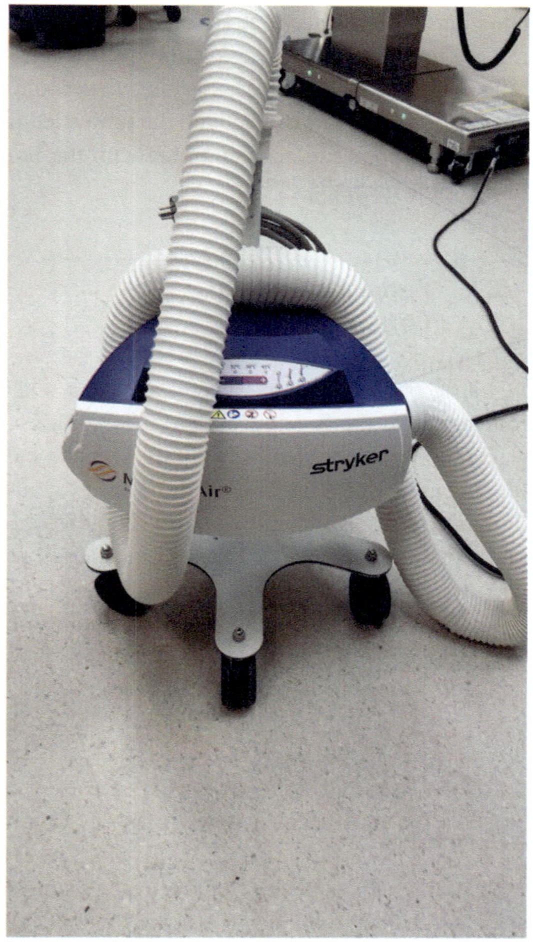

Fig. 13.4 Stryker air conduction warming system. Blower. It enables warming at two different temperatures plus cooling (32 °C)

hypothermia reinforces intraoperative measures, increasing their effectiveness and reducing complications. In the postoperative recovery room, hypothermic patients can actively be rewarmed if cold and hypothermia can continue with the use of warming devices.

13.7 Pediatric Special Considerations

Pediatric patients require special attention. Due to anatomical (body surface area), physiological (metabolic rate and cardiac output), and clinical (coagulation and ventilation) differences, children, neonates, and toddlers, in particular, are prone to rapid heat loss. These considerations and the fact that fluid replacement infusion is typically restricted and controlled (limitations on infused volumes) make certain heating devices and techniques far more important.

13.8 Maintenance of Devices: Special Considerations

Temperature control device maintenance requires special consideration. There are risks associated with malfunction as well as electrical hazards, including electrocution, fire, and burns. Infection control is another significant risk: there is conflicting evidence regarding the risk of surgical field contamination due to air blower systems; companies blame said risk on the purported lower quality of competitor's devices. Fluid warmers operate according to different methods and sets; the risks associated with such devices include air embolism, overheating of the modules, the release of toxic substances, contamination of water solution in the warming chamber, electrocution and surgical field contamination due to splashing.

13.9 Conclusions

The maintenance of normothermia during surgery is a fundamental element for the prevention of complications and the achievement of this goal is considered a standard by many scientific societies. As in other cases, however, only a structured approach subjected to continuous verification of precise quality indicators can positively influence patient outcome.

13.10 Summary Key Points

1. Normothermia should be maintained during anesthesia and surgery. Temperature should be monitored continuously in all operations longer than 30 min for adults and in all children, regardless of duration.
2. Volatile and intravenous (IV) anesthetics markedly impair thermoregulatory control, leading to hypothermia in unwarmed surgical patients. The combination of general and neuraxial anesthetic techniques results in a highest risk of intraoperative hypothermia due to the additive effects of each technique.
3. Pre-warming effectively minimizes initial redistribution hypothermia and should be performed for 20 min immediately before anesthetic induction. Active warming methods are necessary for maintaining normothermia. Forced-air warming is the safest (no wound contamination) and most effective out of said methods, provided that enough skin surface is available. Fluid warming is only effective when large amounts are given.
4. Adverse consequences of hypothermia include coagulopathy, infection, prolonged drug action, thermal discomfort, and shivering.
5. Temperature should be measured during surgery and upon arrival in the post-anesthesia care unit (PACU) or intensive care unit (ICU). Temperature derangements are common in the early postoperative period, and should be promptly treated.

Financial Disclosures The authors reported no relevant financial disclosures.

Suggested Readings

1. Macario A, Dexter F. What are the most important risk factors for a patient's developing intraoperative hypothermia? Anesth Analg. 2002;94(1):215–20.
2. Sessler DI. Perioperative thermoregulation and heat balance. Lancet. 2016;387:2655.

3. Standards for Basic Anesthetic Monitoring. Committee of Origin: Standards and Practice Parameters (Approved by the ASA House of Delegates on October 21, 1986, last amended on October 20, 2010, and last affirmed on October 28, 2016) https://www.asahq.org/~/media/Sites/ASAHQ/Files/Public/Resources/standardsguidelines/standards-for-basic-anesthetic-monitoring.pdf. Accessed 6 May 2016.
4. Checketts MR, Alladi R, Ferguson K, et al. Recommendations for standards of monitoring during anaesthesia and recovery 2015: Association of Anaesthetists of Great Britain and Ireland. Anaesthesia. 2016;71:85.
5. Shirozu K, Kai T, Setoguchi H, et al. Effects of forced air warming on airflow around the operating table. Anesthesiology. 2018;128:79.
6. Madrid E, Urrútia G, Roqué i Figuls M, et al. Active body surface warming systems for preventing complications caused by inadvertent perioperative hypothermia in adults. Cochrane Database Syst Rev. 2016;4:CD009016.
7. Ruetzler K, Kurz A. Consequences of perioperative hypothermia. Handb Clin Neurol. 2018;157:687–97.
8. Torossian A, Bräuer A, Höcker J, Bein B, Wulf H, Horn EP. Preventing inadvertent perioperative hypothermia. Dtsch Arztebl Int. 2015;112(10):166–72.
9. Poveda VB, Oliveira RA, Galvão CM. Perioperative body temperature maintenance and occurrence of surgical site infection: A systematic review with meta-analysis. Am J Infect Control. 2020. pii: S0196-6553(20)30011-0.
10. Kay AB, Klavas DM, Hirase T, Cotton MO, Lambert BS, Incavo SJ. Preoperative warming reduces intraoperative hypothermia in total joint arthroplasty patients. J Am Acad Orthop Surg. 2020;28(6):e255–62.
11. Zheng XQ, Huang JF, Lin JL, Chen D, Wu AM. Effects of preoperative warming on the occurrence of surgical site infection: a systematic review and meta-analysis. Int J Surg. 2020;77:40–7.
12. Kim P, Taghon T, Fetzer M, Tobias JD. Perioperative hypothermia in the pediatric population: a quality improvement project. Am J Med Qual. 2013;28(5):400–6.
13. Brozanski BS, Piazza AJ, Chuo J, Natarajan G, Grover TR, Smith JR, Mingrone T, McClead RE, Rakesh R, Rintoul N, Guidash J, Bellflower B, Holston M, Richardson T, Pallotto EK. STEPP IN: working together to keep infants warm in the perioperative period. Pediatrics. 2020;145(4):e20191121.
14. Soehle M, Dehne H, Hoeft A, Zenker S. Accuracy of the non-invasive Tcore™ temperature monitoring system to measure body core temperature in abdominal surgery. J Clin Monit Comput. 2020;34(6):1361–7. https://doi.org/10.1007/s10877-019-00430-9.
15. Alfonsi P, Bekka S, Aegerter P, SFAR Research Network investigators. Prevalence of hypothermia on admission to recovery room remains high despite a large use of forced-air warming devices: findings of a non-randomized observational multicenter and pragmatic study on perioperative hypothermia prevalence in France. PLoS One. 2019;14(12):e0226038.

Transfusion of Blood and Other Products

14

Ayten Saracoglu, Gamze Tanırgan Cabaklı,
Berk Cimenoglu, and Kemal Tolga Saracoglu

Contents

A. Saracoglu (✉)
Anesthesiology and Intensive Care, Marmara University Pendik Training and Research Hospital, Istanbul, Turkey

G. T. Cabaklı
Department of Anesthesiology and Intensive Care, Marmara University Medical School, Istanbul, Turkey

B. Cimenoglu
Thoracic Surgery, Health Sciences University Kartal Dr. Lutfi Kirdar Training and Research Hospital, Istanbul, Turkey

K. T. Saracoglu
Anesthesiology and Intensive Care, Health Sciences University Kartal Dr. Lutfi Kirdar Training and Research Hospital, Istanbul, Turkey

N. A. Shallik et al. (eds.), *Improving Anesthesia Technical Staff's Skills*,
https://doi.org/10.1007/978-3-030-88849-7_14

14.1 Introduction

The goal of transfusion of blood products is to increase oxygen carrying capacity of blood. Conditions that should be considered before blood transfusion are cardiovascular status, cardiac output, age, anticipated fluid loss, partial and mixed venous oxygen pressure, and blood volume. Oxygen extraction determines the need for transfusion. Cross matching should be performed prior to transfusion. Early stage of this process is called type and screening, which ABO, MN, and P values are evaluated. Febrile non-hemolytic allergic reactions may occur even in autologous transfusion. In this chapter the pearls of transfusion of blood and other products are reviewed.

14.2 Blood Types

Type 0 is considered as universal donor and can donate to recipients with blood types A, B, and AB. Type A can donate to types A and AB. Type B can donate to types B and AB. Type AB can only donate to recipients with blood type AB and if Rh groups match, transfusion is considered 99.9% safe. There is no A or B antigens in blood type 0. Thus, type 0 is universal donor and contains anti-A and anti-B antibodies. Antibodies are present in type 0 Rh (−), however, the amount of antibodies in red blood cell (RBC) transfusion is quite less. Whole blood transfusion, which is rich in plasma, is not recommended because they contain greater amount of antibodies that are present particularly in plasma.

When more than 2 units of 0 Rh (−) RBC are transfused, the maintenance should also be done with 0 Rh (−), because anti-A and anti-B antibodies in 0 Rh (−) suspension may interact with later transfused matched type RBC, causing hemolysis. Transfusion of RBC should be followed the confirmation of anti-A and anti-B levels. When blood broducts are not available, crystalloid and colloid solutions are used for replacement. Of female donors, postmenopausal women without previous transfusion history should be preferred.

14.3 Components of Blood Products

As glycolysis is 30 times slower, blood should be stored in cold. In order to maintain adequate glucose levels, blood products should be kept safe in cold environment. Inadequate level of glucose leads to anaerobic glycolysis causing death of cells. Citrate and phosphate are used as buffers and dextrose is used for energy supply allowing ATP synthesis. Blood can be stored up to 21–35 days (Table 14.1).

14.4 Blood Transfusion and Hb Oxygen Dissociation Curve

Red blood cells maintain vitality after defrosting only when glycerol is added to frozen blood at −79°. Freezing and defrosting procedure reduces antigens in blood and decreases the risk for hepatitis transmission. Leukocyte count decreases and

Table 14.1 Differences between whole blood and red cell suspension

	Whole blood	Red blood cell
pH	~6.73	~6.71
Hb	46 mg/dL	246 mg/dL
K	17.2 mEq/L	76 mEq/L
Na	153 mEq/L	122 mEq/L
Dextrose	282 mg/dL	84 mg/dL
Htc	35–40%	65–75%
Albumin	12.5 g/dL	4 g/dL

2,3 DPG is preserved. P50 is the partial oxygen pressure when 50% of hemoglobin is saturated with oxygen. When P50 value decreases, hemoglobin-oxygen dissociation curve shifts left and the affinity of hemoglobin to oxygen increases. P50 value decreases in stored blood and the affinity of hemoglobin to oxygen increases, which leads to insufficiency in organ perfusion. Therefore, stored blood products older than 15 days should not be preferred. In conditions such as transfusion to newborns or massive transfusion, where oxygen consumption is high, suspensions stored fewer than 15 days should be preferred.

14.5 Blood Transfusion and Coagulopathy

Transfusion induced coagulopathy occurs after transfusion of 6–10 U of RBC in patients without previously known coagulability disorder. It is also related with duration of hypotension time. Without hypotension, coagulapathy is not likely to occur.

The first step of coagulopathy in massive transfusion is the decrease in factor 5 and 8 levels. This is followed by disseminated intravascular coagulation (DIC) and dilutional thrombocytopenia, which can be clinically witnessed as blood leak in operation site and hematuria. Approximately 5–10% of platelets remain in whole blood after 24–48 h. Platelet count should be kept over 50×10^9/L if there is no major bleeding. However, if there is a major bleeding, platelet count over 100×10^9/L should be ensured. Factor 5 and 8 are considered as labile factors. After 21 days, F5 drops to 15% and F8 reduces to 50%. However, in order to avoid bleeding in massive transfusion, at least 20% of factor 5% and 30% of factor8 should be maintained.

14.6 When to Give Fresh Frozen Plasma (FFP)?

FFP should be given if there is active bleeding although platelet count is over 70×10^9/L, PTT is 1.5 times longer and fibrinogen is below 75 mg/dL.

FFP Indications

1. To negate effect of warfarin.
2. To replace factor deficiency.
3. >1.5 fold increase in PT and PTT.
4. Antithrombin 3 deficiency.
5. Thrombotic thrombocytopenic purpura treatment.
6. Massive blood transfusion.

Plasma factor levels can be increased by 30% with 10–15 mL/kg FFP.

14.7 DIC Mechanism

Tromboplastin and toxins cause damaged tissue to release Tissue Plasminogen Activator (TPA). TPA activates plasminogen which causes fibrine breakdown. In other words, TPA causes both coagulation and fibrinolysis. Under normal circumstances, this precise balance is maintained, however, in DIC, this balance is disturbed. Microcirculatory aggregates cause intravascular obstruction which leads to irreversible end-organ ischemia that may progress into multiorgan failure. Extrinsic pathway is activated by TNF and endotoxin. Hence, tissue factor is induced. Intrinsic pathway is activated by F1, F2, F5, F8, and DIC leading to depletion of platelets.

14.8 Diagnosing Bleeding Diathesis

In case of diathesis, first parameter that should be checked is platelet count. PTT, fibrinogen, TEG, or ROTEM should be evaluated. PTT elongation more than 1.5 times is most likely to indicate low levels of factors 5 and 8. In this clinical scenario, FFP should be the first choice in treatment options. Most common reason of bleeding diathesis is thrombocytopenia. When platelet count is lower than 10×10^9/L and bleeding is combated, platelet suspension should be administered. 1 U of platelet suspension contains 70% of platelets in 1 U of whole blood. Fibrinogen levels gradually decrease in stored blood. Dilutional hypofibrinogenemy may also take place. DIC should be kept in mind in cases where fibrinogen levels are lower than 150 mg/100 mL.

14.9 Antifibrinolytic Agents

Epsilon amino capriocacid (EAC) is known to reduce fibrinolysis, however, administrating EAC in DIC may cause thrombosis because DIC itself is related with activated coagulability. However, EAC is indicated when fibrinolysis is encountered after liver transplantation or prostatectomy. Arginine and vasopressin, which are anti-diuretic hormone analogues, increase levels of Factor 8 and von Willebrand factor (vWF). Aprotinine is a serin protease inhibitor that inhibits fibrinolysis and rectifies platelet functions. Tranexamicacid is another antifibrinolytic agent.

14.10 Blood Transfusion Complications

1. *Citrate intoxication:* Hypothermia, hepatic failure, and hyperventilation increases risk for intoxication. Citrate binds with calcium and symptomatic hypocalcemia may occur. Blood pressure decreases, central venous pressure (CVP) increases, contractibility of heart decreases, and ejection fraction of right ventricle decreases. This leads to an increase in CVP and left ventricle end diastolic pressure. This happens when transfusion rate is faster than 150 mL/min or 1 U of blood is transfused faster than 5 min. Ionized calcium cannot be equally distributed in case of inadequate circulation. Citrate can be metabolized after rapid transfusion in patients with normal liver function tests, because calcium can be retracted from bone to blood. Decrease in body temperature from 37 °C to 31 °C slows citrate metabolism by 50%.
2. *Hyperkalemia:* Hyperkalemia incidence increases after blood transfusion performed faster than 120 mL/min. Blood stored for 21 days contains potassium levels up to 30 mEq/L. Hyperkalemia with peaked T wave in Electrocardiogram should be treated with 10% calcium chloride.
3. *Hypothermia:* Decrease of 1 °C in body temperature causes increase in cardiac output by 400%. Hence, hypothermia triggers myocardial infarction.
4. *Acid Base imbalance:* Blood with citrate phosphate dextrose (CPD) is acidic. pH value of CPD solution is 5.5. pH value is balanced to 7 after mixing it with blood. Lactic acid and piruvic acid, which are products of red blood cell metabolism, increase the acidity of solution. pH decreases to 6.9 after 21 days. Carbon dioxide (CO_2) is also a product and blood packs are not permeable to release CO_2. Hence, ventilation should be intact in blood transfusion patients. One molecule of citrate breaks down into 3 molecules of bicarbonate in patients with normal hepatic functions. Heavy increase in bicarbonate shifts the Hb oxygen dissociation curve to the left side and elongates PT.
5. *Hemolytic transfusion reactions*: Even very small amount of blood, like 10 mL, is enough for hemolytic reactions. Mortality rate may be as high as 60%. Receiver's complements and antibodies attack blood components from donated blood, which is called intravascular hemolysis.
6. *Extravascular hemolysis:* This process takes place in reticuloendotelial system (RES) when receiver's antibodies cover but do not harm transfused red blood cells. This antibodies act in extravascular space rather than intravascular space. Fever, chills, and side pain are most common among symptoms. Hemoglobinurea, hypotension, and bleeding diathesis may develop. Serum haptoglobulin, hemoglobin values of serum and urine, bilirubine, and direct antiglobuline values should

be tested as they indicate presence of antibodies binding to transfused red blood cells.

14.11 Treatment

In case of transfusion reaction, transfusion should immediately be stopped and forced diuresis should be performed aiming 75–100 mL/h of urine output. Furosemide and mannitol can be considered. Urine should be alkalinized. Alkaline prevents acid hematin to deposit in distal tubules. Bicarbonate (1 mEq/kg) treatment should be initiated. Urine and plasma hemoglobin, platelet count, PTT, serum fibrinogen values should be tested and blood should be sent back to blood bank for reevaluation. Hypotension should be prevented. Kallikrein and bradykinin are main reasons of hypotension. Complement system gets activated. CVP should be maintained between 10 and 15 mmHg by Ringer Lactate infusion. Hemolytic reaction is triggered by products released by the stroma of hemolyzed red blood cells. Thus, F1, F2, F5, F7, and platelets expire and this would proceed to DIC formation.

14.12 Delayed Hemolytic Transfusion Reaction

It is extravascular and carried out by sensitized antibodies from previous blood transfusion or pregnancy. It is more common in females and develops in 2–21 days. Generally hemotocrite level decreases, jaundice, and hemoglobinurie develop. It often arises from Rh and Kidd system.

14.13 Non-hemolytic Transfusion Reaction

Fever is the most common symptom of hemolytic reaction. Fever, headache, nausea, non-productive cough, hypotension, vomiting, dyspnea, perihilar nodule formation, pulmonary infiltration, and edema on chest X-ray can be observed.

Among allergic reactions, itching, and urticaria can be seen by 3%. It rarely presents with dyspnea and most likely to occur in patients with Ig A deficiency. Washed red blood cell suspension should be given to patients with medical history of Ig A deficiency.

14.14 Transfusion Related Infections

Malaria, Chagas, and Creutzfeldt-Jakob disease may develop. HCV transmission rate is up to 90% in post-transfusion hepatitis and symptoms develop 50–150 days after transfusion. Anicteric post-transfusion hepatitis develops 14–180 days after transfusion. Two fold increase in ALT within 14 days is a pivotal diagnostic sign. Incidences of chronic hepatitis and hepatocellular cancer are 50% and 10%, respectively. HTLV1 is encountered ten times more than HIV. West Nile virus and CMV are carried with leucocytes. Organ transplantation patients should receive frozen-thawed red cell suspension filtered for leucocytes. Thus, passage of antibody-containing cells, such as leucocytes and platelets, is reduced.

Infectious mononucleosis transmission is the reason of post-perfusion syndrome. It is transmitted by blood transfusion. Because blood is stored in +4C, it can act as broth for Yersinia and parvovirus. There is a risk of syphilis if blood is stored at room temperature.

14.15 Transfusion Related Graft Versus Host Reaction

It is an immune reaction of transfused lymphocytes against tissues of the receiver. Generalized rash, leucopenia, and thrombocytopenia may develop.

14.16 Transfusion Related Acute Lung Injury (TRALI)

It is the second most common reason of transfusion related deaths. It can be defined as non-cardiogenic pulmonary edema caused by activity of leucocyte antibodies a couple of hours after transfusion. It takes place approximately 6 h after transfusion. Anti-HLA and anti-granulocyte antibodies are present. Patients suffer from fever and dyspnea. Hypoxia occurs and bleeding may be spotted in endotracheal tube. Especially, FFP is thought to be responsible for this situation. Approximate recovery time is 96 h. Anti-HPA human platelet antibodies may also be responsible along with FFP.

Ocular Side Effects Ocular reactions due to chemical agents in solutions may occur.

14.17 Transfusion Related Immune Modulation

It is related with downregulation of immune functions. Transfusion releated compromised immun function is a risk for recurrent infection in patients undergoing resection for malignities. Viral activation and insufficient lymphocyte response takes place. Increased cytokine production and suppressor response occurs. It is characterized with decreased monocyte and NK counts and increased levels of mediators. Antibody levels against HLA proteins increase. Transfusion should be avoided in patients undergoing transplantation because it shortens the life span of transplanted organs. Suspensions are exposed to −80 °C temperature in order to obtain frozen red blood cell suspension. Blood is purified from leucocytes by leukocyte filters.

FFP is obtained by freezing plasma extracted from whole blood at −20 °C. Similarly cryoprecipitate is obtained by freezing plasma −70 °C followed by defrosting at +4 °C. HTC rates in packed whole blood suspension and red cell suspension are 40% and 70%, respectively. Volume of packed whole blood and red blood cell suspension is 517 mL and 250 mL, respectively.

Blood transfusion should not be performed with ringer lactate because Ca in ringer lactate triggers thrombus formation. Similarly, blood transfusion should not be accompanied by dextrose infusion because dextrose solutions are hypotonic and cause swelling and destruction of red blood cells leading to lysis.

Platelet transfusion should be performed with needles greater than 18 G. Platelets are introduced by specific sets that prevent them to adhere to the filters.

Incidence of platelet solution related sepsis is 1/2000. Platelets should be stored at 24° less than 5 days. Longer storage may cause sepsis. Main sign of this is fever arising within 6 h. Of blood products, the most prone one to infection is platelet solutions. When platelet solutions are cooled, lipid in the cell membrane dissolves to form glycoprotein aggregation. That is why they have to be kept at room temperature rather than cold environment. If platelet solution is exposed to +4 °C, it should be used within 24 h.

Platelet treatment is rarely indicated in immune thrombocytopenic purpura. On the other hand platelet treatment is strictly contraindicated in thrombotic thrombocytopenic prupura. Platelet may be given in case of hemorrhage with platelet dysfunction. If platelet count is below 10×10^9 spontaneous bleeding may occur. Platelet should be given to pediatric patients whose platelet count is below 20,000. ABO compatibility is also sought in platelet transfusion.

FFP contains factor 5 and 8. If it is not used within 20 min after defrosting, these labile factors get wasted. There is no transmission risk of hepatitis B, C or HIV.

14.18 Cryoprecipitate

Cryoprecipitate features factor 8, fibrinogen, vWF, factor 13, and fibronectin. Fibronectin is consist of glycoprotein and helps clearance of RES from bacteria and foreign particles. Fibrinogen saline solutions carry a greater risk of hepatitis transmission than cryoprecipitate. ABO compatibility is not required. Transfusion should not be faster than 200 mL/h. It may be given within 6 h via blood transfusion set. They feature protrombin complex, factor 2, 7, 9, 10. They are used in hemophilia B to fix factor 9 deficiencies.

Similarly ABO compatibility is not required for albumin transfusion. It draws fluid into the intravascular space with an isoosmotic effect.

Dextran 70: Administrating more than 20 mL/kg per day disrupts hemostasis. There is a risk of severe anaphylaxis.

Dextran 40: It is the rheomacrodex that is given to decrease blood viscosity and enhance microcirculation.

14.19 Conclusion

As a conclusion, transfusion of blood and other products is essential for increasing oxygen levels and maintaining adequate tissue perfusion. However, they should be administered under necessary circumstances to patients with appropriate indications. Numerous complications of blood transfusion can be life-threatening.

Regional Anesthesia for Anesthesia Technologists

15

Ahmed Ismail, Ghazi Miladi, and Hamed Elgendy

Contents

A. Ismail (✉) · G. Miladi
Department of Anesthesia, ICU and Perioperative Medicine, Hamad Medical Corporation, Doha, Qatar
e-mail: AIBRAHIM3@hamad.qa: GMiladi@hamad.qa

H. Elgendy
Department of Anesthesia, ICU and Perioperative Medicine, Hamad Medical Corporation, Doha, Qatar

Department of Anesthesia, Al Wakra Hospital, Doha, Qatar

Weill Cornel Medicine, Qatar and Assiut University Hospital – Egypt, Doha, Qatar
e-mail: Helgendy2@hamad.qa

N. A. Shallik et al. (eds.), *Improving Anesthesia Technical Staff's Skills*,
https://doi.org/10.1007/978-3-030-88849-7_15

15.1 Introduction

Regional anesthesia is highly suggested in various and enormous surgical settings due to its crucial benefits in minimizing patient's postoperative agony. It reduces opioids requirements, postoperative pain and decreases length of hospital stay. There is a growing advancement of using technology to enhance success of the regional anesthesia and peripheral nerve blocks. After established use of peripheral nerve stimulator to increase the efficiency of nerve block procedure. Integration of ultrasound machine enables perfect blockade. The assistance that is provided by the anaesthesia technologist to the performing anaesthetist is highly appreciated in the perioperative settings. Careful, vigilant, and professional anesthesia assistant has spurred innovation in the delivery of anesthesia services. The use of multimodal pain management plan enhanced speedy recovery of patients and improved their outcome.

15.2 Patient Education and Preparation

Regardless of patient routine general checkup, an anesthesia history and physical assessment should be performed before any regional anesthesia procedure in order to minimize the associated risks.

15.2.1 Education

- Patient's Rights:
  - Acknowledge the patient's autonomy and dignity and respect his/her privacy.
  - Support the patient's needs and safety.
  - Get Informed Consent for the anesthesia procedure.
  - Brief the patient about the equipment that will be used during the procedure.
  - Consider infection control guidelines.
- Patient must be informed about what is expected to happen after anesthesia such as loss of sensitivity or motricity.

15.2.2 Preparation

- A physical exam must be performed, and good positioning is always required to ensure an adequate anatomy reference.
- Premedication is mandatory for an anxious patient [1].

15.3 Block Room

15.3.1 Block Room Preparation and Setup

Block room is an essential place for performance of the regional procedure with easy access to resuscitation equipment and tools. The use of an appropriate monitor is crucial during performing the regional anesthesia together with using an oxygen source either mask or nasal cannula are mandatory. *If an ultrasound machine will be part of the procedure, it is placed on the side opposite the limb to be blocked.* Adjustment of positioning should be done by the anesthesia technician in a harmony with the performing physician. His job requires fine manipulation of the ultrasound machine, the nerve stimulator, injection of local anesthetic at the direction of the anesthetist together with monitoring of the patient's vitals.

15.3.2 Block Area General Equipment

The anesthesia technician should confirm the room checklist with the attending physician prior to any procedure to ensure a high level of patient safety. The checklist should confirm the availability of medication, consumables, and equipment as well as the planned storage setup for all of these items. A locoregional trolley can be used to store both consumables and medication.

A daily checklist of the trolley should be performed to make sure that all needed items are available such as:

- Antiseptic solution: Chloraprep® (Chlorhexidine gluconate (CHG) 2% w/v and isopropyl alcohol (IPA) 70% v/v) /Duraprep® (CHG/IPA), gauze, dressings drape, marking pen, ruler.
- Hypodermic needles for skin infiltration.
- IV cannulas, which should be inserted before starting any block.
- Ultrasound transducer cover and gel.
- Different types of needles.
- A bundle of medications is including local anesthetics, sedatives, and resuscitation drugs.

High alert medication should be nicely labeled and separately stored to avoid any error.

15.3.3 Emergency Drugs and Resuscitation Equipment

Ultrasound implementation in regional anesthesia practice has enhanced patient's safety and minimized the risk of severe local anesthetic systemic toxicity (LAST) (Table 15.1).

15.4 Equipment for Induction of Regional Anesthesia

15.4.1 Needles

A nerve block consists of locating a volume of local anesthetic close to the nerve. This procedure cannot be performed without an appropriate needle. Actually, we can distinguish many types of peripheral nerves block needles. In addition, an echogenic needle introduced with ultrasound reflecting a beam effect offers a nice view of needle tip and surrounding structures.

Finally, the choice of needles is based on like tip design, gauge, and length.

Table 15.1 Resuscitation equipment and drugs prepared in block area before performing regional anesthesia

Resuscitation equipment	Resuscitation drugs
• Oxygen supply, nasal airway, and O_2 masks • Oral airways of different sizes, laryngeal masks, and endotracheal tubes • Laryngoscopes • Bag-mask ventilation device, Boujie, stylet • Suction • Selection of various size intravenous cannulas • Defibrillator	• Atropine (300–600 µg) • Epinephrine (10–100 µg) • Suxamethonium (40–100 mg) • Ephedrine (5–15 mg) • Phenylephrine (100–200 µg) • Glycopyrrolate (200–400 µg) • Intralipid® 20%

Needle Tip Design During the nerve blockade procedure, the bevel of the needle can impact the extent of damage when especially a needle is closely inserted in the nerve. Within, this framework we can differentiate many types of needles (Fig. 15.1).

Needle Length Needle length varies according to the depth of the nerve and can be easily specified according to blocks types through the use of ultrasound which can exactly show the desired distance. The needle penetration depth can be monitored and calculated using the needle centimeter marks (Fig. 15.2).

Needle Gauge 22 gauge is the common and standard needle size used during nerve block. During insertion, the needle can maintain a straight shape and remain difficult to be blended. This specific size offers an easy advancement when the needle is inserted and it is equally easy to steer during deep blocks. Larger-gauge needles should be used with caution, since they are associated with increased severity of tissue injury and hematoma. Resistance tends to be increased when performing injections with smaller-gauge needles, and it also takes longer for blood to be aspirated back in case the tip is intravascular.

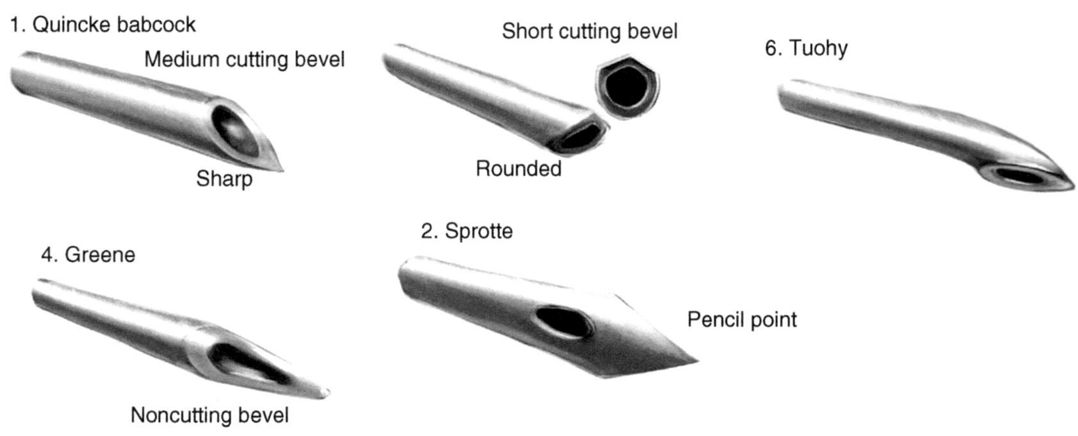

Fig. 15.1 Needle Tip Design used for nerve block. Short beveled needle which has less cutting effect damage, and it may provide better feedback and enhanced feeling for the "pop" that occurs when puncturing through the fascia. However, if it is applied with high pressure, an overshooting can occur and cause a post-traumatic inflammation, myelin damage, and intraneural hematoma. "Source: NYSORA.COM"

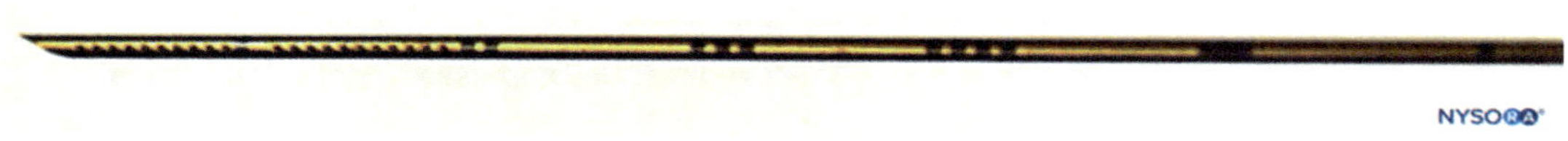

Fig. 15.2 Nerve block needle showing centimeter markings for depth of penetration Monitoring. "Source: NYSORA. COM"

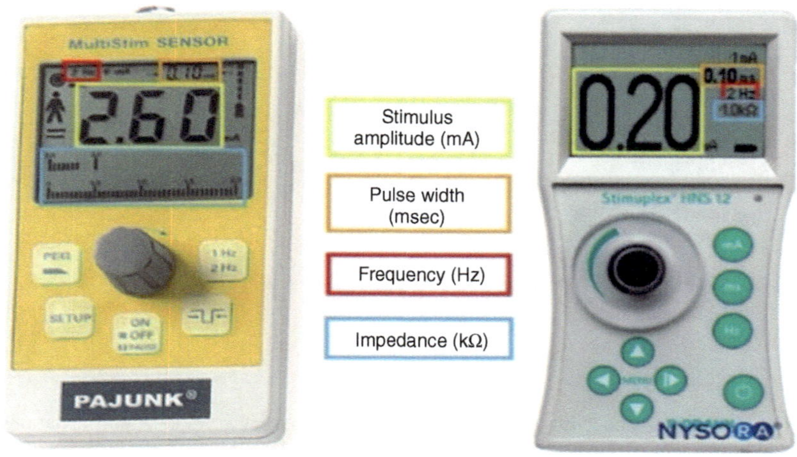

Fig. 15.3 Peripheral nerve stimulators. "Source: NYSORA. COM"

15.4.2 Nerve-Locating Devices

- *Peripheral Nerve Stimulators:* Over a long period of time peripheral nerve stimulator was the fundamental device nerve tracking system allowing measurement of stimulus amplitude, pulse width frequency and electrical impedance.
- *Ultrasound:* The introduction of ultrasound terminology has revolutionized the field of regional anesthesia. In fact, the visualization of nerves and all surrounding structures in real time and with higher resolution has improved block outcomes. Moreover, the combination of both ultrasound and PNS created an objective method of achieving accurate and safe blocks [2, 3] (Fig. 15.3).

15.4.3 Monitoring Devices

Patient Monitoring: It is highly recommended to apply routine monitoring for all patients including those with or without sedation. Furthermore, vigilance remains the best way to predict intravascular injection.

15.4.4 General Monitoring Includes the Following

- Electrocardiogram.
- Noninvasive blood pressure.
- Pulse oximetry.
- Capnography in case of administration of any sedative medication.

15.4.5 Monitoring for Intraneural Injection Paresthesia

15.4.5.1 Electrical Nerve Stimulation

It is no longer used as primary tool to determine nerve location after evolution of ultrasound innovations in regional blocks.

Pressure-Monitoring Device	Left syringe: Uncompressed, containing 10mL of air and 10mL of local anaesthetic. Right syringe: Air compressed by 50% results in exerted pressure of 760mmHg (approx. 15 psi).
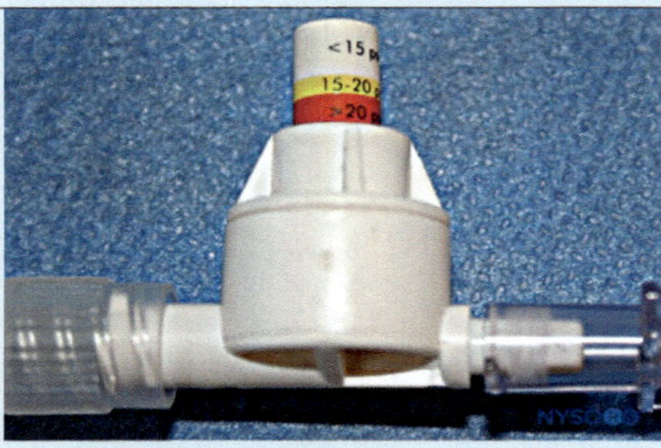	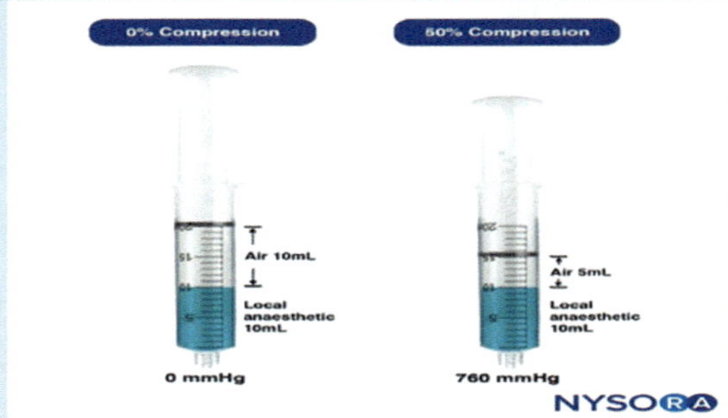

Fig. 15.4 Shows injection pressure monitoring. https://www.nysora.com/foundations-of-regional-anesthesia/equipment/equipment-regional-anesthesia/. "Source: NYSORA.COM"

15.4.5.2 Ultrasound Imaging

It is used with great utility in real-time visualization of the needle tip with a high resolution.

The Above TWO instruments are used to prevent intraneural injection.

15.4.5.3 Injection Pressure Monitoring

On the other hand, monitoring pressure during injection can reflect an adequate placement of the needle. Many studies reported mechanical injuries of neurological tissues because of high pressure intraneural injection with low volumes [4] (Fig. 15.4).

15.4.5.4 Premedication and Sedation

It can be accomplished with small increments of fentanyl and/or midazolam.

15.5 Ultrasound System Preparation and Cleaning

15.5.1 Preparation

The use of high-level technology machines remains a challenge for healthcare practitioners and requiring special recommendations in order to protect ultrasound system, transducer, and accessories.

In fact, applying carefully a compatible acoustic gel and adequate ultrasound probe cover, allow easy transmission and getting high exam quality.

The presence of bubbles between the transducer footprint and the sheath can interfere with the image quality.

15.5.2 Cleaning and Disinfection of Ultrasound System

In reality, it is recommended to proceed for the ultrasound system cleaning after each, but only the transducer can be disinfected to a high level.

On every cleaning process, it is recommended to use the appropriate personal protective equipment (PPE)

- Turn off the machine.
- Unplug the power cord from the outlet.
- Remove the disposable transducer sheath, if applicable.

- Disconnect the transducer from the system and place it where it will not cross clean equipment or surfaces [5].

A highly validated disinfection process is by using of a transducer's cover and a sterile gel as compatible with infection control rules [5].

Tips for the ATs *Damage can occur if the cleaning or disinfection of the ultrasound system will be done in improper way. In our institution, there is a log book to use the US machine indicated details for date, time, both anesthesiologist and anesthesia technologist names.*

15.5.3 Blocks Preparations

- Prior medical history of the patient such as coagulopathy and neurological status should be confirmed by the attending physician.
- Intravenous access should be inserted in all patients receiving a nerve block for a surgical procedure. It should be established to avoid vasovagal events, inadvertent IV injection, and local anesthetic toxicity (LAST) by using promptly the resuscitation drugs.
- Vigilant aseptic technique is crucial during placement and management of regional anesthesia. As with any sterile procedure, hand hygiene, standard precautions, skin preparation, sterile preparation of drugs, sterile draping, and proper technique specific for the block or guidance technology must be used as outline (Fig. 15.5).

15.5.4 Local Anesthetic Systemic Toxicity and Management

Local anesthetics usually work through sodium channel blockade of nerve endings. Two classes of them include amino-amide or amino-ester local anesthetics. When they are used at higher dose or higher concentration leads to local anesthetic systemic toxicity (LAST). It should be managed thoroughly according to the American Society of Regional Anesthesia and Pain Medicine check list (Fig. 15.6).

15.5.5 Contributing Factors

1. Type of LA.
2. Volume and concentration of LA.
3. Level of injection.
4. Speed of injection.
5. Patient's comorbidities.
6. Lipophilicity of LA (more lipophilic LA like bupivacaine have increased risk of toxicity).

15.5.6 LAST Treatment

Presently, the three pillars of LAST treatment consist of seizure management, advanced cardiac life support (ACLS), and prompt administration of a 20% lipid emulsion.

American Society of Regional Anesthesia and Pain Medicine checklist for the treatment of LAST can help guide the treatment process [6].

15.5.7 LAST Prevention

As always, the best treatment is prevention. This is especially true for LAST. For that reason, it is advised to:

- Maintain vigilance,
- Monitor vital signs,
- Communicate with patient,
- Aspirate in every 3–5 ml of LA,
- Inject slowly and avoid high pressure,
- Use of intravascular marker such as 10–15 μg of epinephrine. An increase in heart rate of 10 beats/minute or greater or an increase in systolic blood pressure of 15 mm Hg or greater suggests an intravascular injection.
- Be conservative in dosing of LA: low concentration but optimum dose.

- If signs and symptoms of LAST occur, prompt and effective airway management is crucial to precenting hypoxia, hypercapnia, and acidosis, which are known to potentiate LAST, (I; B)
- Lipid emulsion therapy *(I; B)* :
  - o *Administer at the first signs of LAST, after airway management*
  - o *Timeliness of lipid emulsion is more important than the order of administration modality (bolus vs infusion)*
    - *20% lipid emulsion BOLUS*
      - *100 mL over 2-3 min if patient is over 70 kg*
      - *1.5 mL/kg over 2-3 min if patient is less than 70 kg*
    - *20% lipid emulsion INFUSION*
      - *200-250 mL over 15-20 min if patient is over 70 kg*
      - *0.25 mL/kg/min if patient is less than 70 kg (ideal body weight)*
      - *If circulatory stability is not attained, consider rebolus or increasing infusion to 0.5 mL/kg/min*
    - Continue infusion forat least 10 min after circulatory stability is attained.
    - Appeoximately *12 mL/kg* lipid emulsion is recommended as the upper limit for initial dosing. *(IIb; B)*
    - Propfol is not a substitute for lipid emulsion *(III; B)*
- Seizure control:
  - o If seizutes occur, they should be rapidly halted with benzodiazepines. If benzodiazepines are not readily available, doses of propofol are acceptable, (I; B)
    - Although peopofol can stop seizures, large doses further sepress cardiac functions; propofol should be avioded when there are signs of cardiovascular compromise. (III; B)
  - o If seizures persist depite benzodiazepine, small doses of suceiny leholine or similar neuromuscular blocker should be considered to minimize acidosis and hypoxemia. (I; C)
- If cardiac arrest occurs:
  - o If epinephrine is used, small initial doses (≤1 μg/kg) are preferred *(IIa; B)*
  - o Vasopressin is not recommende (III; B)
  - o Avoid calcium channel blockers and β-adrenergic receptor blockers, (III; C)
  - o If ventricular arrhythmias develop, amiodarone is preferred (IIa; B); treatment with local anesthetics (lidocaine or procainamide) is not recommended. *(III; B)*
- Failure to respond to lipid emulsion and vasopressor therapy should prompt institution of CPB *(I; B)*. Because there can be considerable lag in beginning CPB, it is reasonable to notify the closed facility capable of providing it when cardiovascular compromise is first identified during an episode of LAST.
- *Patients with a significant CV event should be monitored for at least 4–6 h. If the event is limited to CNS symptoms that resolve quickly, they should be monitored for at least 2 h (IIa: B)*
- *Use written or electronic checklists as cognitive aids during the management of LAST. A dedicated reader improves adherence to the checklist. (I; A)*

These recommendarions are intended to encourage optimal patient care but cannot ensure the avoidance of adverse outcomes. As with any practice ad. visory recommendation, these are subject to revision as knowledge advances regarding specific complications.
The class of recommendation and level of evidence for each intervention are given in parenthesis (see Table 1).
Changes from the 2010 LAST practice advisory[1] are italicized.
CPB indicates cardiopulmonary bypas.

Fig. 15.5 Local Anesthetic toxicity management, Adopted from: The Third American Society of Regional Anesthesia and Pain Medicine Practice Advisory on Local Anesthetic Systemic Toxicity Executive Summary 2017: Neal et al., Regional Anesthesia and Pain Medicine, Volume 43, Number 2, February 2018

The presence of LAST prevention kit around the block workspace area can reduce LAST effect. The combination of use of ultrasound and peripheral nerve stimulation remain the best way to reduce the incidence of LAST [1].

15.6 Hypotension: Causes, Prevention, and Management

After successful placement, it is always recommended to maintain vigilance especially the first 10 min which are critical in terms of monitoring cardiovascular response as well as the level of progression of block.

The patient's blood pressure should be taken every 3 min initially, in order to early predict hypotension.

Hypotension is the most frequent immediate adverse effect. It occurs mainly during central nervous system (CNS) blocks.

Decrease of vascular resistance, venous return, and cardiac output are the most common causes of hypotension which can causes nausea, vomiting, and bradycardia.

Hypotension can be treated or prevented by one of the following:

Mechanical Methods A slight head-down position (5–10°) and compressing lower limb are the famous efficient way to increase venous return

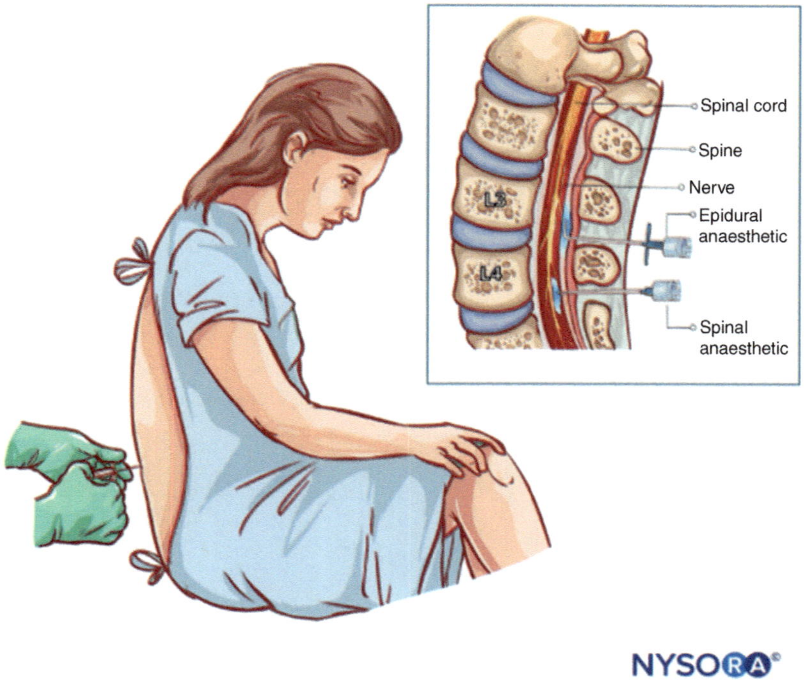

Fig. 15.6 Illustration for position in spinal and epidural anesthesia. "Source: NYSORA.COM"

without altering the spread of anesthetic and the maintenance of an adequate hydration can correct the situation.

Volume Loading The use of crystalloid and colloid as alternative of IV fluid loading is to increase stroke volume and cardiac output.

Vasopressors Ephedrine 5 –10 mg IV boluses, Phenylephrine bolus of 40–160 mcg IV, or infusion of 20–200 mcg/min IV.

15.7 Common Regional Anesthesia Blocks

15.7.1 Introduction

Since late 1800s, regional anesthesia has been started to block the nerve impulses in the peripheral nervous system. At that time, the blocks were performed primarily by using anatomical landmarks; that is, prominent markers (e.g., the lateral malleolus of the ankle). Anatomical variation and practical considerations tended to limit the overall utility of peripheral nerve blockade. Nowadays in the twenty-first century, the use of a nerve stimulator allows a small electrical current to be passed through a block needle. If the needle is in close proximity to a nerve, the stimulus will cause the nerve to send an impulse (stimulate the nerve) and induce any muscles innervated by the nerve to twitch (elicit a motor response). More recently, anesthetists have widely adopted ultrasound-based techniques for block placement as it has several advantages when compared to nerve stimulators or anatomic-based techniques [7].

15.7.2 Indications

A. When patient is sick enough to tolerate a general anesthetic, however, fine regional anesthetic technique can solve the situation without consequences.
B. In combination with a general anesthetic to optimize pain control and the implementation of a perineural catheter can extend postoperative pain control for a few days.

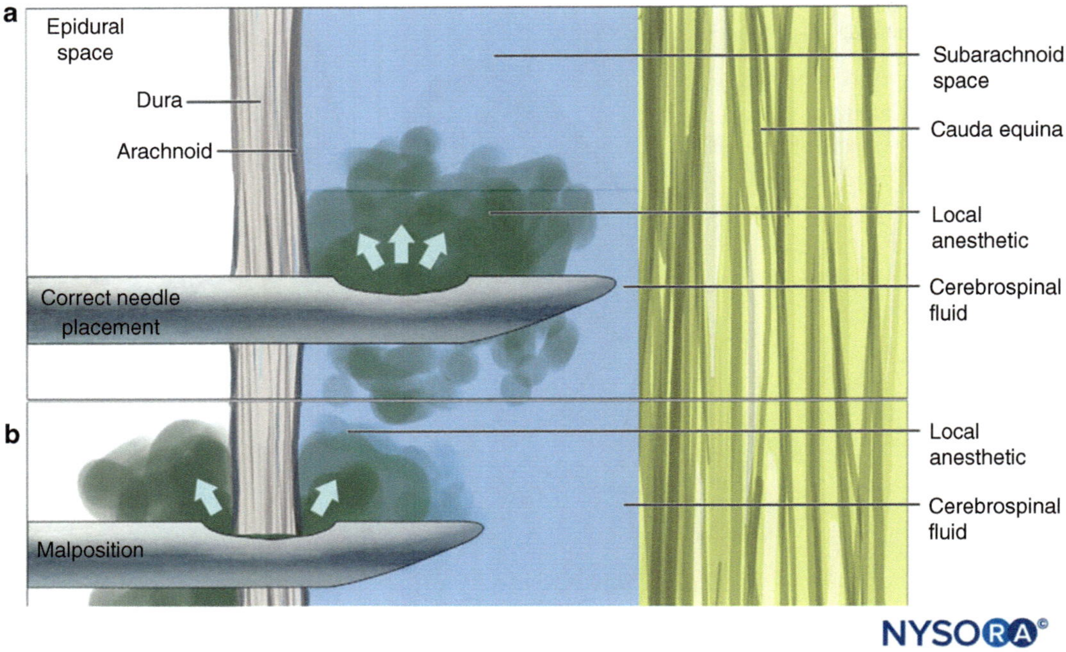

Fig. 15.7 Mechanism for failed spinal anesthesia. Correct needle placement with (**a**) all drug delivered to CSF and (**b**) malposition where some of the drug is lost into the epidural space. "Source: NYSORA.COM"

15.7.3 Contra-Indications

A. Bleeding Disorders: Hereditary or iatrogenic bleeding disorders which includes the use of coumadin or heparin. It initiates epidural hematoma with disastrous consequences. Prior to the procedure, full coagulation profile should be assessed.
B. Pulmonary Function: Some blocks such as interscalene block induce unilateral paralysis of the diaphragm. Another block such as supra calvicular block may precipitate pneumothorax.
C. Pre-existing Nerve Injury: It should be considered carefully as the new block may exacerbate the old previous nerve injury.
D. Local Anesthetic Reaction: when there is an allergy to local anesthetic.
E. Patient Refusal: It is not uncommon for patients to decline a block.
F. Infection of the tissues at the site desired is a contraindication to block placement.

15.8 Central Nervous System Blocks: (Subarachnoid Block and Epidural Block; Fig. 15.7)

Subarachnoid block or spinal anesthesia is a kind of neuraxial regional anesthesia involving the injection of a local anesthetic and/or opioid into the subarachnoid space. Fine needle is commonly used. This block is used mostly for surgeries of the lower half of the body.

Epidural block is performed by injecting local anesthetic into the epidural space to optimize the analgesia effect.

Positioning: There are three different positions which can be established: sitting, lateral decubitus, and prone.

15.8.1 Peripheral Nerves Blocks

It consists of injection of local anesthetic, corticosteroid, and analgesic adjuvant near to the nerve.

Regional Nerve block includes:

- Lower extremity nerve block: Femoral blocks, popliteal, and ankle.
- Upper extremity nerve block: Interscalene, Supra and Infra Clavicular, Axillary, and Wrist blocks.

Positioning The ultrasound view is optimized for the clear anatomical image to obtain a good quality of nerve block.

Tips for the Anesthesia Technologists

- The skilled anesthesia technologist helps the anesthetist to adjust patient's position to open the space between the spinous processes. Careful adjustment of the patient's head after spinal anesthesia to avoid higher spread of the hyperbaric bupivacaine and induce high spinal.
- Handling Intrathecal drugs: It is an important rule of the Anesthesia Technologists.
- Double check with the Anesthesiologist: name of the drug, concentration, and expiry date.
- Drugs must be given under complete aseptic conditions.
- Basic ASA monitors are mandatory during procedures.
- Prepare local anesthetic infusion for patient controlled epidural analgesia (PCEA) and adjust the infusion machine under observation of the physician (Fig. 15.8).

15.9 Upper Extremity Blocks

15.9.1 Interscalene Block

It is the commonest performed block for surgery of the upper arm and shoulder. The ultrasound position is shown in the mid-neck in (Fig. 15.9).

Tips for the Anesthesia Technologists

A. The interscalene block may be associated with hemidiaphragmatic paralysis on the side of the block. It may lead to Horner's syndrome which includes ptosis, miosis, and anhidrosis.

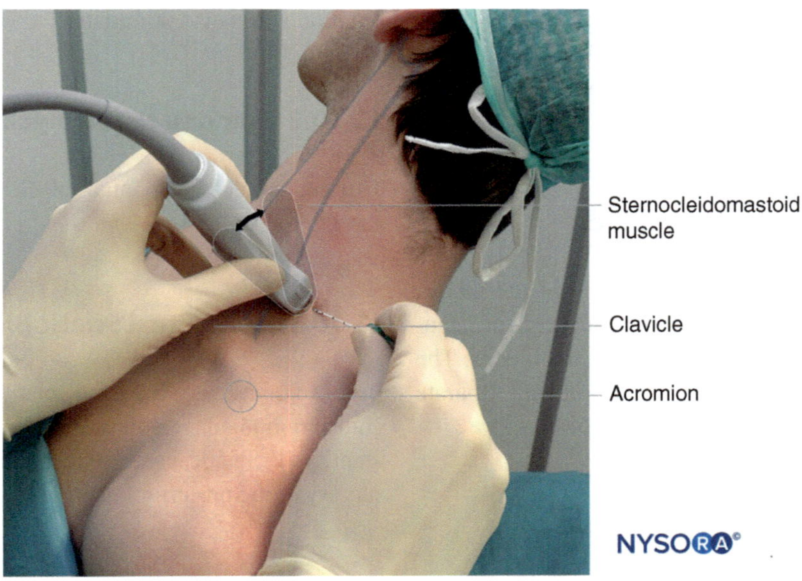

Fig. 15.8 Ultrasound-guided interscalene brachial plexus block: transducer and needle position to obtain the desired ultrasound image for an in-plane approach. The knowledge of external landmarks substantially facilitates and shortens the time to obtain the view necessary for block performance. The transducer is positioned behind the clavicular head of the sternocleidomastoid muscle (SCM) and over the external jugular vein (not seen). The patient is in a semi-sitting position. Tilting the transducer in the caudad direction can facilitate recognition of the brachial plexus (arrow). "Source: NYSORA.COM"

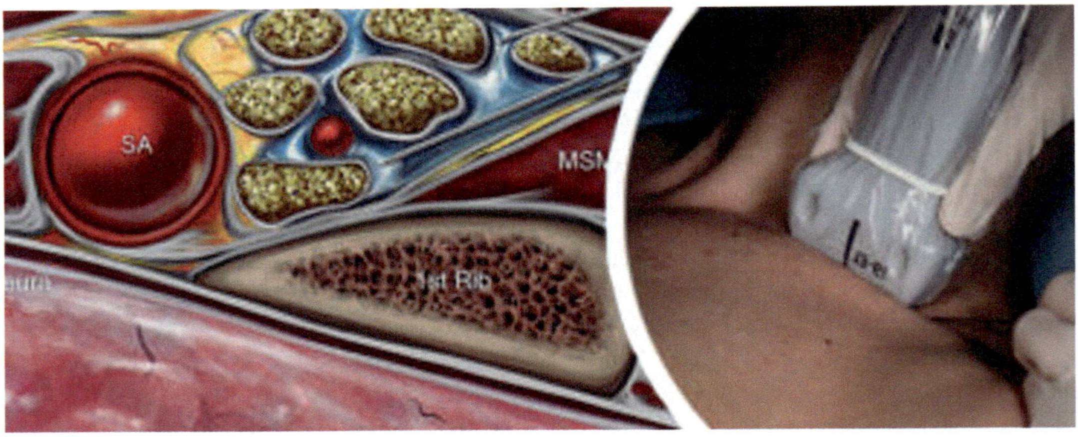

Fig. 15.9 Supraclavicular brachial plexus block. Anesthesia and analgesia for humerus, elbow, forearm, and hand. "Source: NYSORA.COM"

B. Perineural catheter is usually inserted with this block. (1) Leakage and (2) catheter movement are two frequent technical problems can be seen.

15.9.2 Supraclavicular Block

It is a popular block used for surgery of the upper arm, elbow, and hand. This block can be complicated by inadvertent pneumothorax. This can be prevented by use of ultrasound.

15.9.3 Infraclavicular Block

It is commonly used for surgery of the elbow, forearm, and hand. It may have the risk of pneumothorax with other brachial plexus blocks. The musculocutaneous nerve should have a separate block to avoid its sparing (Fig. 15.11).

15.9.4 Axillary Block

It is used frequently for surgery of the elbow, forearm, or hand (Fig. 15.11). The musculocutaneous nerve should be blocked separately as it is commonly splits off prior to this block level (Figs. 15.10 and 15.11).

15.10 Lower Extremity Blocks

15.10.1 Lumbar Plexus Block

It is directed to block nerves arise from the lumbar spine and supply the lower limbs, (Figs. 15.12 and 15.13). Some physicians may perform the block solely using ultrasound; others use a combination with nerve stimulator.

15.10.2 Femoral Nerve Block

This nerve block is a popular block used for knee surgeries (Fig. 15.14).

15.10.3 Subgluteal Sciatic Block

Because of the deeply seated sciatic nerve in the gluteal region, maybe ultrasound is not enough to identify it. Sciatic nerve blocks are suitable for surgery of the posterior knee, lower leg, and foot.

15.10.4 Popliteal Sciatic Block

The popliteal fossa block is a variant of the sciatic block, Fig. 15.15. The block can be placed easily performed with ultrasound, and fairly eas-

Fig. 15.10 Ultrasound image demonstrating an ideal needle path for the infraclavicular brachial plexus block. The blue-shaded area mimics an ideal spread of local anesthetic around the axillary artery (AA) and reaches all three cords of the brachial plexus (the lateral cord [LC], posterior cord [PC], and medial cord [MC]) below the fascia (red line) of the pectoralis minor muscle (PMiM), pectoralis major muscle (PMaM), and axillary vein (AV). "Source: NYSORA.COM"

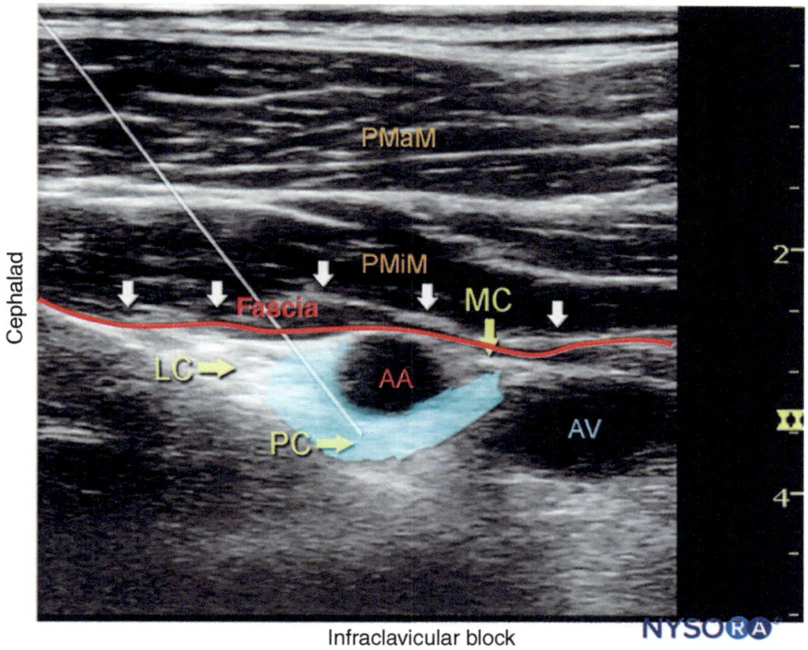

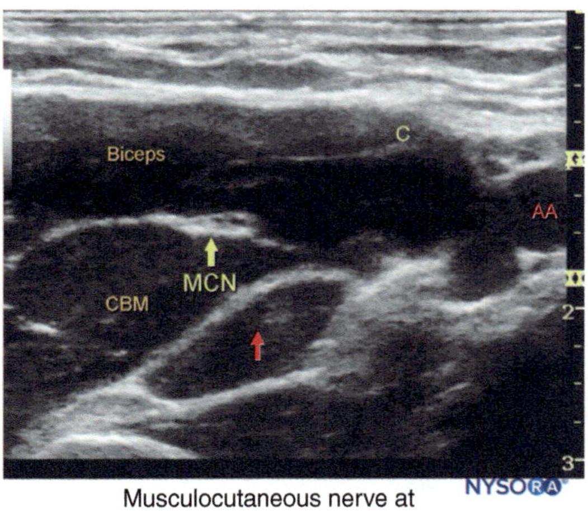

Fig. 15.11 The musculocutaneous nerve (MCN) is located few cms away from the axillary artery (AA) between the biceps and the coracobrachialis muscle. The course of the MCN along the upper arm display frequent anatomic variations. Systematic scanning to identify the nerve and a separate injection of local anesthetic are usually required for a successful axillary brachial plexus block. "Source: NYSORA.COM"

ily using landmarks and nerve stimulation. The popliteal block provides excellent anesthesia for surgery of the lower leg and foot.

15.11 Regional Anesthesia Recommendations in COVID-19 Era

15.11.1 COVID 19 Recommendations for Regional Anesthesia

The American Society of Regional Anaesthesia and Pain Medicine (ASRA) and the European Society of Regional Anaesthesia and Pain Therapy (ESRA) agreed a joint statement during the peak of COVID-19, March, 2020 (Fig. 15.16), [8, 9] to postpone all elective surgeries and procedures in order to minimize the exposure risk of healthcare professionals and keep only lifesaving surgeries and oncology related procedures. They recommended the use of regional anesthesia to overcome the risk of viral transmission among healthcare professionals and preferred it over risk of general anesthesia. It includes preparation and planning of anesthesia, equipment, supplies, and patients' preparations to reduce risk of droplets. It has been described precautions during peripheral nerve blocks and neuraxial anesthesia. A

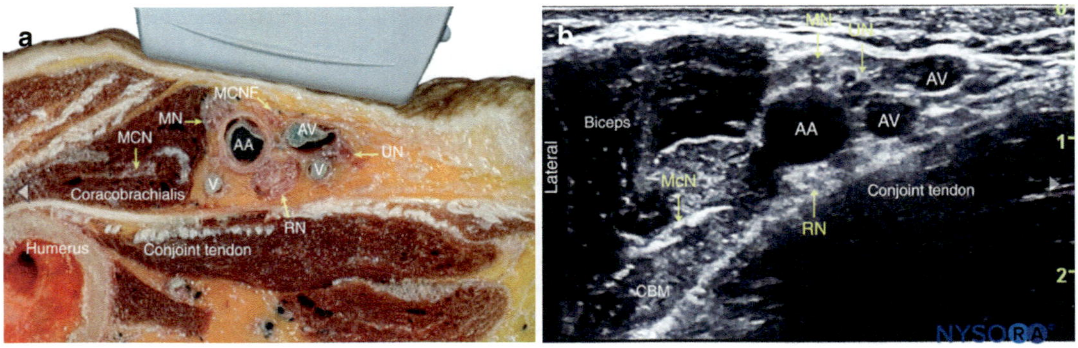

Fig. 15.12 (**a**) Cross-sectional anatomy of the axillary fossa and ultrasound image (**b**) of the terminal nerves of brachial plexus. The BP is seen scattered around the axillary artery and enclosed within the adipose tissue compartment containing the axillary artery (AA), and axillary veins (AV). *MCN* musculocutaneous nerve, *MN* median nerve, *RN* radial nerve, *UN* ulnar nerve, *MACN* medial antebrachial cutaneous nerve, *CBM* coracobrachialis muscle. "Source: NYSORA.COM"

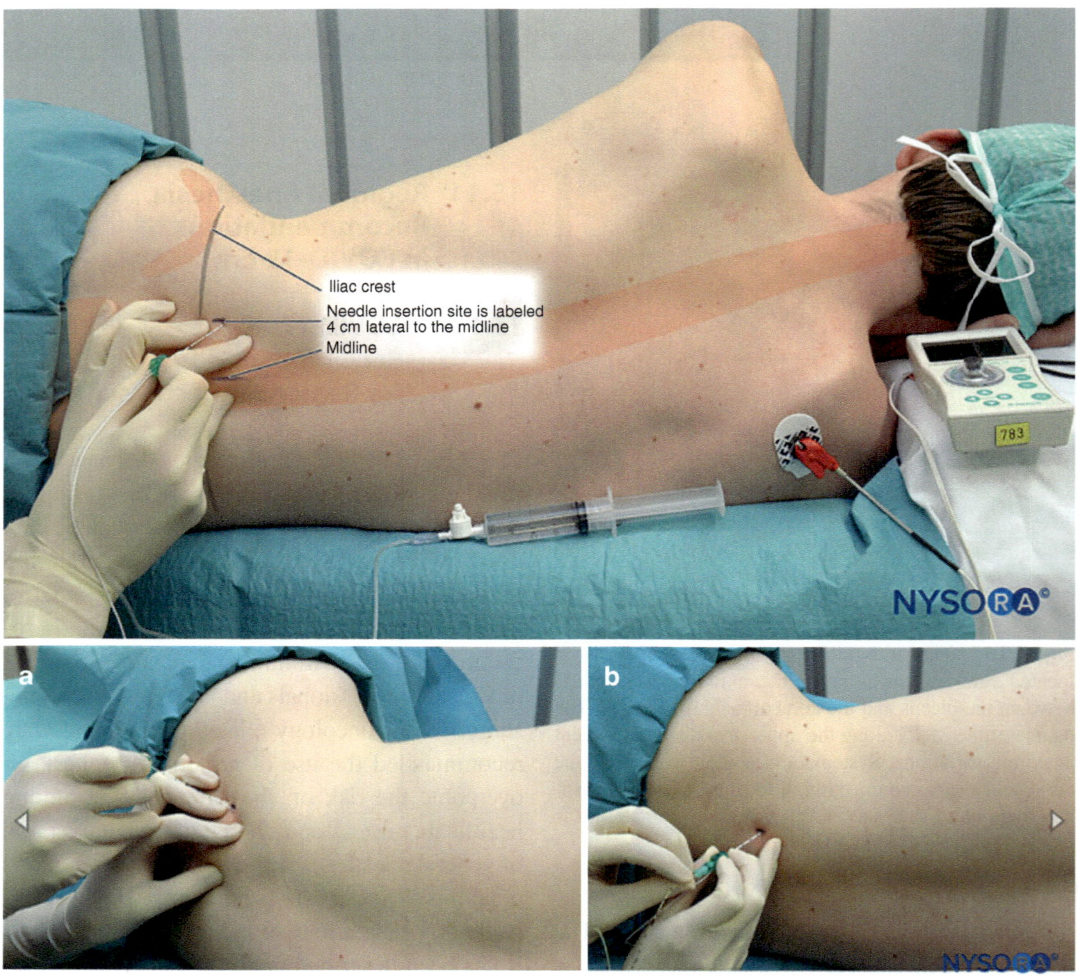

Fig. 15.13 Landmarks for lumbar plexus block. (**a**, **b**) Needle insertion for the lumbar plexus block. The needle is inserted perpendicular to the body plane or with a slight medial orientation (shown) (**a**). Catheter placement technique is preceded by a similar needle technique (**b**). "Source: NYSORA.COM"

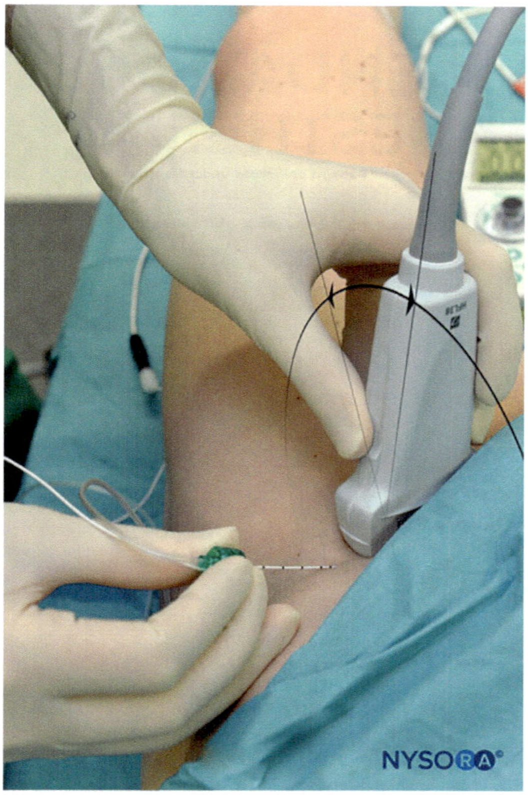

Fig. 15.14 Transducer position and needle insertion using an in-plane technique to block the femoral nerve at the femoral crease. "Source: NYSORA.COM"

Chinese study reported possible transmission rates of COVID-19 to anesthetists even during spinal anesthesia. Many concerns have risen about the variable method of diagnosis of those doctors and patients in this study. Some of anesthetists developed symptoms during their clinical service which mandate further study in this hot topic [10].

15.12 Conclusion

Regional anesthesia is a regenerative and crucial part of anesthesia practice. Recently, it has made great advancements in technology, equipment such as ultrasound and perineural catheters which improved its utility. The ATs should be thoroughly familiar with the techniques and equipment to perform regional anesthesia in order to optimize work harmony in the perioperative settings.

Updated continuous professional development is mandatory for both current and prospective ATs. Providing adequate academic as well as practical tips for regional anesthesia facilitates the collaborative spirit with the attending physicians and improves the quality of their efforts.

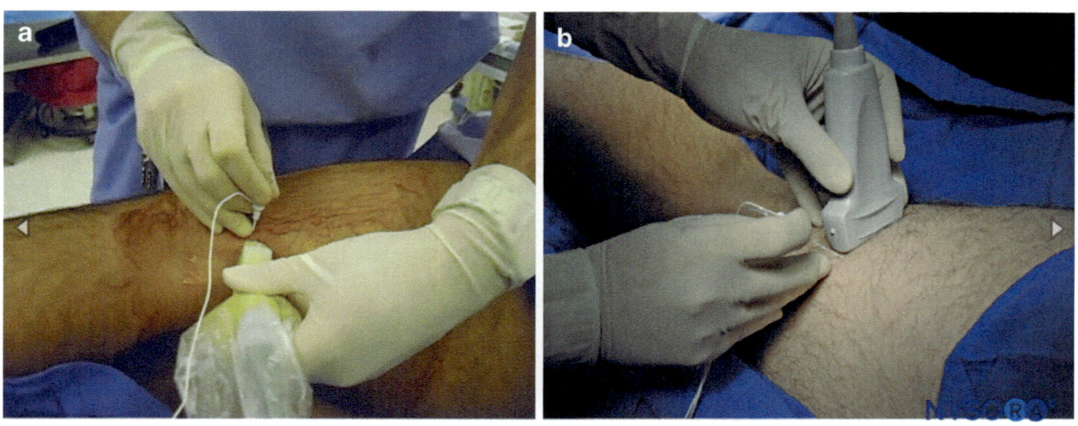

Fig. 15.15 The posterior approach to the US-guided popliteal sciatic block can be performed (**a**) with the patient in the lateral position or (**b**) with the patient prone. (Reproduced with permission from Hadzic A: Hadzic's Peripheral Nerve Blocks and Anatomy for Ultrasound-Guided Regional Anesthesia, second ed. New York: McGraw-Hill, 2011) "Source: NYSORA.COM"

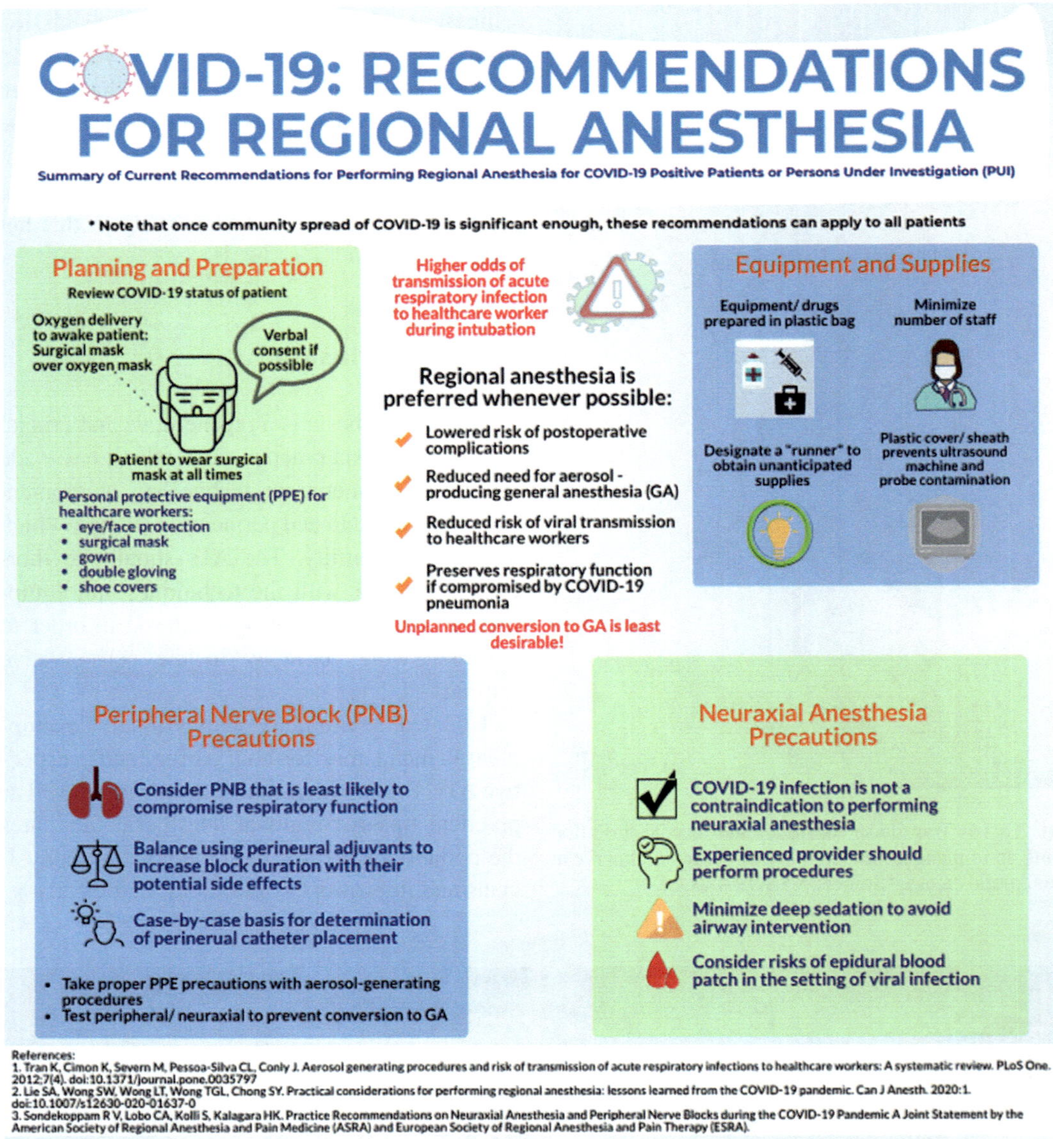

Fig. 15.16 Adopted from: Herman JA, et al. COVID-19: Recommendations for regional anesthesia. J Clin Anesth. 2020 Oct; 65:109885

During COVID-19 crisis, recommendations have been implemented by ASRA and ESRA to prefer regional anesthesia procedures than general techniques. Balance of risk and benefit and established safety for both patients and health care providers should be warranted.

References

1. Woodworth G. The anesthesia technician and technologist manual. Lippincott Williams & Wilkins, a Wolters Kluwer; 2012.
2. Egeler C, Jayakumar A, Ford S. Electronic tutorial for ultrasound-guided regional anesthesia has to

be accurate to be of value. Reg Anesth Pain Med. 2013;38(3):252–3.
3. Shy ME. Ultrasound: the future for evaluating the PNS in humans? J Neurol Neurosurg Psychiatry. 2014;86(4):362.
4. Saporito A, Quadri C, Capdevila X. The ability of a real-time injection pressure monitoring system to discriminate between perineural and intraneural injection of the sciatic nerve in fresh cadavers. Anaesthesia. 2018;73(9):1118–22.
5. Lichtenstein DA. Point-of-care ultrasound: infection control in the intensive care unit. Crit Care Med. 2007;35(5 Suppl):S262–7.
6. Neal JM, Barrington MJ, Fettiplace MR, Gitman M, Memtsoudis SG, Morwald EE, et al. The third American Society of Regional Anesthesia and Pain Medicine practice advisory on local anesthetic systemic toxicity: executive summary 2017. Reg Anesth Pain Med. 2017;43(2):113–23.
7. Labat G. Regional anesthesia: its technique and clinical application. Philadelphia, PA: W B Saunders Company; 1922.
8. Sondekoppam RVL, Lobo CA, Kolli S, Kalagara HK. Practice recommendations on neuraxial anesthesia and peripheral nerve blocks during the COVID-19 pandemic. A Joint Statement by the American Society of Regional Anesthesia and Pain Medicine (ASRA) and European Society of Regional Anesthesia and Pain Therapy (ESRA). 2020.
9. Herman JA, Urits I, Kaye AD, Urman RD, Viswanath O. COVID-19: recommendations for regional anesthesia. J Clin Anesth. 2020;65:109885.
10. Zhong Q, Liu YY, Luo Q, Zou YF, Jiang HX, Li H, et al. Spinal anaesthesia for patients with coronavirus disease 2019 and possible transmission rates in anaesthetists: retrospective, single-centre, observational cohort study. Br J Anaesth. 2020;124(6):670–5.

Transportation of the Anaesthetized and Critically Ill Patient

16

Tahir Imaduddeen and Ahmed Labib

Contents

16.1 Introduction

Transfer of anaesthetized and/or critically ill patient is fraught with difficulties and could be hazardous to the patient and the transport team. Adverse events (AE) during transfer are estimated at 45–79%, whilst serious AE are reported at 4.2–8.9%. Cardiac arrests are infrequently observed, only occurring in 0.38–1.6% of transfers. Another

T. Imaduddeen
Medical Intensive Care Unit, Hamad Medical Corporation, Doha, Qatar

A. Labib (✉)
Weill-Cornell Medical College, Hamad General Hospital, Doha, Qatar

N. A. Shallik et al. (eds.), *Improving Anesthesia Technical Staff's Skills*,
https://doi.org/10.1007/978-3-030-88849-7_16

Canadian report demonstrated AE in only 6.5% in a series of over 5000 urgent ground transfers. AE are associated with increased morbidity [1–4].

AE during transfer arise due to a number of factors which can be broadly classified into patient, practitioner, and transport environment and organizational factors [3, 5].

Patients transported within critical or acute care areas, e.g., the operating room (OR), post-anaesthesia care unit (PACU), the emergency department (ED), or the Intensive care unit (ICU) typically display a rapidly changing and unstable physiology and hence meticulous attention to clinical status and monitoring of vital signs is essential to ensure safety. In addition, several medications and infusions are typically being administered simultaneously including sedatives, analgesics, neuromuscular blocking agents, vasopressors, and/or inotropes. Patients receiving invasive or non-invasive mechanical ventilation require close monitoring of the airway and ventilation throughout the transfer [6, 7].

Team dynamics are particularly relevant to safe transportation and non-technical skills such as situation awareness, effective communication, leadership, assertiveness, and an appropriate team composition are prerequisites for the safe transportation of such patients. Non-clinical AE were as common as clinical AE in a large series of patient transfers [8]. Use of checklists prior to and after transfer is recommended and has been shown to reduce harm and enhance team performance and safety culture [6, 9–11]. Essential aspects to improve safety also include standardization of protocols, use of specialized equipment, and competent personnel [12].

Depending on the platform of transportation, weather, and road conditions, transport environment plays a major role. Ground transfer poses different challenges to fixed- or rotor-wing air ambulance [6, 7, 13].

In addition, in the pandemic era of Corona virus disease of 2019 (COVID-19), patient transfer has become one of the vital services due to capacity, need for isolation or sub-specialty input [14].

In this chapter, we discuss the important factors that provide a safe environment for transportation of patients and how to better prepare for them beforehand.

16.2 Pre-transport Preparation

Patients may be transferred for clinical or non-clinical reasons; within the facility or between hospitals. Examples of clinical indications are intra-hospital transfer to the OR, PACU, ICU, or imaging department. Inter-hospital transfer is typically deployed for specialized service care provision such as cardiac interventions, neurosurgery, or extra-corporeal membrane oxygenation (ECMO) [6, 7].

Non-clinical transfers are mainly for capacity issues or upon family request. Whatever the indication, distance or duration of the transfer; patient and staff safety must be maintained at all times. [6.7].

Both the referring and receiving physicians are responsible for the decision to transfer a patient. Decision to transfer the patient, made by the primary team, must be taken with due consideration of the risks and benefits of the transfer.

Given the potential risk to patient and transport staff, the decision to transfer a patient should involve a senior clinician. Pre-transport planning and preparation is central to safe transfer A methodical approach should be followed and communicated clearly to all parties involved in the transfer [6, 7].

Current guidelines suggest individualized risk assessment and management taking the following points into account:

1. The indication(s) for transfer.
2. Clinical condition of the patient preferably by trends of physiological and laboratory parameters.
3. Equipment, personnel composition of transportation team.
4. The urgency of transfer: emergency vs. urgent vs. elective.
5. The anticipated duration of the transfer.
6. Specific risks related to this particular transfer.

7. Likelihood of further deterioration and/or need for intervention during the transfer.
8. Destination and platform: inter-hospital or intra-hospital (road or air ambulance).
9. Pre-transport resuscitation and optimization in liaison with transport team and accepting facility [6.7].

Some hospitals have developed dedicated transfer teams particularly for severely ill patients such as those with severe respiratory and cardiovascular failure often referred to as "mobile intensive care unit". Dedicated transport team utilization has been associated with reduced adverse events and mortality. [12, 15–18]

Therefore, a systematic approach to facilitate this process can be broken down into the following steps:

1. Identify the patient that meets criteria or requires transfer.
2. Consultation between the referring and accepting consultant.
3. Acceptance and formal endorsement of patient from primary team to transport team.
4. Pre-transfer stabilization, resuscitation, and safety checks.
5. Transfer of the patient.
6. Formal endorsement to the receiving team.
7. Return of transfer team and equipment to base.

16.3 Levels of Patient Care

A thorough understanding of the level of care will enable the referring, transport, and receiving team to decide on the best management approach for the patient.

The UK Intensive Care Society (ICS) states that patient acuity can be categorized into 4 levels. In this classification, level 0 patients do not usually require specialized personnel or equipment whilst level 3 describes the most critically ill multiple organ dysfunction patients [19]. Irrespective of the level of care, patients must be examined, stabilized, and adequately resuscitated before being moved between clinical areas. The transfer team should not feel coerced or under pressure to move the patient as wrong decision could be made. On the other hand, a transfer for immediate life-saving intervention should be accomplished without undue delay whilst ensuring the receiving team is prepared to take over the patient care upon arrival [7]. A systematic approach via a pre-transfer checklist is highly recommended by a multitude of international professional bodies [6, 12, 20]. An example of a checklist is provided in Fig. 16.1.

16.3.1 Pre-transport Stabilization

Prior to transfer, the transport team must perform full clinical examination, review clinical data, laboratory results, and imaging. Patients should be stabilized and resuscitated to minimize possible complications during transport. A balance must be struck in case of an immediate life-saving intervention indication for transport. Involvement of a senior clinician in such scenario is essential [7].

A detailed risk assessment should be undertaken and documented by a senior clinician prior transporting a critically ill patient. This will help inform decisions of urgency, mode of transport, team composition, and skill-mix required for this particular transport [6, 7].

Airway assessment and protection, if needed, should be undertaken before transport. Administration of appropriate sedation and neuromuscular blocking agents is typically indicated for patients undergoing invasive mechanical ventilation [6, 7].

Arterial blood gas analysis should be performed after stabilization of the patient on the transport ventilator and prior to departure, and ventilator settings adjusted accordingly. During transport, oxygen saturation (SaO_2) is used to guide the fraction of inspired oxygen (FiO_2) and end tidal carbon dioxide concentration ($EtCO_2$) guides ventilation [6, 7].

Satisfactory venous access must be secured prior to departure. A minimum of two functional intravenous catheters is recommended. An indwelling arterial catheter is typically indicated

Patient Transportation Checklist

Pre-transport Equipment and Medication Check	
1. Ventilator: a. Pre-use check b. Settings and alarms c. Fully charged d. Extra-battery	
2. Airway set: a. Laryngoscope b. Video-laryngoscope c. ETT d. HME filter e. Bougie f. Stylet g. Bag/mask with PEEP valve h. Suction device i. Full oxygen tank	
3. Monitor: a. Non-invasive blood pressure (NIBP) b. Arterial blood pressure (ABP) c. Electrocardiogram (ECG) d. End tidal CO_2 (Et CO_2) e. Peripheral arterial saturation (SpO_2)	
4. E-Cart: a. Defibrillator b. Fully charged c. Extra-battery	
5. Fluids: a. Crystalloids b. Colloids c. Blood and blood products d. Lines and drains	
6. RSI medication: propofol/fentanyl/midazolam /rocuronium/ketamine/succinylcholine	
7. Vasopressor & Inotropes: a. Norepinephrine b. Phenylephrine c. Adrenaline d. Others:	
8. Antibiotics:	
9. Patient notes, scans and laboratory results	

Fig. 16.1 An example of transport checklist

Pre-transfer Patient Assessment

1. **Airway:**
   a. ETT (Size: mm. Level at the teeth: cm)
   b. HFNC
   c. NRBM
   d. Venturi-mask
   e. Nasal-cannula

2. **Breathing:**
   a. VENT: mode .TV ml. RR /min. PEEP Cm H_2O. PS Cm H_2O. FiO_2 %).
   b. HFNC: flow l/min. FiO_2 %)
   c. NIV: CPAP Cm H_2O: BIPAP: Cm H_2O
   d. Other:

3. **Circulation:**
   a. Vitals: BP mmHg. RR /min. HR /min. SpO_2. %
   b. Blood Gas: pH .pCO_2 .pO_2 .HCO_3 . Lactate . Blood glucose
   c. Access: CVC ☐ ART line ☐ PiCCO ☐ ECMO ☐ Peripheral line ☐

4. **Disability: GCS: /15.** **Pupils:** **Spinal stability:**

5. **Any comments or concerns**

Fig. 16.1 (continued)

in critically ill patients on vasopressor and/or inotrope therapy [6, 7]. Inadequately resuscitated and hypovolemic patients tolerate transport poorly, bleeding should be controlled and intravascular volume should be optimized before departure [6, 7, 13].

Depending on size, physiological impact, and use of invasive ventilation, if the patient has a pneumothorax, it should be drained and a suitable intercostal chest drain inserted. Chest tubes should not be clamped and should be kept below the level of the patient during transport. When indicated, a gastric tube and a urinary catheter should be inserted and secured prior to departure. It is the responsibility of the transport team to ensure the securement and functionality of all catheters and tubes attached to the patient. Prior to departure, the receiving team should be informed of the current patient condition and expected time of arrival [6, 7].

16.4 Modes of Transport

Transport modes are typically ground (road) or air. The selection of mode of transport depends on several factors including the distance, availability of platform and team, urgency, geography, traffic and weather conditions, the nature and condition of the patient, in addition to cost [6, 13].

16.4.1 Ground Transport

Patient transport by road or ground route should be undertaken by the appropriate team and vehicle that meets patient needs.

(a) Stable patients are typically transferred by basic life support ambulance supported by appropriate monitoring and personnel (ward care or level 1).
(b) Critically ill (levels 2 and 3) patients at risk of deterioration and those on continuous infusions, monitoring, and mechanical ventilation should be transported by advanced life support ambulance equipped with appropriate monitoring and clinical team.
(c) The most critically ill patients with severe unstable cardiac or respiratory failure accepted by regional or tertiary centres can be safely transported by specialized retrieval teams utilizing mobile ICUs [13, 15–18].

Compared to aeromedical transfer, ground transporation offers the following advantges: staff familiartity, lower cost, less potentiaol to cause physiological deranagents and shorter time to itintaite and organise. Road transport also provides easier patient monitoring and handling [6].

16.4.2 Air Transport

Aeromedical transport is ideal when access by road is difficult and/or for longer journeys. It can be undertaken by fixed- or rotor-wing air ambulance. Teams should consider the logistic delays for organizing an air ambulance, potential for derangement due to altitude and associated costs. Specialized training and experience are essential requirements for those involved in aeromedical transport due to the particular challenges posed by this mode of transportation such as vibration, noise, loading and unloading of the patient, lack of humidity, and risk of hypothermia.

An aeroplane or fixed-wing air ambulance is usually deployed for long distance inter-hospital or international transfers. Advantages include controlled cabin pressure and lower level of noise and vibrations. Access and egress could be a challenge. Meticulous arrangement, which can take several hours must be in place for ground support and transportation to and from the aircraft.

A helicopter or rotor wing is typically used for shorter transfer distances typically, less than 100 km. Transportation of patients by aeroplane involves loading and off-loading of the patient into a ground ambualnce and shifting of patient between the ground and air ambulance. These two additional steps add to the complexity, potential risks and duration of air transpot. Transporation by helicopter and presence of helipad onsite obviates the need for additional ground transportation. Disadvantages include high level of noise, vibration, non-pressurized cabin, and compact space. When undertaking international air transport, the medical team is advised to ensure validity of entry visa, appropriate clothing for weather, availability of accommodation and some cash in accepted currency.

16.5 Intra-Hospital Transportation

AE are not uncommon during intra-hospital patient transfers [1, 2]. Anesthetized patients that require transportation within a facility should have the same protocols and precautions followed as for any other form of transportation [3, 20, 21]. The primary and the receiving team must be in agreement for the reason of transfer and facilitate the required personnel and equipment to be available at all times of transportation. In many hospitals this is carried out by the anaesthesiologist and anaesthesia technician who is specialized in caring for sedated and intubated patients, who are on vasopressor /inotropic support and require close monitoring of their vital parameters and life support equipment. A typical scenario is when patients are transferred post-surgery to PACU or the ICU. Escort teams must ensure equipment are appropriate for the transfer duration and purpose, e.g., magnetic resonance imaging suite [21].

16.6 Monitoring, Medications, and Equipment

In preparation for the transport, the medical team is advised to go through a transport checklist that validates, accounts for, and estimates all medications, equipment and miscellaneous items that are required during the transportation process. It is essential that transfer teams within a network have a standardized set of checklists, as it will save much needed time in the process and minimize untoward incidents [6, 9–12].

Commonly used drugs include sedatives, analgesics, neuromuscular blocking agents, inotropes, and resuscitation medications. Therefore, before each assigned transport, it is vital to review the list of medications and replenish if needed, to label the medications, lines, and pumps, and to prepare infusions beforehand [7].

Monitors used must be able to display the following data continuously as a bare minimum:

1. Heart rate and electrocardiogram monitoring.
2. Non-invasive blood pressure.
3. SaO_2.
4. $EtCO_2$ in mechanically ventilated patients. This is mandatory in all patients with invasive airway devices. It is recommended to monitor $EtCO_2$ during non-invasive ventilation and other modes of respiratory support to monitor airway patency.
5. Temperature.
6. Audible and visible alarms.
7. The display should be of suitable size and adequately illuminated [6, 7].

Equipment malfunction is the most common AE during transport of patients [2, 6]. Practitioners should be alerted to the artefacts caused by motion and vibrations and their impact on measurements. Alteration of arterial saturation by ambient light and movement is not uncommon. Invasive arterial blood pressure monitoring is more accurate and should be used in critically ill patients, however, vibration and motion may induce inaccuracies. Monitoring of central venous pressure is usually of less value during transport [6].

Transport ventilators should be able to set basic ventilation settings, e.g. positive end expiratory pressure, tidal volume, FiO_2, respiratory rate, and inspiration to expiration ratio. Modes should include pressure and volume control and pressure support. Checks must be done to alarm settings before use [6, 7, 20].

Equipment should be appropriate for use during transport as per manufacturer recommendations. The range of equipment utilized during transport are monitors, infusion pumps, suction, transport ventilators, defibrillators, and warming/cooling devices. These devices are typically battery operable so extra set(s) of charged batteries must be kept on hand [5–7] and the clinical team should know the autonomy of each piece of equipment when they operate from their battery in case they need to be disconnected for a period of time or if there is a power issue with the transport vehicle.

In addition to that, patient trolleys/stretchers used in ICU settings are modified when compared to standard trolleys/stretchers, in that they usually contain side stands to attach infusion pumps and monitors. Although, once in the ambulance it is necessary to keep away any loose equipment around the patient, and that they should ideally be fixed below the level of the patient or in secure locations in the ambulance. No equipment should be kept unsecured on the top of a patient stretcher during transport as this may cause serious injury in case of sudden deceleration. Gas cylinders must also be secured at all times. Standardization of equipment across the network means, there will be less chances of staff unfamiliarity and/or incompatibility of these devices, leads, and monitors. Transport equipment should undergo regular service and maintenance to minimize risk of malfunction during transport [7, 13].

Appropriate restraint (e.g.,5-point straps or harness) should be used to secure the patient to the transport stretcher. A vacuum mattress can be used to support the patient and minimize movement. Care must be taken as restraints can be distressing and uncomfortable, and this should be addressed by appropriate sedation and analgesia and/or reassurance of the awake patient. Adequate padding and protection of pressure areas is recommended specially during longer journeys. Hypothermia is a risk and adequate warming should be provided especially for the critically ill and the old and frail patient. Special attention to cervical spine and other fracture immobilization is warranted in trauma patients [5, 6].

16.6.1 Monitoring During Aeromedical Transportation

Altitude hypoxia secondary to a fall in barometric pressure leads to lower alveolar partial pressure of oxygen. Administration of oxygen or increase of FiO_2 can reverse this effect. Gas-filled cavities will increase in size at altitude due to reduction in barometric pressure. Typical examples are the bowels, middle ear, and endotracheal or tracheostomy tube cuffs [6, 13]. A nasogastric tube should be inserted and connected to free drainage. A pneumothorax must be drained before air transport. Air collections in the mediastinum, peritoneum, or cranium are relative contraindications and should be addressed. Swelling of tissues is not uncommon and splitting of plaster casts should be considered [6, 13]. Temperature and humidity changes are expected therefore appropriate care should be taken to avoid hypothermia and skin dryness [6, 7, 13].

16.6.2 Role of Anaesthesia Technician During Transfer

The anaesthesia technician (or nurse anaesthetist) has multiple of roles and responsibilities. Prior to transfer, the anaesthesia technician supports in resuscitation and stabilization, and assists in pre-transport procedures such as intubation or invasive line insertion. They are responsible for the provision of adequate supply of oxygen, infusions, and medications for the duration of the transfer in addition to preparation and provision of functioning transfer equipment as well as transfusion products.

During transfer, they will monitor the patient, co-ordinate with clinician and support transfer team in patient handling and movement. At transport destination, the anaesthesia technician will have to ensure the patient is appropriately endorsed to the receiving team and collect equipment prior to returning to base. Paramedics carry out a similar role and have been successfully integrated in some countries [22].

16.6.3 Transport Team Safety

Staff safety cannot be over emphasized. The transport team should remain seated and wear a seat belt at all times except when an emergency arises and management cannot be delayed. Appropriate clothing should be worn. Road traffic collisions involving ambulances are not uncommon [6, 7] and transport personnel are encouraged to have personal insurance. The transport team must justify the indication of blue siren or high-speed travel. A case-by-case evaluation and informed decision should be made. Transport of patients should not pose risk to pedestrians or other road users [6, 7].

As we have experienced the devastation brought on by COVID-19, it is of paramount importance that PPE and infection prevention and control practice are strictly adhered to. Use of respiratory protective equipment such as filtering face piece (FFP3) or equivalent is a must. Other PPE include gloves, eye or face protection, liquid-repellent overall/gown, head and footwear. Before and after every transport, the stretcher, equipment, and ambulance used must be properly cleaned and disinfected as per local policy [14, 23].

16.6.4 Operating Room Evacuation and Disaster Management

Whilst patient transportation and safety remain an essential aspect of this chapter, it must be included with unforeseen scenarios where the transport and safety of anaesthetized patients become a challenge. This may include natural disasters such as floods, earthquakes, tornados, to man-made hazards like biological and chemical threats or explosions, to environmental or electrical hazards like noxious fumes leak, electrical fires, and radiation exposures. We must be prepared to protect and provide safe evacuation of anaesthetized patients.

Health care faciliteis are encouraged to develop risk management and mitigation plans such as

Hospital Incident Command System (HICS), which can be activated in any of the aforementioned scenarios. Inter-hospital and intra-hospital collaboration and functional ICU/network communication are vital for the success of this system [24].

In addition to hospital-wide systems, microsystem management within the operating theatre complex should conduct independent disaster preparedness activities to consider issues specific to the OR. Given the diversity of health care practitioners, disciplines, and expertise within the OR, regular training and drills are essential to ensure familiarity and preparedness for these rare but potentially catastrophic events [24, 25].

Recommendations include the following.

- Staff education and training and regular credentialing.
- Facility design must allow emergency evacuation, utilize fire resistant materials, and provide adequate fire exits.
- Fire exits must be kept clear at all times and have clear signage.
- Equipment must include appropriate fire extinguishers, fire alarms and sprinklers, and gas shut-off valves.
- Safe management of fuels and hazardous materials.

In case of emergency evacuation, patient care should continue and basics of monitoring utilized. Individual patient care is a priority. Manual palpation of pulse, portable pulse oximetry, bag-valve mask ventilation, and portable oxygen can buy time. Sedation and/or anaesthesia should be continued by alternative means. Essential monitoring should be applied as soon as possible. After clearance of the emergency, the multidisciplinary team has to decide whether or not to continue the procedure [24–26].

16.7 Documentation and Endorsement

Poor documentation and handover have been reported to increase AE during patient transfer [27]. Clear records and charting of vitals and clinical condition should be maintained at all times [3, 5–7].

The transport team shall be acquainted with these aspects:

1. Patient condition prior to transportation and relevant medical conditions including any recent changes to their clinical status and events. This will give the team a better grasp at what they can expect and be ready to deal with unforeseen complications.
2. Reason(s) for transportation.
3. Imaging studies and relevant investigations.
4. Details of treatment limitations and resuscitation status.
5. Information provided to the patient, family, or carers.
6. The teams involved in referring and accepting the patient.
7. Clinical status and vital signs prior to and throughout transfer. Vital signs should be charted every 5 minutes during transfer.
8. Clinical events and therapy given during transport [5–7].

A formal handover on arrival at destination should take place [28]. Detailed account of transport events should be provided to the receiving team. Documentation shall be standardized within an existing network therefore making auditing and incident reporting done with ease, also duplicates of the documents must be readily available [5–7].

16.8 Training and Competence

Given its complexity and challenges, practitioners involved in patient transport should receive adequate training and be offered appropriate resources as they must be able to demonstrate a range of skills and competencies suitable for their assigned role during transport. Professional and training bodies stress appropriate training and experience of all individuals involved in critical care transportation [6, 7, 29, 30].

Although competencies have been clearly defined for clinicians and nurses, no such syllabus

Transport and Retrieval on ECMO Workshop

Time	Programme
08:00-08:30	Registration
08:30-08:50	Road Transportation on ECMO: What Do You Have to Have? *Senior Paramedic, Ambulance Service*
08:50-09:10	Human Factors in ECMO Transportation: What are the Essential Requirements? *ECMO consultant/Consultant Emergency Medical Service*
09:10-09:30	ECMO Transportation: Current Recommendations and Practice. *ECMO consultant*
09:30-10:00	Panel Qs & As
10:00-10:15	Coffee Break
10:15-10:30	Introduction to Simulation & Equipment
10:30-11:00	Demonstration of Scenario and Debrief
11:00-11:50	First Scenario and Debrief
11:50-12:50	Lunch
12:50-13:40	Second Scenario and Debrief
13:40-14:30	Third Scenario and Debrief
14:30-15:00	Group Discussion: Lessons Learnt & Closure *Course Director*

Fig. 16.2 Typical example of transport training workshop [31]

is available for anaesthesia technician. Attendance to a "transfer course" has been recommended for those to be involved in patient transfers [6, 7]. Many courses are available nowadays offering a combination of didactic teaching and high-fidelity simulation [31]. Fig. 16.2 depicts an example of a such a course. High-fidelity full-scale simulation is regularly used for transport training at our centre (Figs. 16.3 and 16.4).

16.8.1 Research Direction

Establishing a national database for patient transfers would help to understand the trends, timing, and AE during transfer. This would also inform decision makers on service provision and development. Future research should focus on new models of transport teams, e.g., physician assistant or critical care paramedic as well as patient-

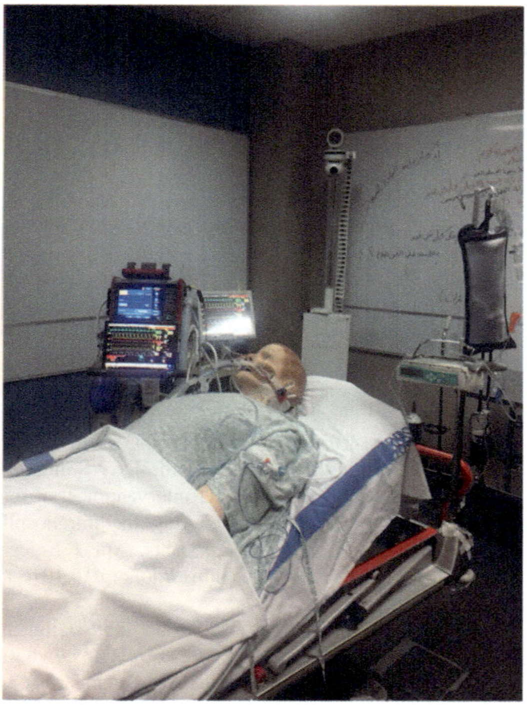

Fig. 16.3 Start of transport scenario with patient simulator in the referring facility

centred outcome. Staff safety, given the COVID-19 pandemic and future other possible health crisis also warrants attention [32].

16.9 Conclusion

1. Transport of anesthetized patient is challenging and needs careful planning and preparation.
2. A thorough clinical examination and stabilization must be carried out before moving the patient.
3. Patients should not be transferred without adequate resuscitation unless it is for a life-saving intervention.
4. The anaesthesia technician or equivalent healthcare professional plays an essential role during all phases of transfer.
5. Only skilled, experienced, and trained medical staff should undertake inter or intra-facility transfers.

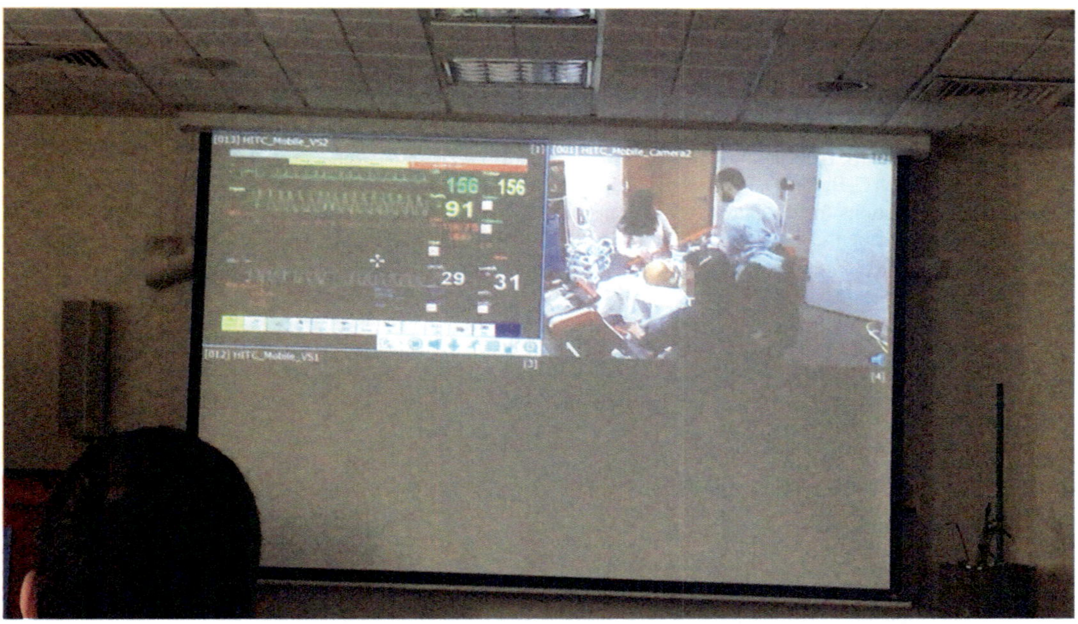

Fig. 16.4 High-fidelity simulation training in transport as seen from the observation room

6. The most appropriate equipment and medical supplies, including medications, need to be selected based on needs, expected transport duration, and pre-empting possible technical and medical issues.
7. The use of transfer checklists improves patient safety and reduces adverse events.
8. Patient safety is everyone's responsivity and clear communication is key to safe patients' transfers.
9. Clear and legible documentation and formal handover are integral to safe transfer.

Acknowledgement We are deeply grateful to our colleagues at the Emergency Medical Service, and ELSO Transport Working Group.

References

1. Jia L, Wang H, Gao Y, Liu H, Yu K. High incidence of adverse events during intra-hospital transport of critically ill patients and new related risk factors: a prospective, multicenter study in China. Crit Care. 2016;20:12. https://doi.org/10.1186/s13054-016-1183-y.
2. Parmentier-Decrucq E, Poissy J, Favory R, Nseir S, Onimus T, Guerry MJ, Durocher A, Mathieu D. Adverse events during intrahospital transport of critically ill patients: incidence and risk factors. Ann Intensive Care. 2013;3(1):10. https://doi.org/10.1186/2110-5820-3-10.
3. Fanara B, Manzon C, Barbot O, Desmettre T, Capellier G. Recommendations for the intra-hospital transport of critically ill patients. Crit Care. 2010;14(3):R87. https://doi.org/10.1186/cc901.
4. Singh JM, MacDonald RD, Ahghari M. Critical events during land-based interfacility transport. Ann Emerg Med. 2014;64(1):9–15.e2. https://doi.org/10.1016/j.annemergmed.2013.12.009.
5. Bourn S, Wijesingha S, Nordmann G. Transfer of the critically ill adult patient. BJA Educ. 2018;18(3):63–8. https://doi.org/10.1016/j.bjae.2017.11.008.
6. The Faculty of Intensive Care Medicine. Guidance on: the transfer of the critically ill patient. London: The Faculty of Intensive Care Medicine; 2019. https://www.ficm.ac.uk/sites/default/files/transfer_critically_ill_adult_2019.pdf. Accessed 20 Nov 2020.
7. The Association of Anaesthetists of Great Britain and Ireland. AAGBI Safety Guideline. Interhospital Transfer. London; 2009. https://anaesthetists.org/Home/Resources-publications/Guidelines/Interhospital-transfer-AAGBI-safety-guideline. Accessed 20 Nov 2020.
8. Beckmann U, Gillies DM, Berenholtz SM, Wu AW, Pronovost P. Incidents relating to the intra-hospital transfer of critically ill patients. An analysis of the reports submitted to the Australian Incident Monitoring Study in Intensive Care. Intensive Care Med. 2004;30(8):1579–85. https://doi.org/10.1007/s00134-004-2177-9.
9. Williams P, Karuppiah S, Greentree K, Darvall J. A checklist for intrahospital transport of critically ill patients improves compliance with transportation safety guidelines. Aust Crit Care. 2020;33(1):20–4. https://doi.org/10.1016/j.aucc.2019.02.004.
10. Brunsveld-Reinders AH, Arbous MS, Kuiper SG, de Jonge E. A comprehensive method to develop a checklist to increase safety of intra-hospital transport of critically ill patients. Crit Care. 2015;19(1):214. https://doi.org/10.1186/s13054-015-0938-1.
11. Choi HK, Shin SD, Ro YS, Kim DK, Shin SH, Kwak YH. A before- and after-intervention trial for reducing unexpected events during the intrahospital transport of emergency patients. Am J Emerg Med. 2012;30(8):1433–40. https://doi.org/10.1016/j.ajem.2011.10.027.
12. The National Institute of Health and Clinical Excellence. London. NICE guideline 94. https://www.nice.org.uk/guidance/ng94/evidence/34.standardised-systems-of-care-for-intra-and-interhospital-transfers-pdf-172397464673. Accessed 12 July 2021.
13. Kulshrestha A, Singh J. Inter-hospital and intra-hospital patient transfer: recent concepts. Indian J Anaesth. 2016;60(7):451–7. https://doi.org/10.4103/0019-5049.186012.
14. Yousuf B, Sujatha KS, Alfoudri H, Mansurov V. Transport of critically ill COVID-19 patients. Intensive Care Med. 2020;46(8):1663–4. https://doi.org/10.1007/s00134-020-06115-1.
15. Uusaro A, Parviainen I, Takala J, Ruokonen E. Safe long-distance interhospital ground transfer of critically ill patients with acute severe unstable respiratory and circulatory failure. Intensive Care Med. 2002;28(8):1122–5. https://doi.org/10.1007/s00134-002-1348-9.
16. Gebremichael M, Borg U, Habashi NM, Cottingham C, Cunsolo L, McCunn M, Reynolds HN. Interhospital transport of the extremely ill patient: the mobile intensive care unit. Crit Care Med. 2000;28(1):79–85. https://doi.org/10.1097/00003246-200001000-00013.
17. Wiegersma JS, Droogh JM, Zijlstra JG, Fokkema J, Ligtenberg JJ. Quality of interhospital transport of the critically ill: impact of a Mobile Intensive Care Unit with a specialized retrieval team. Crit Care. 2011;15(1):R75. https://doi.org/10.1186/cc10064.
18. Campbell CB, Labib A. The development of a mobile ECMO program. Qatar Med J. 2017;2017(1):11. https://doi.org/10.5339/qmj.2017.swacelso.11.
19. The Intensive Care Society. Levels of critical care for adult patients. London, The Intensive Care Society; 2009. https://www.ics.ac.uk/Society/Guidance/PDFs/Levels_of_Care_25_3_21. Accessed 12 July 2021.

20. Warren J, Fromm RE Jr, Orr RA, Rotello LC, Horst HM, American College of Critical Care Medicine. Guidelines for the inter- and intrahospital transport of critically ill patients. Crit Care Med. 2004;32(1):256–62. https://doi.org/10.1097/01.CCM.0000104917.39204.0A.
21. Australasian College for Emergency Medicine, Australian and New Zealand College of Anaesthetists, Joint Faculty of Intensive Care Medicine. Minimum standards for intrahospital transport of critically ill patients. Emerg Med (Fremantle). 2003;15(2):202–4.
22. Campbell CB. ECMO transport: the role of critical care paramedics. Qatar Med J. 2017;2017(1):53. https://doi.org/10.5339/qmj.2017.swacelso.53.
23. https://www.gov.uk/government/publications/covid-19-guidance-for-ambulance-trusts/covid-19-guidance-for-ambulance-trusts. Accessed 12 July 2021.
24. Miles LF, Scheinkestel CD, Downey GO. Environmental emergencies in theatre and critical care areas: power failure, fire, and explosion. BJA Educ. 2015;15:78–83.
25. Hart SR, Yajnik A, Ashford J, Springer R, Harvey S. Operating room fire safety. Ochsner J. 2011;11(1):37–42.
26. Cranshaw J, Gupta KJ. Power failure. In: Allman KG, McIndoe AK, Wilson IH, editors. Emergencies in anaesthesia. 2nd ed. New York: Oxford University Press; 2009. p. 386–7.
27. Ong MS, Coiera E. A systematic review of failures in handoff communication during intrahospital transfers. Jt Comm J Qual Patient Saf. 2011;37(6):274–84. https://doi.org/10.1016/s1553-7250(11)37035-3.
28. Shah Y, Alinier G, Pillay Y. Clinical handover between paramedics and emergency department staff: SBAR and IMIST-AMBO acronyms. Inter Paramed Pract. 2016;6(2):37–44.
29. The Royal College of Anaesthetists. CCT curriculum. London: RCoA, UK; 2010. Available at https://www.rcoa.ac.uk/careers-training/training-anaesthesia/the-training-curriculum/CCT2010. Accessed 18 Oct 2020.
30. Critical Care Network-National Nurse Leads. National competency framework for registered nurses in adult critical care STEP 2 competencies [Online]. London. CC3N UK; 2015. Available from http://cc3n.org.uk/competency-framework/4577977310 Accessed 12 July 2021.
31. Labib A, Alinier G. Transport and retrieval on extracorporeal membrane oxygenation (ECMO): setup and activities of an immersive transport and retrieval on ECMO workshop. J Cardiothorac Vasc Anesth. 2021;35(6):1603–10. https://doi.org/10.1053/j.jvca.2020.11.069.
32. Shehatta AL, Abdussalam AL, Deloso F, et al. Safety oftransport and retrieval of patients on extracorporeal membrane oxygenation during the peak of COVID-19 pandemic in the State of Qatar, Journal of Emergency Medicine, Trauma & Acute Care, Qatar Health Care. Conference 2021:13 http://doi.org/10.5339/jemtac.2021.qhc.1

Index

N. A. Shallik et al. (eds.), *Improving Anesthesia Technical Staff's Skills*,
https://doi.org/10.1007/978-3-030-88849-7

GPSR Compliance

The European Union's (EU) General Product Safety Regulation (GPSR) is a set of rules that requires consumer products to be safe and our obligations to ensure this.

If you have any concerns about our products, you can contact us on ProductSafety@springernature.com

In case Publisher is established outside the EU, the EU authorized representative is:

Springer Nature Customer Service Center GmbH
Europaplatz 3
69115 Heidelberg, Germany

Batch number: 10732801

Printed by Printforce, the Netherlands